Dr Apple's
Symptoms
Encyclopaedia

Dr Apple's Symptoms Encyclopaedia

The reassuring guide to self-diagnosis

Dr Michael Apple
Dr Jason Payne-James

Contributing editors:
Dr Robin Fox
Dr Hugo Hammersley
Dr George Moncrieff
Dr K.S. Pandher

Kyle Cathie Limited

This new revised 2007 edition published by
Kyle Cathie Limited
122 Arlington Road, London NW1 7HP
general.enquiries@kyle-cathie.com
www.kylecathie.com

Conceived, designed and produced by
Duncan Petersen Publishing Ltd
C7, Old Imperial Laundry, Warriner Gardens, London, SW11 4XW

10 9 8 7 6 5 4 3 2 1

ISBN 978-1-85626-748-9

Editorial director Andrew Duncan
Editor Jacqui Sayers
DTP editor Jacqui Sayers
Index Marielle Kalamboussis

A CIP catalogue record for this title is available from the British Library.

Printed and bound by Printer Portuguesa, Portugal

The authors

Dr Michael Apple gained a first in medicine at Birmingham University and has been in general practice since 1980. He was Chairman of the Medical Writers Group of the Society of Authors from 2005 to 2006 and besides this guide, has written several best-selling medical guides and many newspaper and magazine articles.

Dr Jason Payne-James qualified in 1980 at The London Hospital Medical College. He trained in surgery and gastroenterology. He is a Forensic Medical Examiner for the Metropolitan Police service and the City of London Police, and regularly acts as an expert witness in court. He has co-edited, co-authored and contributed to a number of books inlcuding *The Encyclopaedia of Forensic and Legal Medicine* (2006 winner of The Society of Authors/RSM/Medico-Legal Society prize for the best medicolegal publication).

The editors

Dr Robin Fox is a general practitioner in Bicester, Oxfordshire. He is a tutor for the Royal Free and University College Medical School and Oxford University and was previously a lecturer in medical education. He is currently an editorial advisor to *The British Medical Journal*.

Dr Hugo Hammersley studied medicine at Birmingham University then held hospital posts in medicine, surgery, paediatrics, obstetrics and gynaecology, and anaesthetics. He then trained in general practice and is now senior partner in a practice in central Oxford. He is a tutor in General Practice at the University of Oxford and doctor to several of the Oxford colleges.

Dr George Moncrieff has been working as a general practitioner since 1985, and has been training in general practice since 1989. He is also an examiner for the Diploma in Child Health for the Royal College of Physicians. His areas of expertise include dermatology, and he is GP representative for the National Eczema Society's Scientific Committee.

Dr K S Pandher is a GP principal and a tutor at the University of Oxford. His special interests include ophthalmogy (he trained in the speciality) and dermatology, and he is an accredited colposcopist at the Department of Gynaecology at the Oxford Radcliffe Trust. His main non-clinical commitment is the education of medical professionals and the development of e-learning. He has published papers on eye conditions, and colposcopy in the management of cervical abnormalities.

Contents

Introduction

Every patient carries her or his own doctor inside.
– Albert Schweitzer, French philosopher and physician (1875-1965)

We all like to feel well, so much so that we take our bodies for granted until something goes wrong. Then we enter the uncertain world of symptoms. Some symptoms matter, some don't – the skill is to tell the difference. And it is at this point that knowledge, such as found in this book, really begins to count, because of course it helps us understand what is going on; only then can we begin our journey to recovery.

However, *Dr Apple's Symptoms Encyclopaedia* aims to do a little more than just provide the facts. It aims to *make sense* out of symptoms – an ambitious task since the subject is so huge. We believe that this can, nonetheless, be done by revealing how a doctor thinks when faced by patients telling their stories. How does a doctor think? By ranking the possible diagnoses in terms of probability – which is exactly what has been done in this book.

We, the authors and editors, believe we will have achieved our goal if this book helps people to engage positively in the process of diagnosis; and, with luck, put their illnesses and subsequent management in to perspective.

The approach

This book has been designed to be extremely easy to use. Please read what follows carefully, as there are two different ways to use the book, depending on whether you want to arrive at a diagnosis based on your symptoms (see 1-3) or find out more about an illness you may already have (see 4).

For the first time ever in a popular medical guide, all the symptoms you could reasonably expect to encounter are put into perspective. A diagnosis may be possible in the presence of only some of the symptoms listed with bullet points. It is not necessary to experience all the symptoms in order to confirm a diagnosis.

We divide the diagnoses into:
• What is **probable**: the common causes of the symptom such as would immediately spring to a doctor's mind. Most of these probable diagnoses occur commonly: doctors see them regularly.
• What is **possible**, once the probable causes have been excluded. Some of these diagnoses are not uncommon, but they may well require testing to establish them without doubt.
• **Rare** causes: it would be misleading to define how rare. The frequency of these diagnoses is extremely variable. Unless your symptoms happen to match closely the features listed, these diagnoses are unlikely.

Extensive testing may be required to establish these diagnoses and in some cases doubt may remain.

Using this book

1 Mostly, you will find it best to start with your symptom or symptoms (though perhaps not always – see paragraph 4, following page). If it is easy to put a name to the symptom, such as headache or painful wrist, look for this in the index, which lists all the symptoms, and which will refer you straight to the relevant page number.

2 If your symptom is not quite so obvious, or easily defined, you need to decide if it can be isolated to a single part of the body – such as the knee, or abdomen – or whether it is a 'general', whole-body symptom, such as fever, or weight loss.

In the case of symptoms clearly occurring in one part of the body, or in one system of the body, for example the digestive system, turn straight to the relevant section and look through it. You will find that:
• Each part of the body has its own section, clearly identified with a heading.
• The sections are arranged in a logical order, starting at the top of the body (with the eyes) and moving downwards towards the feet. It ends with 'general' symptoms which cannot be easily isolated to any one part of the body or any one of the body's systems.

The abdominal symptoms are an exception to this rule.

• Within each section, the order generally echoes that of the book as a whole: the specific come first, and the general come last. Also, symptoms which are obvious to others – revealed by clear visual signs such as a rash or a limp – are put first. Inwardly experienced symptoms, or those which only you are likely to know about, such as loss of sense of smell, come last within a section.

The psychological and nervous symptoms in The Brain and Nervous System are an exception to this rule, following an alphabetical sequence.

In addition, symptoms are grouped like with like, so that, for instance, a common cold, shivers, chills and sweating all occur within the same few pages.

Simply browse through the relevant section looking for the symptom, or combination of symptoms that fits your condition; and if necessary follow the cross-referencing, which has been introduced to avoid too much unnecessary repetition.

3 If your symptom or symptoms cannot be isolated to a single part of the body, go to the 'general' symptoms section, which comes last in the book. (We use single quotes around the word general because although such symptoms may appear to be general, they may well, on closer inspection, be specifically related to a problem in one part of the body, or one of the body's systems.)

Within this last section of the book, symptoms are again ordered like with like, and as far as possible they proceed to from the obvious and noticeable to the 'internal' and private. But this classification is not so easy to apply to general symptoms and to give additional help with symptom-finding in this section, the black bands up the edges of each page give extra help to what is covered on these pages.

4 The second way to use this book is when you already know, or suspect, that you have a particular illness, and want to find more information about its symptoms. Simply look up the illness or disease in the index, which will send you straight to the page(s) where it is covered.

Medical terms

Certain medical or neo-medical terms are used so often in this book that explaining their meaning every time would be too space-consuming. They are:

Acute

Occurring now; a sudden appearance or exacerbation.

Anxiety

'Fear spread thin'; feelings of dread and worry.

Benign tumour

A lump which is not cancerous.

Chronic

A disease or illness either lasting a long time or present for years.

Circulatory disease

Disease of the arteries or veins which carry blood around the body.

Cyanosis

Bluish skin colouration caused by lack of oxygen in the tissues.

Cyst

A sac within the body, usually fluid-filled; may also appear as a swelling in or on the body.

Diagnostic

Unique to; aiding the diagnosis.

Follicle

Glandular structure under skin from which a hair grows.

Immunosuppression

The immune system is the body's defence system against infection and other insults; if it is supressed, by either illness or drugs, its normal function is limited or rendered less effective.

Indigestion, acidity

Both terms are used to describe discomfort after eating.

Lesion

A mark; a cut; a wound.

Malaise

Feeling generally unwell.

Malignant

Cancerous.

Nodule

A lump or swelling generally felt on the body's surface.

'Non-specific'

Usually describes a symptom which does not signify any disease in particular.

Palpable

Can be felt by hand.

Phlegm

Sticky mucous, produced typically in the lungs as a response to infection.

Rigor

A sudden shaking episode, typically accompanied by a fit of shivering.

Sepsis

Infection.

Systemic

Affecting all of the body's systems; widespread rather than local.

Tumour

A growth, often a lump, either benign or malignant.

Using this book

The eyes, nose and ears

The eyes: introduction

The eyes are extraordinary structures: delicately built, yet durable, and highly sensitive. Just as remarkable are the mechanisms within the brain that interpret the visual impulses travelling to it from the eyes.

Even now, our understanding of how the eyes work is only sketchy. The study of the eyes is one of the most specialized branches of medicine. There are, however, only a few common symptoms of eye disease – symptoms such as blurred vision or a red eye. Most family doctors have a useful working knowledge of eye disease, enough to make a confident diagnosis of everyday problems, but detailed assessment of more serious eye conditions should be for an eye specialist. Eye problems are common in modern life. Children are especially prone to eye infections; adults to eye injury; and the elderly to deteriorating eyes.

Report all but the most trivial eye problems to your doctor, especially pain or blurred vision. If there is eye disease such as glaucoma in your family, you should have regular eye checks.

For symptoms on:

The nose – see pages 50-57.
The ears – see pages 58-72.

Retina
Optic nerve
Bones of the skull
Eye muscle
Eyelid
Cornea
Pupil
Lens

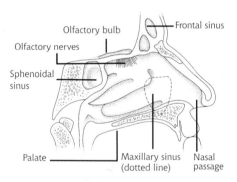

Olfactory bulb
Frontal sinus
Olfactory nerves
Sphenoidal sinus
Palate
Maxillary sinus (dotted line)
Nasal passage

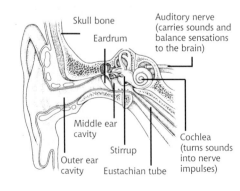

Skull bone
Auditory nerve (carries sounds and balance sensations to the brain)
Eardrum
Middle ear cavity
Stirrup
Cochlea (turns sounds into nerve impulses)
Outer ear cavity
Eustachian tube

Skin changes around the eye

Brief colour changes are probably due to minor infections. Here are other possibilities to explain more long-lasting colour changes.

Probable

◆ Injury

Any injury causing bruising of the forehead, or above the eye, will result in a blue/black eye, as the blood in the bruise tracks down the face to settle around the eye. In other words, a black eye need not be caused by injury directly to the eye area.

- At first, redness and pain.
- Black eye appears after a few hours.
- Fades over seven to ten days.

◆ Eczema

The skin of the eyelids and below the eyes is especially sensitive.

- Red, itchy skin.
- Dry and Flaky.

Those suffering from eczema elsewhere on the body are particularly prone to this problem. It is commonly caused by an allergy.

The skin around the eye is so delicate that it can react, for example to make-up, fragrances or even nail varnish. Such a reaction is described as dermatitis. Often, an allergy test is needed to confirm the cause.

◆ Xanthelasma

- Yellowish, slightly raised nodules, usually on the skin on the nasal side of the eye, or around the lower eyelid, in adults.
- Painless.
- Grow very slowly.
- Similar nodules may be found on elbows, hands and knees.

If you notice these, have a cholesterol check, since xanthelasma can be a sign of raised blood fats.

◆ Milia

These are small, pinhead-sized white-yellow spots on the skin near the eye. They are very common and entirely innocent. Essentially, they are simply blocked grease glands and can easily be pricked out with a sterile needle.

Rare

◆ Rodent ulcer (also known as basal cell carcinoma)

A slow-growing skin cancer often found on the face, by the bridge of the nose or the outer margin of the eye's orbit. Commonest in the elderly.

- Begins as a slightly raised spot, which can ulcerate.
- Sometimes crusts as it grows, but usually has a pearly appearance.
- May bleed.

Cure can virtually be guaranteed if treated early.

The Eyes

Ring around cornea

Probable

◆ Corneal arcus

A white circle around part or all of the cornea, common in the over-60's. Typically most marked in lower half of the cornea. If seen in a younger person, it may be associated with raised blood cholesterol, which should be checked. Otherwise it is of no significance.

Possible

◆ Iron ring

Grinding or hammering can cause a tiny fragment of metal to become implanted in the cornea. This is instantly painful and will cause marked watering of the eye. If the fragment is not completely removed (or left for many hours), a brown ring stain may be left on the cornea.

◆ Copper ring

Also called Kayser-Fleischer ring.
A green-brown ring associated with the rare condition of Wilson's disease, in which copper builds up in the body. A childhood disease.

- Liver disease (swelling, easy bruising, jaundice).
- Tremor of the limbs.
- Dementia.

  Early detection and treatment means a good outlook.

◆ Calcium

In conditions where the the calcium level in the blood is abnormally high, a chalky white deposit can develop as a fine line at the junction between the cornea and the white of the eye. This can be quite irritating and cause redness of the eye. Important to have a blood test to measure the calcium level.

Red and painful eye

Never ignore this symptom, which may be a sign of sight-threatening disease. Seek immediate medical attention.

Probable

◆ Severe conjunctivitis

The conjunctival membrane covers the white part of the eye. Inflammation causes a mass of red blood vessels running over the eyeball.

It is highly contagious, so tends to spread rapidly around close contacts.

- Initially, itching.

- Both eyes become red.
- The redness is greatest around the outer part of the eyeball.
- Bright light is mildly irritating.
- A yellow discharge.
- Crusted eyelids.

  Antibiotic eye drops or ointment are often recommended and probably render bacterial causes less contagious.
Sometimes the symptoms are confined to one eye only; in which cases a doctor will need to exclude other diseases.

The Eyes

◆ Arc eye

Can be described as acute keratitis – see below. Prolonged use of an arc welder, without adequate tinted eye protection, can result in this miserable condition, often several hours after exposure.

- Intense weeping from both eyes.
- Light aversion resulting in the patient keeping their eyes tightly closed.
- Red eyes.

There is little treatment other than pain relief, padding the eye and drops to relax the iris. The condition is fortunately self limiting and symptoms usually settle after a few hours. Few people make the mistake a second time.

A very similar condition can occur from exposure to natural ultraviolet light, for example when skiing without UV eye protection ('snow-blindness').

Possible

◆ Acute iritis

This is inflammation of the coloured part of the eye, the iris, or associated structures.

Iritis is not a final diagnosis in itself, since it can be caused by many diseases, in particular arthritic disorders and connective tissue disorders.

- Usually only one eye is affected.
- Moderately painful and red.
- Redness is greatest around the coloured iris.
- The pupil is smaller on the affected side.
- Vision is reduced, blurred.
- The pupil may appear irregular after

repeated attacks.

- In severe cases, a milky collection of pus can collect in front of the iris behind the cornea.

◆ Acute keratitis

Once again, this is not a final diagnosis, but a complication of several diseases affecting the cornea of the eye. The commonest are rosacea , an ulcer on the cornea, or injury.

- Rapid onset of symptoms.
- One eye affected.
- No change in vision.
- Profuse watering; blinking.
- Light irritates the eye.

There are now highly effective anti-viral drugs to counter the Herpes virus which is often the cause of this problem, but early treatment is essential.

Sometimes steroid eye drops are recommended, so referral to a specialist is recommended.

Rare

◆ Acute glaucoma

The eyeball contains fluid which circulates via tiny channels. In glaucoma, this fluid builds up pressure, causing changes in the field of vision. However, the changes usually happen so gradually that nothing is noticed until a late stage in the disease. For this reason, screening for glaucoma is strongly advisable in anyone with a family history of the problem, and anyone over the age of 60. Sudden, rapid rise in pressure can, on rare

The Eyes

The Eyes

occasions, occur because of blockage in the channels, or perhaps if a drug dilates the pupils. This is acute glaucoma.

The early symptoms of glaucoma are:

- None at all.
- Possibly vague aching in the eyeball.
- Haloes around lights at night.
- Tunnel vision – see page 40.

Acute glaucoma is a medical emergency which causes:

- Sudden, excruciating pain in the eye.

- Vomiting as a result of the pain.

Indeed, sometimes the patient is just generally unwell with vomiting, and the eye symptoms can be overlooked, resulting in the diagnosis being missed. Also causes:

- Redness around the iris.
- A hazy cornea.
- Vision severely reduced.

Urgent treatment is needed to reduce pressure within the eye and to save sight.

Slightly reddened eye, or red eye without pain

These are unlikely to signify any serious underlying cause, unless there is also blurred vision, or light hurts the eyes.

Probable

◆ Conjunctivitis

An infection of the conjunctiva, the thin membrane that covers the white of the eye.

- Eyes may feel itchy or sore.
- Redness appears rapidly, due to many dilated blood vessels.
- The redness is least next to the coloured iris, greatest at the sides of the eyeballs.
- Discharge of yellow.
- Eyelids may be crusted.

Conjunctivitis is usually a straightforward diagnosis, but be cautious if redness affects only one eye, when other possibilities need to be considered. Antibiotic eye-drops or ointment are usually effective.

Contact lenses are frequently a cause of eye problems. Keeping soft lenses in your eyes for prolonged periods means you are 17 times more likely to have an eye infection or conjunctivitis. It is much better to use short-use, hard, gas permeable lenses. Exposure to the air is crucial for the cornea's oxygen supply. A contact lens acts as a barrier and can result in damage to the surface cells of the cornea if the barrier remains in place for too long.

A frequent cause of infection is inadequate cleaning of lenses or, equally important, the lens case, or from out of date fluid.

◆ Allergy

Recurrent, mildly red eyes raise the possibility of allergy. Common causes of allergies (allergens) are pollens or animal dander.

- Mildly red, itchy eyes.
- May be seasonal, typically associated with sneezing and a runny nose.
- May be related to exposure to allergens.
- Discharge, if any, tends to be clear and not yellow.
- Under-surface of eyelids may appear grainy.

Several effective anti-allergy treatments can help, though for some this becomes a long-term problem.

◆ Irritant

Smoky atmospheres and air pollution can cause a reaction in the eye, resulting in a sore, red conjunctiva.

Possible

◆ Subconjunctival haemorrhage

An extremely satisfying condition for a doctor to diagnose, since the patient can be totally reassured that no harm will come of it.

- Painless, so the condition is often pointed out by someone else.
- One eye has a bright red patch, which is essentially just a minor bruise. This remains bright red for a few days as the blood is oxygenated from air contact.
- The patch may cover half or more of the white of the eye.

- Stops short at the iris.
- Fades away towards the sides of the eye.

It may look alarming, but it is simply due to bleeding from a tiny blood vessel and will fade away over a couple of weeks. In the elderly, it may be prudent to check the blood pressure.

If, however, it occurs after a blow to the head, expert assessment is needed to check whether there is damage to the eye further back in its socket.

◆ Feverish illness

Many febrile illnesses will give slightly red eyes.

Rare febrile causes:

Measles typically causes a viral conjunctivitis affecting both eyes.

Other features include a troublesome cough and a rash which first starts on the head and neck and spreads down the body over a few days. The lesions are raised, reddish bumps which fade to leave a brownish mark.

◆ Kawasaki disease

- Usually a young child (aged 2-5 years).
- Very high fever.
- Bumpy red rash.
- Sore throat and dry cracked lips.
- The glands in the neck can become quite large.
- Both eyes become red and sore, but no discharge.

The Eyes

After a few days there may be some peeling of the skin on the hands.

Needs urgent hospital admission to prevent long-term complications.

Rare

◆ Scleritis/Episcleritis

• One part of the white of the eye is red.

• Prominent blood vessels are seen to cause the redness.

• Slight discomfort.

• Often recurrent.

This condition is notable since it tends to be associated with other diseases, especially joint problems.

It needs further investigation.

◆ Meningitis

A few red flecks suddenly appearing on the whites of the eyes may be the earliest signs of meningitis in a baby or child. There may also be:

• A high-pitched cry.

• If old enough, the child will complain of a terrible headache.

• Drowsiness.

• Photophobia.

• A bulging, soft spot (fontanelle) on the baby's scalp.

• A red rash elsewhere on the body, which doesn't blanch if pressed under a glass tumbler (glass test).

Severe meningitis can occur without any of these signs, so the absence of one of these features, in an ill child, should not be relied on to exclude this life-threatening condition.

This is a medical emergency: rush the baby or child to hospital.

Abnormally small pupils

The pupils are the apertures through which light enters the eyes. Their size is controlled by nerves which make the pupils open and close. Those nerves are affected by changes within the brain and, surprisingly, these nerves run through the chest. It is not always obvious whether one pupil is abnormally small or the other pupil is abnormally large.

It is normal for both pupils to become smaller in bright light. In the elderly, the pupils tend to be smaller than those of young adults.

A young person, unconscious, and with pupils like pin points, should immediately arouse suspicion of a narcotic drug overdose.

Probable

◆ Long-sightedness

Small pupils are normal in the long-sighted.

• Both pupils are small.

• The pupils react briskly to light and dark.

Possible

◆ Drugs

Many drugs, and typically pilocarpine and timolol eye drops used to treat glaucoma (page 42), constrict the pupils. Small pupils may also be a side effect of the powerful narcotic painkillers such as morphine, dihydrocodeine and pethidine or drugs of misuse such as heroin.

◆ Iritis

See page 33. Suggested by finding:

* Affected eye may have a small, irregular pupil.
* Pain.
* Redness around the iris.
* Reduced vision.

Rare

◆ Horner's syndrome

A combination of:

* One abnormally small pupil.
* Partially drooping eyelid on that side.
* Decreased sweating on the same side of the face.

The significance of Horner's syndrome is that it demonstrates a problem in one of the nerves controlling the pupil somewhere along its route from the brain, down the chest and up again to the eye.

Damage to the nerve could be caused, for example, by a brain disease (such as multiple sclerosis), a lung tumour or enlarged glands within the chest; So although Horner's syndrome is uncommon, its significance is great and all the more so if there are associated symptoms such as:

* Chest pain.
* Coughing blood.
* Unsteadiness of gait.
* Blurred vision.

◆ Brain-stem stroke

An unconscious person (usually middle-aged or older) with bilateral pin-point pupils may have sustained a stroke in this critical part of the brain.

* Irregular or very reduced breathing.
* Extreme sweating.
* Incontinence.

The patient should be rushed to hospital by emergency ambulance.

Enlarged pupils

Young people typically have larger pupils and their size gradually reduces with age.

Probable

◆ Emotion

Both pupils will dilate in response to emotional triggers such as fear, excitement and anxiety. Accompanying symptoms include:

* Rapid pulse.
* Thumping heart beat.
* Dry mouth.

- 'Stars' in the eyes; but this is controversial.

◆ Drugs

Commonly prescribed eyedrops such as atropine and homatropine, are used to treat iritis and are intended to dilate the pupil.

Possible

◆ Third nerve palsy

See page 27. The third nerve is one of three nerves controlling eye movements. It also carries nerve fibres controlling pupil size. If the nerve is damaged:

- The eye turns outwards.
- The eyelid droops.
- The pupil enlarges.

◆ Injury

A blow to the eyes severe enough to damage its internal structure will upset movement of the pupil.

This is a particular risk in games using a small ball such as squash.

- Probably bruising around the eye.
- Enlarged pupil, unreactive to light.
- Blurred vision is likely (the lens can become dislocated, or there can be a bleed within the eye).

Clearly, this needs immediate treatment.

◆ Coma

A severe head injury or other serious disease affecting the brain, such as a stroke, may cause dilated pupils.

- Deep unconsciousness.
- Breathing irregular and shallow.
- No response to painful stimulus.

At the worst, dilated pupils in both eyes which do not respond at all to light signal brain death.

◆ Adie's pupil

A harmless condition.

- One enlarged pupil, which constricts in reaction to bright light, but more slowly than usual.
- Vision and health otherwise normal.

◆ Blindness

Depending on the cause of blindness, the pupil in a blind eye may be larger than its companion because the normal reflex response to bright light is absent.

Indeed, any condition that diminishes the perception of light in an eye (for example, corneal scar, cataract, detached retina, or damage to the optic nerve) will result in the affected eye not responding rapidly to a direct light.

Rare

◆ Irritation of nerves to eyes

The same process which produces Horner's syndrome (page 19) can, in its early stages, stimulate the nerve, causing a dilated pupil.

Accompanying symptoms which raise suspicion therefore include:

- Chest pain.
- Coughing blood.
- Unsteady gait.
- Blurred vision, numbness of hands.

Irregular pupils

Normal pupils are round or slightly oval, but minor irregularities are common.

Their significance depends on the individual's overall state of health.

Probable

◆ Normal variant

Minor degrees of irregularity are almost certainly of no importance and may well be hereditary.

- No pain or visual disturbance.
- No change with passing of time.
- Otherwise sound health.

Possible

◆ Iritis

See page 33. A small, irregular pupil is a particular feature of this painful condition, especially after repeated attacks.

Rare

◆ Multiple sclerosis

A neurological disease often beginning in early adult life.

- A common initial feature is sudden loss or blurring of vision in one eye.
- Numbness and weakness of different parts of the body.
- Tremor, unsteady gait.

A definite diagnosis of multiple sclerosis can only be made once the individual has experienced further changes in the brain or spinal cord. Often this never happens, or may happen only after several years have passed.

◆ Syphilis

Years ago, small, irregular pupils would immediately have brought very late stage, untreated syphilis to mind.

Other features would be:

- Brief, severe limb pains.
- Unsteady gait.
- Loss of pain sensation in joints, leading to gross distortion of knees, ankles.
- Drooping eyelids on both sides.

Enlarged eyeball

Probable

◆ Hyperthyroidism

Strictly speaking, this causes not enlargement, but protruberance of the eyeballs.

- Both eyeballs affected, though not always symmetrically.

- Sweating, weight loss.
- Fine tremor, hyperactivity.
- Racing heart beat.

Though treatment controls the general effects, the eyes often remain a little protuberant.

The Eyes

Rare

◆ Tumour

- Progressive swelling of one eyeball. (children or adults).
- Squint, loss of vision, pain.

Only after expert assessment can treatment be decided.

◆ Congenital glaucoma

Raised pressures inside the eye gives rise to a child with:

- 'Bull eyes'.
- Cornea appears to bulge.

◆ Thrombosis

A risk in cases of meningitis and severe dehydration.

Blood clots in the structures behind the eyes rapidly causing:

- Painful protruding eyes.
- Restricted eye movements.
- Eyes that look swollen.

Doctors often check the eyes as a matter of routine because the eye may be an indicator of disease elsewhere in the body, for example jaundice or anaemia.

The possible and rare causes of coloured patches and are really very infrequent.

Probable

◆ Pterygium

A sheath of blood vessels and accompanying tissue grows out along the white of the eye towards the cornea.

The term derives from the Latin for flies' wings – to which the condition does have a superficial resemblance. It is thought to be caused by long-term exposure to the elements (especially wind), so is most common in cyclists and sailors.

- Appears usually in the middle aged.
- Small, triangular-shaped white tissue, blood vessels within.

- The broad base points away from the cornea.

A pterygium rarely causes anything other than a cosmetic problem, or possibly slight irritation; but can be removed if it threatens to grow over the cornea.

◆ Pinguecula

The name derives from a tern meaning 'to do with grease'. These yellowish discolourations are again little more than cosmetic nuisance.

Usually only found in the elderly.

- Yellow, opaque raised lumps in the white of the eye.
- Triangular-shaped, with the broad base closest to the cornea.

Possible

◆ Scleritis

In between episodes of inflammation, these groupings of blood vessels simply form a flat, discoloured area to one side of the eyeball.

See page 18.

Rare

◆ Growths

Any of the lumps and bumps – warts,

cysts, moles and cancers – that grow on skin anywhere in the body may appear on the white of the eye.

Diagnosis is a specialist matter. Report any recently noticed spot to your doctor.

Remember, the appearance of any of these on the eye is very rare.

Discharge from eyes

Eyes may discharge tears or pus, or often a combination of both.

Probable

◆ Conjunctivitis

- Red eyes develop over a day or so.
- Constant discharge of small amounts of yellow pus.
- Eyelids stick together in the mornings – with crustiness.

Minor infections settle by bathing the eyes with tepid water; severe infections, especially in children, need antibiotic drops. See also page 16.

◆ Allergy

Suggested by a combination of:

- A clear discharge from both eyes.
- Itching.
- A blocked nose with clear nasal discharge and sneezing.
- May be seasonal (hay fever) or may be perennial (for example, due to animal dander).

See also page 403.

Possible

◆ Blocked tear duct

In babies up to one year of age, this is common cause of a constantly running eye and sometimes of repeated episodes of conjunctivitis.

The tear duct is too narrow for tears to drain normally into the nose. (Newborn babies cannot normally produce tears, so this usually becomes seen after about one month of age.)

- Usually only one eye is affected.
- Eye runs tears even when the baby is perfectly well.

Most babies grow out of this by their first birthday.

If necessary, it is possible to dilate the tear duct by probing it (does not need full hospital admission).

◆ Ectropion

A lower eyelid sags and turns outwards so that tears spill over; common in the elderly.

The Eyes

Rare

◆ Gonorrhoea

Not long ago, gonorrhoea was common enough to consider it as a reason for a baby to develop a heavy discharge from the eyes. Now it is a rarity in the developed world. It affects new-born babies. Untreated, it causes blindness.

- Profuse yellow pus surrounding the eyes and under the eyelids.
- Swollen eyelids, making it difficult to open the eyes.

Constant twiching movements of the eyes

Technical term: nystagmus. It is not always an abnormality, as some people show a few beats of nystagmus if they look to the extreme of their gaze.

Probable

◆ Cataract

This is an opacity of the lens, sometimes visible as a pupil with white-grey glint. Gradually worsening vision.

Usually a disease of later life, but can be present at birth (see opposite). Standard treatment is to replace the cataract with an artificial lens.

◆ Injury

Any serious injury to the cornea will leave an opaque patch, which may obscure vision, depending on its position.

Possible

◆ Congenital

Several unusual inherited conditions can cause a cataract or lead to deterioration of the cornea during childhood.

Diagnosis only established by a specialist examination.

Rare

◆ Trachoma

Though rare in developed countries, this infection is one of the commonest causes of blindness.

- Swollen eyelids.
- Under surface of eyelids is granular.
- Gradual opacity of the cornea.

◆ Vitamin A deficiency

Or Keratomalacia.

Worldwide, this is a serious and avoidable cause of blindness, especially in children.

- Rare in developed countries.
- Hazy cornea with a thickened, coarse appearance.
- Night blindness.

◆ Infection

Yet another hazard to vision now confined mainly to undeveloped countries.

Possible sources of infection are parasites, gonorrhoea and syphilis, complications of each giving rise to a clouded cornea.

◆ Acute glaucoma

Gives a clouded cornea, but in a red, excruciatingly painful eye (see page 15).

◆ Tumour

In young children, the earliest sign of a tumour within the eye may be an opaque pupil. The 'red-eye' effect of flash photography is not seen, and the pupil of the affected eye has a white or black appearance instead.

- Rarely, both eyes are affected.
- May be hereditary.
- A newly-appeared squint is also cause for suspicion.

  Needs urgent hospital treatment.

Cataracts

A cataract is an opacity within the lens of the eye. It cuts down the amount of light that can enter the eye and what ever light does not enter is made hazy and blurred. An early cataract will not cause any symptoms and will only be spotted on examination of the eye; but a mature cataract is visible as a whitish haze on the lens. Between these two stages there will be variable symptoms.

Most cataracts are the result of ageing. Occasionally they occur following injury or disease. On rare occasions, a child can be born with a cataract as a result of a rare metabolic disease, or certain infections in the mother during pregnancy.

Probable

◆ Ageing

Most people over 60 will have some opacity of the lens, but if it does not interfere with vision, it is probably best left alone.

- No other general disease.
- Vision deteriorates slowly.
- Eyes are pain free.

  Cataract surgery is highly effective.

◆ Injury

A penetrating injury to the eye (most commonly a high-velocity fragment, for example from hammering or drilling) can damage the lens and trigger cataract formation.

- The size of the opacity remains unchanged.
- Disturbance of vision depends on its size.

Possible

◆ Diabetes

Those suffering from this condition have an increased risk of developing cataracts in later life.

◆ Steroids

Steroids are invaluable drugs, used in the treatment of many diseases including severe asthma, joint diseases and inflammatory eye diseases such as iritis (see page 33). However, their long-term uses can cause many side-effects, including early formation of cataracts. This problem is most likely to result from long-term use of high doses of oral steroids. However, it can also even result from steroid eye drops, which should only be prescribed under specialist supervision.

Rare

◆ Congenital rubella

Rubella – 'German measles' – caught during the first four months of pregnancy will cause multiple abnormalities in the developing baby.

These include:

* Cataracts.
* Mental retardation.
* Heart disease.
* Deafness.

  These tragic consequences are avoided by routine vaccination of girls against the disease.

◆ Metabolic or congenital disease

Several unusual conditions may explain cataracts in children, usually in association with failure to thrive and, with some, epilepsy or developmental delay.

Twitching eyelid

For some reason this symptom generates much anxiety. It is not clear why this should be so. Although Hollywood uses it as cinematic shorthand for an impending nervous breakdown, it is harmless.

* Brief repeated twitching.
* Same lid is affected.
* Worse when tired or stressed .
* Rarely lasts for longer than a few days.

Drooping eyelids

Probable

◆ Ectropion

Sagging of the lower eyelids, very common in the elderly.

* The red under-surface of the eyelid is exposed.
* Tears spill out easily on the cheek.
* Increased risk of conjunctivitis.

  Really bad cases can be corrected by a simple operation.

Possible

◆ Bell's palsy

A paralysis of the facial nerve.

* The lower eyelid on the affected side droops.
* Sudden onset.
* The face sags on that side.
* The eye cannot be completely closed.

The Eyes

Normally, when the eye closes, the eyeball looks up into a resting position, with the cornea out of harm's way. In this condition however, a rather disturbing feature is that the eye looks towards heaven whenever the patient blinks.

Recovery takes time and is often incomplete.

Medical assessment is a priority, as this is most commonly caused by the *Herpes simplex* virus. Early, aggressive treatment can significantly improve the recovery.

It is also necessary to exclude a stroke, which can result in a very similar weakness, but with a subtle difference.

◆ Congenital

The probable diagnosis in a child with drooping upper eyelids.

- Normal eye movements.
- Normal muscular power.

Rare

◆ Third nerve palsy

Refers to the third cranial nerve which is damaged (for example by pressure).

- Paralysis involves one eye only.
- Eye turns outwards.

- Enlarged pupil.

Specialist investigation is needed to determine the underlying cause, which may be a brain tumour, diabetes or an enlarged artery in the brain pressing on the nerve.

◆ Myasthenia gravis

A treatable condition causing rapid tiring of the muscles. Drooping eyelids are an early feature.

- Both upper eyelids are an early feature.
- Both upper eyelids are affected.
- Muscles elsewhere grow fatigued abnormally fast, sometimes resulting in slurred speech, swallowing difficulties or double vision.

◆ Syphilis

The late stage of untreated syphilis (which may be up to 20 years or more after the first infection) causes widespread nerve disorders.

- Tingling feet.
- Brief shooting pains in the limbs.
- Unsteady movements.
- Pain sensation is diminished.
- Drooping eyelids on both sides.

Eyelids inflamed or itchy

Localized inflammation probably due to infection.

More generalised itching is usually allergic.

Probable

◆ Blepharitis

An irritating condition in which the margins of the eyelids just by the roots of

The Eyes

the eyelashes become chronically inflamed.

- Constant raw appearance.
- Crusting near the eyelash roots.
- Flaking skin on eyelids.
- Irritation.

The problem is often associated with eczema elsewhere on the body. All doctors have their favourite treatments, a sure sign that none guarantees a cure, but hot saline soaks are probably as good as anything.

This common condition may be thought of as a type of dandruff (see dermatology section) affecting the eyelids. Some people find it helps to wash their eyelids nightly with a diluted solution of shampoo on a cotton bud.

◆ Allergy

- Both eyelids are involved, causing a persistent mild irritation and desire to rub.
- Skin is slightly reddened.
- Dry, flaking skin.
- Often causes eczema elsewhere.

This is another minor but annoying condition, often caused by an allergic contact reaction. Possible triggers include hair spray, eye make-up or even nail varnish, but the reason often remains obscure, even after allergy testing.

The skin around the eye is so delicate that it reacts to minimal exposure, even though other areas of the skin tolerate triggers without a problem (for example, nail varnish).

Possible

◆ Insects bites

A common reason in the summer and autumn.

- Localized, raised red bump.
- Itchy for a few hours.

◆ Pubic lice

Lice will happily make a home in any hairy area which has the right density of hair, and this happens to include the eyelids. A diagnosis to be delivered with tact.

- Tiny round insects seen adhering to the root of the eyelashes.
- May also inhabit the eyebrows.

Treatment is to suffocate the lice with a copious application of vaseline.

Rare

◆ Trachoma

A Third World infection causing:

- Swollen eyelids.
- Grainy red under-surfaces of the eyelids.

One of the most common preventable causes of blindness. See also page 24.

Lumps on eyelids

Probable

◆ Stye

Infection at the root of a single eyelash.

- Often preceded by a day of mild discomfort.
- Pus may appear.

The most important treatment is regular, hot saline soaks. Antibiotic drops may help.

◆ Infected meibomian cyst

The meibomian glands are helpful little structures which produce a greasy lubricant for the eyelashes. Infection reaches them via hair roots.

The important difference between this condition and a stye is that the lump is behind the root of the eyelash, on the flat part of the eyelid.

It can be felt and seen as a small, pea-like lump below the skin.

- Pain, redness inside an eyelid.
- Small, tender lump appears.

Treatment same as for a stye, although an oral antibiotic is often required. Often an unsightly lump remains, which may need to be removed later.

Possible

◆ Molluscum contagiosum

A long name for a benign, wart-like condition, that appears in mini-epidemics among children.

- Small, rounded, slightly raised lumps which usually dimple in the centre.
- Likely elsewhere on body.

Harmless, though cosmetically a nuisance.

Best left to clear spontaneously, as messing about with them can make the virus spread.

Rare

◆ Dacrocystitis

Infection in the tear duct, which drains tears from the inner corner of the eyelid into the nose.

- Pain, swelling near bridge of nose.
- Skin becomes red and tender.
- Pus discharges from eye.

A fairly serious condition that needs early treatment. See also page 31.

◆ Rodent ulcer

A slow-growing form of skin cancer, commonest in the elderly who have led an outdoor life.

- Begins as a small, pearly lump.
- Grows slowly.
- Centre may ulcerate and bleed.

Considered curable, but needs attention as early as possible.

See also *Swollen Eyelids*, below.

The Eyes

Swollen eyelids

The loose skin of the eyelids easily swells to an alarming degree, but rarely for any serious reason.

Probable

◆ Allergy

An allergic reaction of the skin of the

The Eyes

eyelids to various agents, including fragrances, make-up, hair spray and nail varnish. Often, the cause remains unknown. Usually both eyes are affected.

- Painless.
- Mild itching, flaking skin.
- Looks worse after sleep, because swelling worsens when lying flat.

◆ Stye

Though a stye is a boil at the root of an eyelash, large ones do cause generalised swelling of the rest of the eyelid.
See also page 33.

- Only one eye affected.
- Treatment as for a stye.

◆ Blepharitis (chronic)

Prolonged inflammation of this kind, described on page 27, eventually makes the eyelids permanently slightly swollen.

Rare

◆ Orbital cellulitis

A spreading infection involving the skin of the eyelids and the surrounding parts of the face.

- Confined to one eye.
- So much swelling that the eyelids cannot be opened.
- Red tender eyelids.
- Malaise, fever.

Needs vigorous and immediate treatment with antibiotics to prevent it spreading deeper behind the eye.

◆ Nephritic syndrome

A very rare condition nowadays, most commonly due to an immune reaction in the kidneys following a streptococcal infection.

- Swelling around the eyes, with (initially) a markedly reduced amount of dark urine being passed.
- Loin pain.

This needs urgent assessment, usually in hospital.

Pain or aching in the eye area

Probable

◆ Eye strain

This familiar symptoms arises after hours of close work, especially under poor or glaring light, especially if appropriate corrective glasses are not worn.

- Vision is undisturbed.
- Aching in and around eyes.
- Relieved by a few hours' rest.

Recurrent eye strain means that you should have an eye test, or consider adjustment to the lighting where you work.

◆ Nasal congestion

Along with common cold there is often:

- Aching behind and around the eyeball.

* Blocked, runny nose.
* Mild headache.

   The symptoms settle after a few days.

◆ Conjunctivtis

Gives a prickling sensation, together with:

* Red eyes, worst around the margins.
* Mildly irritated by light.
* No loss of vision.
* Often a crusty deposit on the eyelashes.

Possible

◆ Glaucoma

See page 42. This serious, but treatable condition frequently causes no other symptoms than a vague ache in and around the orbit.

   It is easily detected with a simple eye check by an optician.

◆ Dacrocystitis

An infection in the tear duct at the inner corner of the eye.

* Pain and swelling.
* A red lump appears.
* Eye runs with tears and pus.

   Early treatment with antibiotics is advisable.

◆ Flu-like illness

Aching in the eyes is frequent accompaniment to a feverish illness, including the common cold, or flu.

* Vision unaffected.
* Slight redness of eyes.
* Fever, aching muscles.

Within a few days the underlying cause is clear.

◆ Sinusitis

A very common cause of aching in and around the eyes.

* Usually develops after a common cold.
* Pain or pressure felt across the forehead and in the morning.

   Sinusitis responds to steam inhalations. Occasionally, a steroid nasal spray or an oral antibiotic may be necessary.

Rare

◆ Tumour

Needs to be considered in case of persistent pain, especially with:

* Children.
* Bulging eye.
* Disturbed vision.
* Newly appeared squint.

The Eyes

Dry eyes

A constant feeling of irritation in the eyes and frequent, mild conjunctivitis.

Probable

◆ Ageing

The eye's natural ability to lubricate itself

with tears decreases with age. 'Artificial tears' in the form of eye-drops are effective, but have to be used regularly.

◆ Regular use of a visual display unit

This can cause uncomfortable or dry eyes. There is static electricity between the eyes and the screen. Dust is attracted to the eyes and can cause irritation. Tip: have your own anti-static wipe and uses it to keep the area around your work-station as free from dust as possible.

Possible

◆ Dry atmosphere

Many people complain of dry eyes during the winter, when the central heating is on, after spending time in an air-conditioned atmosphere.

Rare

◆ Sjögren's syndrome

Tear production by the tear gland is dramatically reduced, as well as reduced saliva production in the mouth leading to a dry mouth.

It may be associated with rheumatic disorders or with auto-immune disorders, giving rise to:

- Joint pains.
- Swollen joints.
- Rashes.

Blood tests are usually necessary to establish the diagnosis.

Feeling something in the eye

Considering how much dust flies around the average street, it is remarkable how rarely anything gets into the eyes.

- A sudden, prickling feeling in one eye.
- Rapid blinking.
- Tears, aversion to light.
- Mild discomfort.
- The feeling that you must get something out of you eye.

Probable

◆ Foreign body

Typically dust. Often a helper can see and remove the foreign body. But beware of a foreign body involving high-speed fragments, for example while hammering concrete or drilling.

Continuing symptoms, or signs of infection, deserve specialised examination in case a foreign body has lodged deeper into the eye.

◆ Conjunctivitis

It is common, during the early stages of conjunctivitis before the redness is noticeable, to feel that something is lodged in the eye.

Some cases of conjunctivitis may actually begin with small foreign body, which then creates infection.

Possible

◆ Ingrowing eyelash

A constant feeling of irritation in one part of the eye suggests that you should scrutinize the eyelids for this frequently overlooked cause.

The Eyes

◆ Allergy

A recurrent feeling of irritation may be caused by allergy:

- Mild redness.
- Itching, rather than pain.
  See also page 23.

◆ Stye

An infection at the root of an eyelash.

- Visible as a yellow swelling.
- The eye becomes red.
- Swelling of the eye lid is common.
  See also page 30.

Moderate to severe pain in eye

With the exception of an obvious foreign body, any such degree of eye pain needs expert assessment since neglect may damage sight.

Probable

◆ Foreign body

Dust, grit or in-growing eyelashes cause irritation out of all proportion to the size of the foreign body.

- One eye affected.
- Sudden onset, feeling something in the eye.
- Intense irritation and watering.
- Light irritates the eye.
- Vision unaffected, though may be blurred by tears.
  The eye's own protective mechanisms sweep out the foreign body in most cases.

◆ Ulcer or abrasion of cornea

An ulcer can quite easily occur on the delicate cornea, due to damage from a foreign body or from infection. The symptoms are:

- Intense discomfort in one eye.
- Builds up over a few hours.

- Light causes much discomfort.
- Redness around the iris (the coloured part of the eye).

Possible

◆ Iritis

An inflammation of the iris; it may be associated with a variety of rheumatic disorders, which need to be considered in recurrent cases.

- One eye affected.
- Redness, greatest around the coloured area.
- Marked aversion to light.
- Blurred vision.
- Small pupil on affected side.
  Treatment with eye drops, though quite straightforward, is necessary to prevent permanent damage to the iris.

◆ Episcleritis

Irritation in one part of the eye:

- Redness in one obvious area of the white of the eye.
- Prominent blood vessels.
- Pain is moderate.

The Eyes

- Moderate aversions to light.
- Vision is unaffected, apart from blurring due to tears.

◆ Shingles

Every doctor has a tale to tell of being fooled by early stages of this condition, which is caused by the chicken pox virus.

- At first, discomfort around one side of the face with no skin changes.
- After a few days, the rash appears.
- Crusting sores develop over the eyelids, side of the nose and forehead.
- Accompanied by severe pain.

If spots appear on the side of the nose or inside the nose, there is an increased chance of the eyeball being infected.

The worry about this otherwise harmless condition is ulceration of the cornea. Fortunately, there are now powerful anti-viral drugs which reduce this possibility, but they need to be given early in the illness.

Rare

◆ Acute glaucoma

See page 15.

◆ Retrobulbar neuritis

Inflammation of the optic nerve, especially associated with multiple sclerosis.

- Rapid loss of vision in one eye.
- Moderate pain when the eye is moved.

◆ Thrombosis

A blood clot in the skull behind the eyes, causing:

- Sudden pain behind both eyes.
- Eyes to protrude.

◆ Corneal ulcer

A possibility if only one eye is inflamed. These uncommon infections begin with:

- Itching in one eye.
- Intense photophobia.
- Redness, mainly around the coloured iris.

Contact lens wearers should be especially aware of this problem, which can arise from overuse of the lenses.

A doctor will check for an ulcer using a fluorescent stain. The usual cause is the Herpes virus. Specialist assessment and early vigorous treatment with anti-viral eye drops is essential.

Eyes abnormally sensitive to light

Any existing irritation of the eyes will cause some discomfort in bright light. Persistent or severe sensitivity to light is termed photophobia, and can be a symptom of:

Probable

◆ Conjunctivitis

Mild redness around the outer parts of the whites of the eyes, plus:

- Sticky discharge.
- A mild gritty feeling in eyes.

Antibiotic eye drops or ointment is usually advisable, if only to reduce contagion as much as anything. See page 16.

◆ Allergy

Recurrent photophobia suggests an allergy, especially in someone with other signs of an allergic constitution, such as:

- Eczema.
- Runny nose: sneezing on exposure to pollens, animal hair.
- Itching eyes on exposure to dust or in specific environments.
- Vision is not affected, other than by the watering produced by the allergy.

Treatment is typically a combination of anti-histamine tablets and anti-allergic eye-drops.

Possible

◆ Iritis

See page 33.

◆ Damaged cornea

A picture similar to iritis, but with:

- Less severe pain.
- Redness around the cornea.
- History of abrasion or ulcer in the eye.

Needs appropriate treatment.

◆ Measles

An increasing rarity in developed countries, where vaccination programmes are leading to its eradication, measles is still found in the Third World, where it can kill up to 20 per cent of children.

Aversion to light is prominent feature in the days before the rash appears.

- High fever for four days.
- Bloodshot eyes.
- Runny nose cough.
- Blotchy red rash appears being the ears and spreads over whole body.
- Temperature remains high for another three to four days.

Rare

◆ Meningitis

Aversion to light is a significant symptom of meningitis, but there will usually be associated symptoms, including:

- Headache.
- Resistance and pain on attempting to bend the neck.
- Nausea.
- Drowsiness, or confusion.
- In babies, a bulging, soft spot on top of the skull.

If you suspect meningitis, don't delay seeking medical advice.

◆ Albinism

Due to lack of pigment, albinos have a special sensitivity to bright lights.

Nystagmus (abnormal eye movements, see *Constant twitching movements of the eyes*, page 24) and squint are also common features.

Blurred vision

The everyday experience of the world being somewhat out of focus can nearly always be put down to just that – in other words you need spectacles.

Temporary blurring will result from any eye irritation causing tears to flow, for instance conjunctivitis.

Persistent or recurrent blurring may result from the following:

Probable

◆ Uncorrected vision

With time, the power of the lens of the eye changes, as does that of the muscles that change its shape in order to focus in on objects at different distances from the eye.

• A very gradual change.

• Can be corrected with spectacles.

Adults are aware of the process. This may not be so in children who may not realize that they have a problem: hence the importance of eye tests in childhood.

Possible

◆ Macular degeneration

A process of deterioration of part of the retina in the elderly, causing loss of fine vision to a variable degree, not correctable with glasses.

See page 41.

◆ Cataract

The interference with light caused by the cataract may be misinterpreted as blurred vision.

See page 25.

◆ Effects of drugs

Many drugs affect the muscles in the eye, causing blurred vision.

It is a question of relating the symptoms to taking the drug.

Common culprits include those drugs given to control bladder function, and anti-depressants.

Rare

◆ Diabetes

Swings in the blood stream's sugar level can cause blurred vision.

• A temporary symptom, fading within minutes.

Undiagnosed diabetes causes thirst, excess urine production and tiredness.

Distortion of vision

Objects look too small, or too large, and straight lines appear curved.

Not a common symptom and, if persistent, needs expert assessment.

Probable

◆ Unknown cause

The sensation of distortion of size or shape sometime happens for just a brief moment. An object may suddenly seem to be distant.

- Vision otherwise unaffected.
- Recovers within moments.

Possible

◆ Detached retina

Light fading on the crinkled, detaching retina is seen as distorted.

- Preceded by many floaters – see page 39.
- The classic symptom is often described as a 'curtain coming down to obscure the sight.'
- Many flashing lights.

  Seek medical help immediately, since early intervention can prevent loss of vision. See page 44 for further details.

Rare

◆ Distortion of the retina

Just as the distortion of the screen distorts the film projected on it, so distortion of the retina has the same effect.

This may be caused by tumours, bleeding or inflammation.

- Other symptoms of retinal detachment, above.
- A bulging eye.
- Loss of vision.
- In children a white appearance to the lens.

The Eyes

Double vision

Movements of the eyes are delicately co-ordinated by an automatic process of the brain. The process has to be learned, accounting for the alarming gyrations of the eyes that occur in new-born babies until they have developed the necessary coordination.

Once achieved, we experience stereoscopic vision beyond the dreams of Hollywood. When things go wrong, we start seeing two of everything since the brain is no longer able to merge the output from the two eyes into one image. Don't confuse this symptom with blurred vision which raises quite different possibilities.

Probable

◆ Using extremities of gaze

It is normal to experience double vision if the eyes are swivelled to the extreme left or right, up or down.

◆ Paralysis of eye muscles

The eye is moved by six muscles each of which turns the eye in a particular direction. Paralysis of any of those muscles results in double vision because of the affected muscle is unable to move the eye as well as the other eye can move.

The pattern of weakness gives a clue

as to which muscles are affected, being some combination of:

- The affected eye turning inward or outwards.
- Eyelid may droop.
- Pupil on that side may be wider than the unaffected side.

Many cases are unexplained. A head injury is a common cause and will be obvious.

Other possibilities are meningitis, infections and botulism, but these give rise to further dramatic symptoms which overshadow the double vision, for instance:

- Severe headache.
- Confusion, drowsiness.
- The eye hurt by light.

Possible

◆ Multiple sclerosis

A disease of the nervous system often beginning in early adult life.

Double vision results from partial weakness of the eye muscles.

- Vision may also be blurred.
- Slight discomfort in the eye.
- Unsteadiness in walking.
- Tremor or weakness in the arm or legs.
- Numbness of the limbs.

The double vision usually recedes over a few weeks.

Rare

◆ Displacement of eyeball

Caused by something pushing the eye forwards and interfering with its movements.

Bleeding behind the eye, or thrombosis, would be suggested by:

- Sudden onset.
- Pain in the eye(s).
- Eye(s) suddenly protruding.

Graves' disease, associated with an overactive thyroid gland, or a tumour behind the eye, would produce:

- Slower onset of symptoms.
- Gradual protrusion of one or both eyes.
- Sweating, rapid pulse and weight loss.

◆ Myasthenia gravis

An unusual disease in which the muscles anywhere in the body tire rapidly. Eye symptoms are an early feature.

- Eyelids droop.
- Double vision may occur in any direction of gaze.
- Both eyes are affected.

The diagnosis is established by the individual's reaction to certain injected drugs.

◆ Disease of one lens

The apparently impossible symptom of double vision affecting one eye may, in fact, though rarely, be due to disease in one lens which splits the image as a prism does.

The Eyes

Flashing lights

Caused by individual light receptors firing off the retina.

Probable

◆ **Normal**

Flashing lights are frequently experienced after a blow to the head or after suddenly getting up from a squatting position, when blood flow is briefly disturbed.

• Both eyes affected.
• You feel light-headed, briefly.
• Return to normal within seconds.

Possible

◆ **Migraine**

Flashing lights shimmering in one section of the field of vision are a typical warning of the onset of migraine.
See also page 45.

• Usually both eyes are affected.
• Nausea.
• Headache.
See also page 101.

Rare

◆ **Detached retina**

See page 44.

• One eye affected.
• A shower of flashes.
• Numerous floaters.
These symptoms need urgent specialist attention.

The Eyes

Floater – floating spots before the eyes

The interior of the eye is a liquid, in which it is normal for clumps of cells to float around, hence the term 'floater'.

An alternative medical term is muscae volitantes, meaning 'flying flies'.

Probable

◆ **Normal**

A floater is probably harmless if:

• There are only one or two.
• Vision is otherwise normal.
• The eye is painless.

Possible

◆ **Severe short-sightedness**

This can cause the release of more than usual numbers of floaters.

Rare

◆ **Detached retina**

See page 44.

Before complete detachment, warning signs include:

• Large numbers of floaters.
• Shower of lights.

If you have these symptoms, you need urgent specialist attention.

◆ Damage to retina

Inflammation or bleeding within the eye causes:

- Many floaters in one eye.
- Blurring of vision.
- Pain.
- Redness.

Treatment depends on the causes.

Seeing haloes around lights

This happens if the cornea becomes waterlogged, as in glaucoma, or if something within the lens is scattering the light.

Probable

◆ Glaucoma

See page 42.

- Haloes, seen especially at night.
- Tunnel vision.

Untreated, glaucoma progressively destroys sight, producing little by way of symptoms until the disease is well advanced. So it is important to have you eyes checked if a close relative suffers from glaucoma, while those over 60 should be checked anyway from time to time.

Possible

◆ Cataract

See page 25. The haziness in the lens acts like a prism: it scatters light so that objects appear to be surrounded by haloes and rainbows.

Tunnel vision

Loss of the outer field of vision: you seem to look at the world through a tube. The brain is so adaptable that the condition can progress remarkably far before you notice a problem.

Probable

◆ Glaucoma

Suggested by the combination of:

- Tunnel vision.

- At night, bright lights appear to be surrounded by haloes.
- Sometimes, aching in eyes.

See page 42.

Possible

◆ Retinitis pigmentosa

See page 47.

The Eyes

◆ Migraine

- Symptoms develop over a few minutes.
- Visual field appears to shrink.
- Followed by severe headache, nausea.
- Vision recovers.

Rare

◆ Brain tumour

Can cause tunnel vision by increasing the pressure inside the brain, or by a direct destruction of the parts of the brain required to interpret vision.

There are likely to be other symptoms such as:

- Severe headache, typically on waking at night.

- Persistent nausea.
- Change of personality.
- Altered awareness.

◆ Syphilis

Years after infection, the widespread damage wrought by this disease also causes a multitude of symptoms including:

- Severe shooting pains in limbs.
- Unsteady gait.
- Drooping eyelids.
- Loss of pain sensation in limbs. Leading to grossly deformed joints.
- Some degree of mental disturbance.

The Eyes

Blindness

There can be no glossing over the fact that many causes of blindness remain untreatable. It is, therefore, of little consolation – but nonetheless important – to know which causes of blindness are treatable, or at any rate controllable. People with high blood pressure, diabetes or a family history of glaucoma should take special care of their eyes and heed any warning signs, including flashing lights, and pains in the eyes and temples.

Probable

◆ Cataract

A white patch seen in the lens of the eye and nearly always due to the ageing process.

- Very gradual loss of clear vision.
- The awareness of light is not lost, only clarity.

Cataract surgery is surely one modern medicine's unqualified successes.

See page 25.

◆ Macular degeneration

The retina of the eye is made up of a sandwich of light sensitive elements. The macula is a small area of the retina where these elements are most concentrated and where the sharpest vision is achieved.

'Degeneration' means, literally, decrease in function – part of the natural process of ageing.

This is commonest cause of deterioration of eyesight in the elderly.

Disease in the macular has a serious effect on vision, but does not cause total loss of sight. The usual reason for its deterioration in the blood supply or the nerves to, or in, that area.

Unfortunately, little can be done to halt established degeneration, but recent advances can help some people with macular degeneration.

- Gradual, painless loss of vision.
- Central vision deteriorates making reading, for example, impossible.
- Vision, especially close vision, is blurred and not improved with spectacles.
- Outer vision is unaffected.
- Objects may look distorted or small.

There is never complete loss of vision, because the outer parts of the retina are spared.

◆ Diabetic eye disease

One long-term effect of diabetes is degeneration of blood vessels within the retina. This causes loss of vision that can be gradual or sudden, depending on the pattern of degeneration. Diabetics, therefore, need regular checks on their retinas. It is possible to treat blood vessels which appear diseased with a laser beam. There are no symptoms of this condition: it has to be assessed by an expert.

◆ Glaucoma

Raised pressure inside the eye, a common condition which should be screened for in the elderly and earlier in those with family history of glaucoma. The features on blindness caused by this insidious disease are:

- Painless.
- Peripheral vision is lost, giving rise to tunnel vision.
- Occasionally, aching in the eyes.
- At night, bright lights appear to be surrounded by a halo.

Possible

◆ High blood pressure

This may increase the likelihood of macular degeneration (see page 41) and should be treated. Mild to moderate high blood pressure has no symptoms. Very high blood pressure over a long period may cause:

- Severe headaches.
- Symptoms due to strain on the heart such as breathlessness, ankle swelling.
- Palpitations or chest pain.

◆ Choroiditis

The choroid is one of the layers in the sandwich that makes up the retina. Inflammation in the choroid results in a gradual, but permanent, loss of vision corresponding to the site of damage.

The reason for most cases of choroiditis is unknown, although there is proven association with toxoplasmosis, an infection that causes an illness similar to glandular fever. Syphilis used to be a more common cause.

- You may recall an episode of disturbed vision in one eye.

The Eyes

- You then become aware of an area of blindness in that eye.
- Only one eye affected.
- The area is fixed, and neither grows nor shrinks.

◆ Retinitis pigmentosa

A degenerative condition affecting the retina and so called because of the dark pigment that is visible over the retina through an opthalmoscope.

This tends to be an inherited condition and nothing can be done to stop it.

- Symptoms begin in adolescence.

- Gradual loss of the peripheral field of vision, leading eventually to tunnel vision.
- Night blindness.

Rare

◆ Trachoma

Worldwide, trachoma is a common cause of blindness, but it is rare in the developed world.

The infection causes:

- Extremely sore, puffy eyes.
- Running eyes.
- Scarring of the cornea, resulting in partial or total blindness.

The Eyes

Sudden blindness

Unusual, but when it does occur, this usually has a serious underlying cause.

Probable

◆ Blockage of central retinal artery

This artery supplies blood to the back of the eye.

Blockage may occur because of a tiny blood clot or because the artery constricts to the point where it cuts off blood flow:

- Sudden, total blindness.
- No pain.
- One eye affected.

If the blockage is a result of a spasm of the artery, there is a change of vision returning after an hour or so. Otherwise, there is no treatment.

It is important to search for the causes that may threaten the sight of the other eye, for example, a source of blood clot in the heart or temporal arteritis, see page 44.

◆ Blockage of the central retinal vein

This vessel carries blood away from the eye. Blockage is usually caused by pressure from a diseased retinal artery, which runs very close to the vein.

- The elderly, and those with diabetes or high blood pressure, are at increased risk.
- Loss of vision is rapid, but not instant, as in arterial blockage.
- Usually, light can still be seen.

Sometimes partial vision returns, though this can take a few weeks.

◆ **Detached retina**

It may come as a surprise to know that the retina is not firmly attached to the back of the eye, but is held in place by the pressure of fluid within the eye.

The retina can tear, allowing fluid to leak behind it and to peel it off the back of the eye. A blow to the head may also dislodge the retina, or, rarely, a tumour growing at the back of the eye.

- Most common in the very short-sighted.
- Multiple flashing lights may be a warning of detachment.
- A shadow appears to fall over the field of vision. Sometimes described as a curtain falling over the field of vision.

With early treatment, the retina can often be anchored back into place.

◆ **Amaurosis fugax – mini-stroke**

This is, in fact, a blockage of the central retinal artery; however, the blood clot rapidly dislodges.

- Sudden, painless loss of vision in one eye.
- Vision returns after a few minutes.

Your doctor must search for the site where the blood clots originate. It is usually in the carotid artery, which runs up the neck.

◆ **Stroke**

A stroke is caused by blockage of blood flow within the brain. If the blockage happens to involve the part of the brain that processes information from the eyes, the result is blindness.

- Sudden, painless onset.

- Vision is usually lost in both eyes at once.
- Sudden paralysis of one side of the body.
- In severe strokes, unconsciousness follows.
- The exact nature of the loss of vision can give a clue as to where in the brain damage has occurred.

See also *Blind spots*, page 46.

Possible

◆ **Temporal arteritis**

This cause of blindness should be better known because it is treatable.

It is almost always confined to people over 55 or 60 years of age.

- The artery on the side of the scalp becomes exquisitely tender, making brushing the hair or wearing a hat intolerable.
- The blood supply to the muscles used for chewing can be compromised, so the individual has to stop eating every few minutes.
- General malaise.

The condition responds dramatically to steroid drugs, which can save sight if the condition is recognised in time.

It is associated with a condition known as polymyalgia rheumatica (See page 447) which also only occurs in the elderly.

- Gradual appearance of a vague weakness and malaise.
- Muscular tenderness, especially around the shoulders and neck.

◆ Migraine

Visual disturbances, including temporary blindness, are common in migraine. Commonest in, but not confined to, the young and middle-aged.

- Shimmering lights in the eyes.
- Nausea.
- One-sided temporary blindness.
- Possibly slurred speech, loss of use of one hand.
- As symptoms fade, a severe headache begins.

The first time this happens, it may seem like a stroke. Many doctors recommend further tests, since occasionally there is a cause for the migraine within the brain.

◆ Optic neuritis

Inflammation of the optic nerve, usually in a young adult.

- Sudden loss of vision in one eye.
- Usually, the loss is confined to the central field of vision, so the individual can still see 'at the edges of vision'.
- The eye may ache.
- Recovery after a few days.

Optic neuritis can be a warning sign of multiple sclerosis.

Other underlying causes may be syphilis, diabetes and lack of B vitamins.

◆ Vitreous haemorrhage

Bleeding into the fluid within the eyeball. Associated with diabetes, and with general arterial disease.

- Mild cases give rise to multiple floaters – see page 39.
- Otherwise painless partial loss of vision in one eye.

The condition is confirmed by looking at the interior of the eye with an opthalmoscope.

There is rarely any treatment. The outcome depends on the size of the bleed and any underlying disease.

◆ Acute glaucoma

See page 15.

Suggested by the sudden onset of:

- Excruciating pain in one eye.
- Vomiting.
- Red eye.
- Glazed appearance of the eye.

Requires emergency treatment.

Rare

◆ Methyl alcohol

Drinkers of methylated spirits are at risk of sudden blindness in one or both eyes. It may be total.

◆ Injury

A head injury can cause sudden blindness by damaging the part of the brain involved in vision, or by causing retinal detachment – see opposite.

◆ Hysteria

Blindness of psychological origin is suspected if the back of the eye appears normal and if electrical tests show that visual stimuli are reaching the brain.

The individual has usually exhibited other odd physical symptoms, such as:

- Unexplained paralysis.
- Loss of speech.
- Abnormal gait.

- Does not show expected emotional reaction to blindness, when for most people it is a devastating event.

There is often a previous psychotic history.

Blind spots

You may become aware of an area of your field of vision where the vision is dim or absent altogether. Wherever you look, that patch remains fixed in relation to the rest of your visual field. This is known as a scotoma.

A scotoma that suddenly appears draws attention to itself, whereas a slowly enlarging scotoma can be entirely overlooked until it is of considerable size – you are aware only of unspecific blurring of vision.

Scotomas in both eyes are usually due to damage to the optic nerves somewhere in the brain. A scotoma in one eye is nearly always due to a cause within that eye.

A scotoma should not be confused with the blind spot which everyone has: an area of absent vision which might possibly be noticed if one eye is covered and an object slowly moved to the side. There is a point at which the object briefly disappears from vision. This corresponds with the part of the retina where the optic nerve leaves the eye and where, therefore, there are no visual receptors.

Probable

◆ Macular degeneration

Age-related deterioration of the eye causing a fixed area of dim or absent vision. See page 41.

- One eye affected more than the other.
- A loss of vision in the centre of the field.
- The area of loss may increase very slowly.

◆ Stroke

A stroke affecting the back of the brain causes:

- Loss of part of the field of vision.
- Both eyes are affected.
- Other features of a stroke, such as paralysis, confusion.

See also page 377.

◆ Injury

A blow to the head severe enough to damage the eye or brain may cause loss of vision.

- Usually both eyes are affected.

Possible

◆ Pituitary tumour

The pituitary gland is a structure in the brain which lies close to the nerves coming from the eyes. Any tumour in the gland presses on those nerves, producing a blind spot.

- Painless.
- Loss of the outer field of vision.
- Mild headache.

There may be other symptoms as a result of abnormal hormone production: for example, excessive height, absent periods, breasts constantly leaking milk.

Rare

◆ Poisoning

Tobacco, ethyl alcohol and lead are some of the many poisons that may affect the optic nerve.

- Gradual loss of the central field of vision.
- Vision is generally dimmed.
- Loss of vision may be abrupt after a binge.
- Recovery depends on how longstanding the damage is.

◆ Cartoid aneurysm

Caused by the effect of pressure from a swollen carotid artery within the brain, which presses on the optic nerve.

- A blind area in the outer field of vision.
- Affects one eye at first.
- Gradually involves both eyes.

The Eyes

Night blindness

Probable

◆ Retinitis pigmentosa

See page 43.
Suspected in a young adult with:

- Night blindness.
- Tunnel vision.

Possible

◆ Severe short-sightedness

- Difficulty seeing in poor light.
- Blurred vision helped by glasses.

◆ Congenital

Occasionally, poor night vision is present from birth.

Rare

◆ Vitamin A deficiency

Vitamin A is required for vision, this being the basis for the parental wisdom that eating carrots, a rich source of Vitamin A, will help night vision.

It is a fair bet that this explanation will leave children unimpressed and carrots uneaten, but children should at least be aware that lack of this vitamin is a major cause of blindness in the Third World.

- Night blindness is an early symptom.
- The eyes appear leathery, and the lenses clouded.
- Given soon enough, high doses of Vitamin A save sight.

Colour blindness

A condition affecting about one in 12 males and about one in 200 females. In the commonest form, red-green vision is partly or completely absent; less commonly, blue-green vision is affected. Total absence of any colour vision is very rare.

So adaptable is the brain that it is possible to reach adult life without any suspicion of a problem. The individual appears to distinguish colours by noting subtle differences in brightness and greyness; context also helps – for example, the lowest traffic light is green, because that is what everyone else calls it. The writer has even known a successful colour blind interior designer. Normal colour vision is needed in certain occupations – typically pilots and train drivers – where it is essential to see colour absolutely correctly.

Occasionally, someone with previously normal colour vision finds it deteriorating for one of the following reasons:

Probable

◆ Cataract

This common problem, typically experienced as haziness in the lens, does not really destroy colour vision but makes colours less easy to distinguish.
See page 25.

◆ Damage to retina

Many retinal diseases can affect colour

vision by damaging the receptors responsible for seeing colour.

Other symptoms, considered fully elsewhere in this section, can include:

• Gradual loss of vision.

• Sudden loss of vision.

• Blind spots.

It is not possible to be more specific without medical assessment of the eye, optic nerve and the parts of the brain responsible for vision.

Possible

◆ Malnutrition

Lack of vitamins and protein needed for the visual receptors can cause colour vision to deteriorate.

It is a possibility among the severely malnourished, alcoholics, those with wasting diseases or the mentally disturbed.

There is likely to be also:

• Night blindness.

• In children, failure to grow.

• Hair loss, loss of skin colour.

• Swollen ankles.

Rare

◆ Toxic drugs

• This includes a massive over-use of tobacco, and alcoholism.

• Overdosage of digoxin, as used in heart disease, can make the world look yellow or green.

Squints

A squint is the result of the eyes being out of alignment: they appear to point in different directions. Often a squint is suspected as an impression rather than definitely seen: you may have a feeling on looking at someone that their eyes are not quite in line. If that someone is a child, please do not ignore that feeling, for squint is an important symptom and should never be ignored.Forget the old wive's tale of children growing out of a squint: it does not happen. What does happen is that the child experiences double vision and gradually its brain learns to ignore the vision from one eye in an effort to overcome the defect. If unrecognised, this leads to permanently damaged vision in one eye.

Symptoms which suggest a squint are:

- Obvious deviation of one or both eyes.
- Head held in an unusual posture to compensate.
- Squint noticed if child is tired.

The assessment and treatment of squint is a complex area. In most cases the cause is either muscle imbalance or different strengths of lens of each eye. Both causes are treated by surgery or glasses.

Probable

◆ Muscle imbalance or inequalities of vision

If the head is held at an unusual angle, it suggests the likelihood of muscle imbalance underlying the squint. You may also notice that one eye cannot turn beyond a certain point. Otherwise, it is likely that one eye is long-sighted, or less commonly, short sighted compared to the other. Usually, however, it is a matter of specialist assessment to differentiate these problems.

Possible

◆ Prominent skin folds

In children, the folds of skin by the bridge of the nose may be unusually wide, giving the impression that the eyes turn in. Even if this happens to be the case the child should still be checked.

Rare

◆ Nerve palsies

It has been mentioned (see *Paralysis of the eye muscles*, page 37) that six muscles control the movements of the eyes. Each muscle is subject to paralysis for a variety of reasons. Nerve palsy is probably the cause if there is:

- A drooping eyelid.
- Changes in size of the pupil (see pages 18 and 19).

Nerve palsies have a variety of causes, which themselves need further investigation.

◆ Tumours of the eye or socket

These can occur at all ages, producing a squint by pressure on one eyeball. So don't ignore a newly acquired squint, especially in children.

- The eye protrudes more and more.
- There is a pain behind the eye.
- The pupil may appear white if the tumour is inside the eye.

Nose an odd shape

There is, of course, no such thing as a 'normal' shape for a nose.

The 'one-off' factors that can deform it are considered here.

Probable

◆ Injury

Typically, the nose is flattened or made crooked (you may hear doctors describe the latter as 'deviation'). This is likely to be accompanied by swelling and bleeding and indicates a fracture of the nose bone.

It is normal to wait for a week to allow swelling to go down before deciding whether the nose needs straightening by surgery.

• Nasal bone fracture.

• Flattening of the nose.

• Deviation of the nose.

• Swelling.

• Bleeding.

Possible

◆ Rhinophyma

Also known as 'potato nose' or 'bottle-nose'. Caused by over-activity of the sebaceous gland of the nose. It takes some years to develop.

It is relatively common, affecting men more often than women, and is usually seen in older age groups and in those with a high alcohol consumption.

• Large, bulbous nose.

• Purplish red in colour.

• Irregular 'pitted' surface: the pits mark the entrances to the glands.

Can be treated easily by surgery and long-term antibiotics can be given to reduce occurrence.

Rare

◆ Nasal septal necrosis

A blow to the nose may not break the nasal bones, but instead damage the nasal septum (a thin layer of cartilage separating the two sides of the nose). Pressure from a blood clot under its mucous membrane covering causes:

• Headache.

• Local pain at the tip of the nose.

• Apparent widening of the tip of the nose.

• Loss of sensation over the skin of the nose.

• Destruction of septal cartilage over a matter of weeks, causing the nose to dip at the bridge.

◆ Leprosy

Causes collapse of the nose due to septal ulceration.

• This is one of several obvious symptoms which will be apparent.

◆ Cancer of the nose

Any irregular sore on the nose that enlarges over months or years, that bleeds, ulcerates or is painful could be malignant. Enlargement of local lymph nodes suggests malignancy.

Reddened nose

Probable

◆ Staphylococcal infection

An infection of the skin in a part of the nose.

- Local swelling.
- Local redness.
- Local pain.
- Local heat.

  May require antibiotics.

Possible

◆ Acne rosacea

A rash caused by over-activity of the sebaceous glands.

- Associated with facial flushing.
- Redness from small blood vessels.
- Rash covers nose, brow, face and chin.
- Small pustules may be evident.
- May persist for years.

  Treatment is available, usually with antibiotics for the long term, but can be difficult.

◆ Erysipelas

A bacterial skin infection.

- Associated with a break in the skin.
- Often near eye, nose or mouth.
- Fever.
- Malaise.
- Hot, reddened swelling all over affected area.

The sinuses

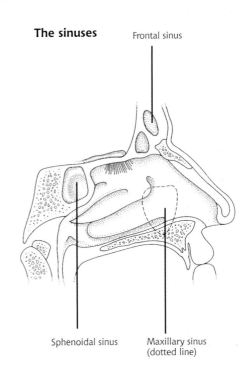

Frontal sinus

Sphenoidal sinus

Maxillary sinus (dotted line)

The Nose

- Painful.
- Blisters may appear..

  You need to see a doctor soon. Antibiotics will treat this effectively if given at an early stage.

◆ Rhinophyma

See page 50.

Streaming nose

Probable

◆ Common cold

There are many different types of common cold virus. As you throw off each new one, you develop a natural immunity to it. Children often have a 'perpetual runny nose'. This is because they are being exposed to new viruses every day at school. The elderly rarely get colds for they have built up immunity to so many of the viruses.

◆ Vasomotor rhinitis

Some individuals suffer from over-reaction of the nasal lining. This leads to an excess of the usually small amounts of 'normal' nasal discharge. Some treatments taken as nasal sprays, which can be obtained from pharamcies, may help this condition. Its features are similar to those of allergic rhinitis.

◆ Allergic rhinitis

In the same way that hay fever is caused by pollen, many allergens can cause a running nose. Locally applied steroid nasal sprays can be effective in preventing the reaction.

Possible

◆ Sinusitis

Nasal discharge will often be yellow or green, sometimes thick. There may be an associated headache.

◆ Foreign bodies

• Discharge is foul-smelling and on one side only.

The foreign body needs to be removed by a doctor.

◆ Nasal polyp

Polyps – which are benign, fleshy growths – can appear inside the nose. As well as obstructing the nasal passages and blocking the nose, they can cause an increase in the volume of secretions, which will appear as a runny nose.

Treatment is medical management (use of topical nasal steroids) or surgical removal of the polyps.

◆ Drug withdrawal

A clear, runny discharge is a common symptom when withdrawing from a 'hard' drug such as heroin, or its substitute, methadone.

Other signs include:

• Running eyes.

• Sweating.

• 'Goose flesh'.

• Yawning.

• Stomach cramps.

• Diarrhoea.

Rare

◆ Cancer of the nose

Any tumour of the nose or in the spaces around the nose may cause a nasal discharge.

Recurrent nosebleeds or bloody streaks in the discharge may be a feature.

Discuss with your doctor.

The Nose

Nosebleeds

Also known as epistaxis. A particularly common problem in children, although most adults have episodes of bleeding from the nose at some time. There are many causes, some due to local disease and some indicative of systemic, or 'whole body', disease.

Most nosebleeds can be treated by continuous, firm pressure across the fleshy part of the nose just below the bridge. Pressure should be maintained for as long as ten minutes in severe cases. Sit forward with the head supported and breathe through your mouth. Local application of ice at the bridge of the nose may also help.

Only in rare cases is medical or surgical intervention required, but see your doctor or local hospital emergency department about any profuse or prolonged bleeding.

Probable

◆ Minor infection

The commonest cause of persistent and recurrent nosebleeds is a minor nasal infection. This brings blood vessels very close to the surface on the inside of the nose. The slightest disturbance will then set off a nosebleed. Antibiotic ointment used inside the nose over a few days can have dramatic results.

◆ Nose picking

Probably the commonest cause in children. The finger, or the fingernail, damages an area of skin, known as Little's area, situated at the entrance to the nose.

- Occasionally, profuse bleeding.
- Often occurs at night.
- Almost always cures itself after applying pressure.
- May be recurrent.

◆ Injury

If the nose is clearly deformed or misaligned as a result of a blow, see a doctor. There could be an underlying fracture.

◆ Common cold

Nosebleeds are a surprisingly frequent symptom of common colds. The inflammation compromises the fine blood vessels.

Repeated nose-blowing to clear mucus may also bring on bleeding.

Possible

◆ Foreign body

A toddler or young child pushes a bead or some other small object into a nostril, which remains unrecognized for days, weeks or months. Inflammation develops, causing:

- Discharge from one nostril; it may be
- Purulent – yellow-green.
- Possibly bloodstained and smelly.

Removal may require a general anaesthetic.

◆ Chronic sinusitis

The linings of the bony sinuses become chronically infected.

The Nose

The naso-pharynx

Naso-pharynx

- Profuse discharge back into throat, rather than out through the nostrils.
- Obstruction of the nose.
- Head pain, particularly in the forehead or under the eyes.
- Loss of sense of smell.
- Nosebleeds, often with excessive noseblowing.

◆ **Drug-induced**

A number of drugs, typically warfarin, which thins the blood, and some drugs used to treat arthritis may cause nosebleeds.

If nosebleeds occur while you are taking warfarin they may indicate that you are taking too much – consult a doctor.

◆ **Benign tumours, including nasal polyps**

These can bleed from time to time, particularly after nose-picking or blowing.

- Obstruction of the nose.
- Associated sinusitis.
- Discharge of mucus.
- Loss of sense of smell.

Rare

◆ **Hereditary haemorrhagic telangiectasia**

See page 79.

◆ **Disorders of blood clotting**

The commonest are Factor 8 deficiency (true haemophilia), Christmas disease and von Willebrand's disease.
Common features include:

- Persistent bleeding after minor cuts and abrasions.
- Marked bruising.
- Bleeding after extraction of teeth.
- Bleeding into joints, causing eventual degeneration.
- Spontaneous bleeding including nosebleeds.

Simple blood tests will determine whether thre is any abnormality of clotting.

It is particularly important to know if you have a disorder before dental treatment if in doubt, check.

◆ **High blood pressure**

In the middle-aged and elderly.

An otherwise fit individual who suddenly gets recurrent nose-bleeds must have blood pressure measurements and tests to check clotting ability.

The Nose

◆ Cancer of the nose

There are several potential symptoms:

- Obstruction of the nose.
- Discharge from the nose.
- Associated sinusitis.
- Nose-bleeds.

    It is *very* rare for anyone to present nosebleeds to their doctor as a symptom of cancer of the nose.

Nasal-sounding speech

Any disease or injury that blocks the nose or distorts the nasopharynx will alter the quality of the sound produced. Commonest of the causes are the common cold; septal deviation (page 56); 'adenoids' (page 56); and injury.

Less common, but worth considering, are: cleft palate (page 80); a foreign body (page 53); chronic sinusitis (page 53); and benign tumours, including polyps (page 54).

Snoring and sleep apnoea

An all-too-common problem, rarely reported to doctors by snorers.

It happens when the tongue obstructs air flow, setting up vibrations of structures in the mouth, particularly the uvula (the fleshy, wriggly bit that hangs down between your tonsils), soft palate and tongue. Most common in drinkers, the obese, the over-40's and males, and those with nasal obstruction or misshapen noses. Sleeping on the side, rather than the back, will probably help. If you find your partner's snoring is making you seriously dissatisfied with him (or her), you will not want a doctor to tell you to be understanding because snorers cannot help it. However, you should be interested in the fact that some snoring, some of the time, is inevitable.

Exceptionally severe, persistent snoring justifies surgery. A modern operation known as a uvuloplasty, which reshapes the soft palate at the back of the mouth, can transform the lives of severe snorers.

For less severe cases, one trick that is said to work is to sew a hairbrush inside the back of your pyjama jacket. This wakes you when you roll on to your back – the snoring position. Also try adjusting pillows and bedding, changing the ventilation in your bedroom and eating bedtime snacks – all of which are said to have made a difference to some people's snoring.

Sleep apnoea is defined as an episode when breathing stops during sleep. This can occur many times a night and the resulting sleep deprivation causes day-time lethargy, poor concentration, poor memory and falling asleep.

The person is usually overweight and has a short, thick neck.

In children the tonsils may be so large that they meet or 'kiss' in the middle.

This needs referral to a specialist.

The Nose

Breathing through the mouth: a blocked nose

The effects of an obstructed nose depend somewhat on the cause, but may include:

- Pain in the nose.
- Discharge from the nose.
- No sense of smell.
- Breathing through the mouth.
- Snoring.
- Dry mouth.
- Bad breath.

For details, see the sections concerning those symptoms. Causes of obstruction include:

Probable

◆ Adenoids

Perhaps the commonest reason for 'mouth breathing'. The adenoids are lymph tissue lying at the back of the nose and pharynx near the soft palate. They are prone to acute or chronic infection.

Acute infection gives:

- Pain behind nose.
- Catarrh.
- Nasal obstruction (due to enlargement).
- Enlarged neck lymph nodes.

Chronic infection gives:

- Enlarged adenoids.
- Chronic catarrh.
- Persistent cough.
- Breathing through the mouth.
- Ear infection, possibly leading to impaired hearing.

Both types of 'adenoiditis' cause alteration in the quality of speech. As the adenoids perform no essential function, removing them is a common and usually very helpful operation: common, of course, in childhood.

This operation used to be carried out frequently. Current understanding of how both the adenoids and the tonsils develop is that there is a natural shrinkage of these tissues as a child reaches his or her tenth birthday. An operation can be avoided if symptoms are not too troublesome.

◆ Septal deviation

The septum is the thin layer of cartilage separating the tow sides of the nose. 'Deviation' may occur during birth (one to two per cent of babies have permanently deviated septa). It may also occur as the result of injury at a later age. The result is obstruction of one or other of the nostrils, either partially or completely. See *Nose an odd shape*, page 50.

◆ Injury and common cold

See page 50; and page 423.

◆ Vasomotor rhinitis and allergic rhinitis

See page 52.

Possible

◆ Foreign body, chronic sinusitis, benign tumours including nasal polyps.

See pages 53 and 54.

Painful nose

This is such a general symptom that analysing it in its own right is not helpful. There will always be some other accompanying factor(s) to pin it down. Is there nasal discharge or bleeding? Is the speech affected? Is the nose misshapen? Does the nose itch? Has the sense of smell gone? These are all covered in detail in neighbouring pages and will give proper insight into 'pain in the nose'.

Tingling nose; sneezing

Look for an outside cause first: is it the smell of a houseplant, or an animal? Or a chemical? Or chilli powder or pepper? Some people sneeze in bright sunlight.

There are many different causes, a large number unique to individuals. Failing these, consider *Vasomotor rhinitis*, or *Allergic rhinitis*, page 52.

No sense of smell

Probable

◆ **Smoking**

◆ **Common cold**

◆ **Vasomotor rhinitis**

◆ **Allergic rhinitis**

These diagnoses are either self-evident or covered in detail elsewhere: see page 52. With a common cold, the loss is transient; vasomotor rhinitis and allergic rhinitis cause intermittent loss, which may become long-term.

Possible

◆ **Obstructive lesions of the nose**
See *Breathing through the mouth*, opposite.

◆ **Breathing through the mouth**
See opposite page.

◆**Sinusitis**
See page 53.

Acute sinusitis may lead to transient loss and chronic sinusitis to long-term loss.

Rare

◆ **Head injury**
A blow to the head may sever the filaments of the cranial nerve in the roof of the nose. As the nose is pushed in, or the forehead struck, there is a bony displacement which can cut the nerve responsible for sensing smell, causing permanent loss of smell.

◆ **Meningioma**
A tumour of the sheath covering the brain. It can press on the olfactory nerve (responsible for smell), causing progressive loss of smell and other symptoms, such as headache.

◆ **Frontal lobe tumour**
This can cause pressure on brain tissue involved in sensing smell, and it can damage the pathways conducting sense of smell. Loss is progressive and other symptoms will be apparent.

The Nose

The ear: introduction

This organ has something in common with an iceberg: there is so much more to it than you see.

There are three parts to the ear: the outer, the middle and the inner ear.

The visible ear is cartilage, covered with skin, and it is subject to any of the problems that affect skin elsewhere: bruising, infections and eczema.

Hidden from view is the eardrum, which guards the inner ear, a beautifully intricate structure that turns sound waves into the electrical impulses for transmission to the brain.

The inner ear also contains the fluid-filled semi-circular canals which give you your sense of balance and orientation. Then there are the passages connecting the inner ear to the back of the throat: they allow equalization of air pressure on both sides of the eardrum, without which you experience pressure or 'popping' in the ears.

Skin, nerves, bones, fluid: little wonder that there are many minor diseases which can afflict the ear, and a few serious ones.

Bleeding ear

Blood from the ear, usually mixed with pus, is a common symptom, not often due to a serious cause.

Probable

◆ Middle ear infection

This problem is inescapable in childhood, occasional in adults and usually accompanies a common cold. The eardrum becomes red and bulges.

If the drum bursts, pus and blood ooze from the ear for a few days.

- Pain in the ear for a day or two.
- Then, suddenly, a smelly, bloodstained discharge.
- The pain goes.
- The discharge lessens over a few days.

There is evidence that most ear infections are viral in nature. Most will settle with analgesia, and doctors do not like prescribing antibiotics for the first three days.

The eardrum nearly always heals, but your doctor will want to watch progress in order to be certain.

Possible

◆ Boil

Just like a pimple elsewhere, a boil in the canal of the ear may burst, discharging a few specks of blood.

- An extremely tender spot, just inside the ear canal.
- Bursts after a day or two.
- Symptoms then rapidly vanish.

◆ Polyp

These fleshy lumps can form deep inside the ear if there is recurrent infection.

The Ears

They are painless, but may ooze or bleed and can be seen through an instrument for seeing inside the ear.

◆ Injury

A severe blow to the head may rupture the eardrum and cause bleeding.

Rare

◆ Cancer

Growths within the ear canal or within the inner ear are unusual.

- Intense, persistent pain in the ear.
- Constant discharge of pus mixed with blood.
- Partial paralysis of one side of the face.

Boil in the ear

Probable

◆ Boil

Boils form at the root of the tiny hairs lining the ear canal. They cause pain out of all proportion to their tiny size because the skin of the ear canal is unable to stretch much without intense pain.

- Localized, throbbing pain.
- You may be able to feel a tender lump.
- Reaches a peak after a day or two.
- Discharges small amounts of blood and pus for a couple of days.

  Will usually clear by itself, but antibiotic drops help.

  Sometimes oral antibiotics are necessary.

Possible

◆ Herpes simplex

A cold sore in the ear canal will give symptoms similar to a boil, but:

- The pain is more prolonged and recurrent.
- The sore is filled with clear fluid, rather than pus.

◆ Ramsay-Hunt syndrome

See page 63.

Lumps and bumps on the ear

Probable

◆ Resolved boil

Meaning the aftermath of a boil.

- Initially, pain and redness from the boil.
- May discharge pus.
- Becomes smaller over a few days.
- Firm lump left at the site.

  Usually the lump disappears, but this can take months.

◆ Cauliflower ear

This is the permanently enlarged, fleshy,

misshapen ear left after injury. It results from permanent scarring of the cartilage that makes up the external ear and is an occupational hazard of boxers and rugby players.

Possible

◆ Auricular appendage

A small, painless outgrowth between the ear canal and the cheek.

It is present from birth, harmless and removable.

◆ Wart

Can occur on the ear as on other parts of the skin.

- Appears rapidly, then stops growing at about 5 mm in length.
- The end is rough, with black spots.

Removable, but a complete cure can be difficult.

Rare

◆ Gout

A disorder of body chemistry leading to the appearance of crystals of uric acid in many parts of the body, especially the joints.

- Firm, irregular lumps called tophi in the outer ear.
- These become extremely painful.
- Pain in other joints, classically the big toe.

◆ Tumours

A slow-growing skin cancer can involve the ear.

- Begins as a small, crusted spot.
- Develops a rolled edge.
- May bleed.
- Does not heal.
- Gradually enlarges.

Can be treated. See a doctor.

Discharging ear

Probable

◆ Ear infection

See page 64.

- Gives pain, pus and blood for a few days.

◆ Otitis externa

Meaning eczema of the skin lining the ear canal. The skin of the ear canal is as prone to eczema as is skin elsewhere in the body.

Aggravating factors include swimming-pool chemicals, poking about in the ear with pencils or earbuds, and even medicated ear drops. Frequently, bacteria or fungi invade the eczema, giving a mixed picture of infection and irritation which it is difficult to cure.

- Intensely itching ear canals.
- Persistent, thin, watery discharge.
- Discharge thicker if infection occurs.
- Pain on pulling the ear signifies an infection.

Treatment is with anti-fungal, anti-inflammatory ear drops and oral antibiotics.

Possible

◆ Chronic otitis media

Literally, chronic infection of the inner ear, with pus discharging for weeks on end through a hole in the eardrum. There is usually a previous history of repeated ear infection.

*   Yellowish discharge.
*   Quantity varies from day to day.

Treatment involves eradicating infection, getting air into the ear and, eventually, repairing the hole in the eardrum.

Rare

◆ Cholesteatoma

This is a mass of abnormal cells which forms usually as a result of recurrent ear infections. The cells destroy surrounding tissues, so causing symptoms of:

*   Deafness.
*   Discharge.

*   Vertigo.

Treatment consists of surgically removing the cholesteatoma and refashioning the inner ear. This is a complex operation.

◆ Polyp

A fleshy, non-cancerous growth arising from a cholesteatoma and causing discharge, sometimes bloodstained.

◆ Rupture of eardrum

Caused by injury and resulting in:

*   Deafness, which may be partial or total.
*   Ringing in ears.
*   Bloody discharge.

An injury serious enough to fracture the skull near the ear means that the fluid which surrounds the brain may leak out of the ear.

This significant condition causes the above symptoms plus:

*   Painless, persistent leakage of clear fluid.

Earache

Pain in the ear is usually caused by a relatively minor problem within the ear. It nonetheless keeps doctors on their toes because it can be a symptom of disease elsewhere.

Probable

◆ Ear infection

See page 64.

*   Pain, pus and discharge arising over a few hours or days.

A routine symptom in children with common colds.

◆ Eustachian catarrh

This condition may be described by your doctor as Eustachian tube dysfunction.

If fluid builds up inside the inner ear, it muffles hearing. This condition is common for a few days or weeks after a common cold. Chronic catarrh is also familiar to those who suffer from hay fever or sinusitus. It is particularly important to pick up in childhood since it can cause deafness severe enough to interfere with speech and to hinder progress in school.

- Hearing is muffled.
- A feeling of pressure inside the ear.
- Yawning relieves pressure temporarily.
- In children, delay in learning to speak.

Adults rarely need any treatment other than decongestants; children suffering deafness may need surgery to drain the fluid.

The Eustachian tube

The Eustachian tube is a ventilation pipe which goes from the back of the throat to the inner ear. Air passes through the tube to equalize the pressure on either side of the eardrum. This is why swallowing relieves popping ears.

The tube is narrowest during childhood and it is then that most problems occur.

◆ Wax

A block of hard wax may eventually become painful and give rise to muffled hearing. People vary enormously in how much ear wax they produce and often recognize for themselves when so much has built up that they need their ears cleared by syringing. If possible, however, leave your ears alone.

The ear is a self-cleaning organ. It is rarely necessary to have ears syringed.

Small hairs move the wax to the outer ear where it can be wiped away.

Avoid cleaning your ears with cotton buds – it causes more problems than it cures. Always try simple earwax softening drops first, and try to allow the ear to clear naturally. Ear syringing is rarely required.

◆ Boil

See page 59.

A pimple in the ear canal, causing a remarkable amount of pain for such a small object.

Possible

◆ Throat infection

A throat infection (including tonsillitis) may seem obvious and recognizable, but often the throat symptoms are overshadowed by earache. Common in young children.

- Sore throat.
- Pain on swallowing.

If there are white patches on tonsils, it may signify tonsillitis.

◆ Teeth problems

The large molar teeth, if decayed, may cause aching which appears to radiate into the ear.

In children, eruption of the back teeth can cause a combination of symptoms easily taken for an ear infection:

- Feverish, unhappy child.
- Rubbing ear.
- Dribbling.

◆ Mastoiditis

The mastoid bone is the prominent swelling behind the ears and it was once common for ear infection to spread into that area.

With the use of antibiotics, this is now unlikely.

- Pain behind the ear.
- Tender, red swelling of the mastoid bone.
- Fever and malaise.
- Heavy yellow discharge from the ear.

The condition urgently needs surgical drainage of the mastoid bone.

◆ Perichondritis

Occasionally, the outer ear, which is made up of cartilage, becomes inflamed, typically after a knock, or in cold weather.

- Throbbing pain over part of the outer ear.
- Skin is reddened.

Symptoms settle of their own accord over a few days, just occasionally needing antibiotic treatment.

Rare

◆ Rodent ulcer (Basal cell carcinoma)

A form of skin cancer that can occur anywhere on the ear or in the ear canal.

- Starts by looking like a small sore that does not heal.
- Grows very slowly.
- May bleed and cause pain.

Cured by treatment given at an early stage.

◆ Tic douloureux

The medical term for this is trigeminal neuralgia.

An unpleasant condition arising from irritation of the nerve which supplies feeling to much of the face and the ear. The cause is unknown. Commonest in the late middle-aged and elderly.

- Sudden, severe shooting pains across ear, face, nose.
- Pains set off by eating, the cold or other triggers.

There are several drug treatments for this miserable, though harmless illness.

◆ Ramsay-Hunt syndrome

This is a form of shingles which can be a puzzling cause of pain.

- Pain in one side of throat and the ear on that side.
- Hearing may seem hyper sensitive.
- Loss of taste on that side of the tongue.
- Small, crusting spots appear in the throat and ear after a week or two.

◆ Cancer of the ear

Cancer of the ear canal or inner ear is unusual.

- Intense, prolonged pain.
- Bloody discharge.

◆ Cancer of the tongue

It is important to check the back of the tongue in cases of persistent earache where there appears to be no cause within the ear itself.

- A persistent, shallow ulcer on the back of the tongue.
- Commonest in smokers.
- Gradually enlarges, with pain and bleeding.

◆ **Cancer of the tonsil**

Another unusual cancer, most common in old age.

- One tonsil is enlarged.
- Earache.
- Pain on swallowing.

Ear feels 'full'

A familiar sensation, variously described as fullness, cotton wool between the ears, pressure in the ears, muzziness in the head.

The basic features are slight deafness and muffled hearing due to some physical obstruction to hearing.

The causes are often obvious and readily treatable.

Probable

◆ **Eustachian catarrh**

See *Earache*, page 61.

Caused by build-up of fluid within the inner ear as after a common cold; treatment, if needed, consists of decongestants and aromatic inhalations.

◆ **Wax**

Probably the commonest cause of a slight feeling of fullness, often accompanied by dizziness, discomfort, mild earache, see page 62.

Simple earwax softening drops often allow the ear to clear naturally.

◆ **Infection**

Rather than causing the painful picture described elsewhere (see, for example, *Earache*, page 61), infections sometimes run a less obvious course with:

- Vague mild discomfort.
- Fluctuating, mild deafness.
- Feeling of pressure in ear.

The diagnosis has to be made by a doctor or nurse who can see the eardrum.

Possible

◆ **Hay fever**

Causes fullness as a result of swelling of the lining of the nose and ears.

- Seasonal sneezing, sore eyes.
- Persistent runny nose during the pollen season.
- Often associated with eczema and asthma.

Rare

◆ **Chronic otitis externa**

Severe cases give rise to chronic swelling of the ear canal, which also becomes blocked up with debris.

Cleansing is needed for a long time. See page 68.

Deafness or hearing difficulties in adults

Adult deafness or loss of hearing is, to a large extent, a normal part of the ageing process. The hearing loss can gradually worsen, unnoticed, until it interferes with work or social relationships, at which point it is suddenly seen as a 'new' problem. Special attention should always be given to sudden deafness, deafness affecting one ear only or when it is associated with pain, giddiness (vertigo), or ringing in the ears (tinnitus).

Probable

◆ Wax

An extremely common cause for a mild degree of hearing loss.

- Often causes sudden, partial hearing loss.
- 'Blocked' feeling in ears.

◆ Chronic otitis media

Long-term infection within the ear leads to:

- Deafness.
- Persistent discharge of pus-like material.
- Sometimes pain and vertigo.

Treatment is meticulous cleansing of the ear in a specialist clinic.

The sudden appearance of pain and vertigo calls for urgent specialist assessment: this could indicate a deterioration of the condition. Normally, continuous cleansing of the ear will allow healing.

◆ Otosclerosis

A condition causing increasing stiffness of one of the bones that transmits sound waves from the eardrum.

- Often runs in families.
- Commonest in women, and gets worse in pregnancy.
- Progressive deafness, starting in early adulthood.
- Ringing in the ears – tinnitus – is common.

Surgery can help, but usually a hearing aid is the simplest treatment.

◆ Presbyacusis

This is the familiar hearing loss that comes with age, caused by degeneration of the pathway that turns sound waves into electrical impulses for transmission to the brain.

- Typically noticed in late 60s.
- Both ears affected.
- Pain-free.

Possible

◆ Mèniére's disease

Suggested by repeated attacks of deafness along with vertigo and ringing in the ears – tinnitus.

◆ Acoustic trauma

Repeated loud noise damages hearing. It is said, however, that five years of exposure is needed for any significant damage to occur, by which time the most dedicated disco-goer may well have moved on to embroidery.

The Ears

Actually, discotheque deafness is usually temporary; but prolonged and repeated exposure to loud noise can result in some loss of hearing. Ringing in the ears is common after hearing loud noises. Workers exposed to loud noise should wear ear protection and have regular hearing checks.

> Prolonged use of personal stereos at high volume damages ears. The direct application of earphones, delivering high volume sound, has been shown significantly to affect young people's hearing.If others around you can hear it – it is too loud.

◆ Arteriosclerosis

Poor blood flow to the arteries supplying blood to the ear can cause a range of symptoms, usually confined to the elderly.

- Fluctuating deafness, giddiness, ringing in the ears.

Symptoms may vary, depending on the position of the neck. There is no specific treatment.

Rare

◆ Infection

Deafness is a rare and unpredictable complication of certain infectious illnesses, notably measles and mumps. It is also a possible consequence of meningitis and syphilis.

Children who have recurrent ear infections may have decreased hearing. See also *Hearing difficulties in children*, opposite.

◆ Acoustic neuroma

A slow-growing tumour on the nerve of hearing. Though rare, it is suspected frequently on the basis of the following suggestive symptoms:

- One-sided progressive deafness.
- One-sided tinnitus.
- Vertigo.
- Later numbness of face, unsteadiness.

A brain scan allows for quite precise localization, improving the chances of successful removal by surgery.

◆ Skull fracture

Could damage the nerve of hearing and disrupts the delicate bones that transmit sounds, causing sudden loss of hearing.

◆ Drugs

The nerve of hearing is sensitive to several drugs, the commonest of which is aspirin taken in overdose.

- Tinnitus (ringing in the ears) is an early warning sign.
- Giddiness.

◆ Paget's disease

A not uncommon condition of later life in which:

- Bones become tender.
- Bowing of the legs.
- Enlargement of the head.

The deafness is caused by a squeezing of the nerve of hearing by enlarged bone. This disease is frequently unrecognized until characteristic signs are noticed on an X-ray.

The Ears

Deafness or hearing difficulties in children

Hearing difficulties in childhood are difficult to detect, but every effort must be made to do so. Specialised testing of the new born is becoming increasingly routine. Suspect a hearing problem if there is no startled reaction to sudden, loud noises, or if, as he or she develops, the baby does not turn to a sound. Later, delay in starting to speak should arouse suspicion. Later again, a schoolchild's performance may deteriorate for no obvious cause; once more, consider the possibility of loss of hearing.

You cannot be too careful.

Probable

◆ Wax

Simple to detect, and simple to remedy with drops to soften the earwax.

Most specialists advise against syringing in young children.

◆ Serous otitis media

A common reason for hearing loss in children who have recurrent ear infections leading to a build-up of fluid within the inner ear.

The condition is also known as glue ear because the fluid can be thick and sticky. The condition often cures itself over a few months.

The symptoms are:

- Deafness, which may be partial or total.

- Occasional pain in ear. Certain typical changes in the appearance of the eardrum will alert a doctor to the condition.

As a remedy, grommets may be inserted.

Possible

◆ Congenital

Always to be considered in children born deaf, in whom there may have been a failure of development of the organs of hearing.

Sometimes deafness runs in the family; sometimes the mother has been exposed to drugs which damage the ear (see below) or has had German measles – Rubella.

There are also many syndromes in which deafness is one of several abnormalities, but this is a matter for specialist assessment. In most cases of congenital deafness, however, no cause can be found.

Rare

◆ Congenital rubella – German measles

A rarity since vaccination has become generally available. Rubella contracted in the first four months of pregnancy wreaks havoc on the developing child. As well as deafness, it can cause:

- Poor development of the brain and mental retardation.

- Cataracts.

- Heart defects.

The Ears

This tragic outcome is rare thanks to national immunization programmes against Rubella.

Check on your Rubella immunity before you get pregnant.

◆ Infection

Deafness is an unusual and unpredictable complication of certain infectious illnesses, notably measles and mumps, both of which are increasingly rare, thanks to immunization.

It may also be a consequence of meningitis.

◆ Neonatal jaundice

Severe jaundice in the days after birth can cause brain damage, including deafness. Hence the vigorous treatment given to babies who develop the condition.

◆ Drugs

The nerve of hearing is sensitive to several drugs, the commonest of which is aspirin taken in overdose.

Another is gentamicin, now reserved for life-threatening disease such as meningitis, where the risk of damage to hearing is outweighed by the risk to life.

Tinnitus (ringing in the ears) is an early warning sign.

• Giddiness.

If a potentially harmful drug has to be used, blood levels will be monitored to avoid damage.

◆ Congenital hypothyroidism

An under-active thyroid gland, giving a child with:

• Coarse features.

• A gruff cry.

• Enlarged tongue.

In many countries there are screening programmes to detect this curable illness as early as possible in new-born babies.

Itching ear

Probable

◆ Otitis externa

A form of eczema affecting the skin of the ear canal. Common in adult life, typically in those with eczema elsewhere.

• Intense itching.

• Skin of ear canal and ear itself is flaking, crusting, swollen.

• Ear feels wet, with a thin, clear discharge.

Like any other skin, that of the ear can become sensitised to chemicals. Common among these are chlorine in swimming pools, hair spray and the antibiotics in the very drops used to treat otitis externa.

Possible

◆ Fungal infection

Organisms known as fungi can invade skin already broken down by otitis externa.

The Ears

- Symptoms of otitis externa.
- Black spores may be visible in the discharge.

Treatment is with anti-fungal drops.

Noises in the ear

Noises other than ringing in the ear are very common and very rarely due to worrying underlying causes. They nearly always pass within a fortnight.

Many cases remain unexplained, the symptoms going as mysteriously as they came. If noises occur in a particular location, check for a cause as simple as the hum from central heating, power lines or similar noise source.

See also *Ringing in the ears*, page 70.

Probable

◆ Eustachian catarrh

Blockage caused by fluid building up inside the ear, often experienced with a common cold.

- Muffled hearing.
- Popping or crackling inside the ears.
- Slight discomfort from a feeling of pressure in the ears.
- Swallowing gives temporary relief.

◆ Acute inner ear infection

Causes noises for similar reasons as does acoustic catarrh (see above).

- Rapid onset of pain.
- Deafness.
- Crackling inside ears. Antibiotics are usually given for this condition.

Rare

◆ Heart murmur

The sound arising from a diseased valve in the heart may be heard inside the head when there is no competing noise.

- A whooshing noise.
- In time with heart beat.

Needs to be assessed by a doctor.

◆ Anaemia

If extreme, anaemia is said to cause noises in the ear. This symptom is likely to be overshadowed by other features of anaemia such as:

- Pallor.
- Tiredness.
- Sore tongue.
- Dizziness on standing.

A blood test will quickly confirm the diagnosis.

The Ears

Tenderness behind the ear

Immediately behind the ear is a bone known as the mastoid, felt as a prominent swelling. Pain and swelling in this area is always to be taken seriously.

Probable

◆ **Acute ear infection**

Although the infection is confined to the middle ear, occasionally there is a mild degree of tenderness over the mastoid bone. Middle ear infections are usually treated with an antibiotic, which should prevent further spread.

Possible

◆ **Mastoiditis**

Though now uncommon, this was once a feared consequence of ear infections, since infection can spread from the mastoid region into the brain.

- Begins with an ear infection.
- Redness, swelling over mastoid bone.
- Yellow/green discharge from ear.
- Fever, pain, malaise.

  Urgent surgical treatment is needed.

Ringing in the ears – tinnitus

Of all ear diseases, this causes most misery – because of its persistence. It is usually described as a ringing noise, but sometimes it is lower-pitched than that, more of a hum. As an occasional symptom it is quite common, no more than a nuisance.

Chronic tinnitus is another matter. Treatments vary from drugs to devices that mask the sound, but there is no real cure. Brief episodes of tinnitus may be caused by a blow to the head, wax in the ears, a foreign body, infection or sudden changes in air pressure. Prolonged cases may be due to the following:

Probable

◆ **Otosclerosis**

This is a common cause of deafness. See page 65. Tinnitus tends to be the earliest symptom of the condition, which is due to increasing stiffness of one of the bones that transmit sound.

◆ **Mèniére's disease**

The classic symptoms of this disease are varying combinations of:

- Tinnitus.
- Vertigo.
- Deafness.

◆ **Presbyacusis**

Hearing loss as part of the ageing process is frequently accompanied by tinnitus. See page 65.

Possible

◆ **Arteriosclerosis**

The blood supply to the brain and ear arrives via major arteries in the neck

The Ears

which, with age, can get furred up. This is thought to underlie cases of tinnitus in the elderly associated with:

- Giddiness on standing up.
- Giddiness set off by head movements, especially looking up.
- Deafness.

It helps to take your time when getting up and to avoid sudden, extreme movements of the neck.

◆ Drugs

Common drugs which can cause tinnitus include aspirin, quinine and streptomycin.

◆ Psychological

Occasionally, tinnitus or other noises in the ears are actually hallucinations in someone suffering from serious mental

disease. Suspicion aroused by reports of:

- Bizarre noises.
- Voices commenting on the individual's activities.

The individual may also appear:

- Unusually suspicious.
- Moody to an exaggerated degree.

This situation needs sensitive, expert assessment.

Rare

◆ Paget's disease

A disease of bone which can squeeze the nerve of hearing, resulting in:

- Deafness.
- Tinnitus.

See also page 66.

Vertigo

Vertigo means a sense of rotation. Giddiness is a mild form of the same symptom. They are frequently caused by disorders of the ear, although the connection may not be obvious since there may be no other features of ear trouble such as pain, discharge or tinnitus. For that reason, vertigo/giddiness is covered in detail elsewhere in this book. See *The brain and nervous system, 348-382.*

The following conditions are, however, relevant to the ear.

Probable

◆ Catarrh

The congestion which accompanies a

Auditory nerve (carries sound and balance sensations to the brain)

Outer ear canal

Middle ear cavity

cold often also causes mild giddiness for a few days.

- Nasal congestion.
- Slight pressure in ears.
- Mild deafness and ringing in the ears – tinnitus.

◆ Labyrinthitis

A common, alarming, but harmless condition, occurring in mini-epidemics. It may be due to a viral infection of the balance organ which is sited in the ear, but is increasingly thought to be due to shifts in crystals that line sensitive structures within the ear. The nerve endings that normally transmit messages telling us how we are balanced become inflamed and send off inaccurate and confusing messages. This causes acute loss of balance and intense true vertigo, with the room spinning round.

- Abrupt, disabling vertigo: you may even find it impossible to stand up.
- Usually noticed on attempting to get up in the morning.
- Nausea or vomiting are common.
- Vertigo returns each time you move your head.

This is a panic-inducing illness: but be reassured that the symptoms will fade over two or three weeks. Minor recurrences are possible for several months afterwards.

◆ Ménière's disease

Vertigo can be an early symptom of this condition.
Later there is:

- Ringing in the ears – tinnitus.
- Deafness.

Possible

◆ Chronic otitis media

See page 65. Persistent yellow or green discharge from one ear, together with:

- Discomfort.
- Deafness.

Needs specialized treatment to clean the ear and to eradicate infection.

◆ Otosclerosis

A cause of deafness in middle life, but as early features there can be:

- Tinnitus.
- Vertigo.
- Wax.

A convenient scapegoat for many ear problems, perhaps too convenient. However, if there is just mild giddiness, with no other symptoms except that the ears are full of hard wax, it is reasonable for a doctor to suggest clearing the wax with drops to soften it, or, if necessary, syringing the ears, to exclude wax as a cause of vertigo.

Rare

◆ Acoustic neuroma

See page 66. This growth on the nerve of hearing is suspected if, as well as vertigo, there is progressive:

- One-sided deafness.
- One-sided vertigo.
- One-sided tinnitus.

The Ears

The mouth, face, head, throat & neck

See the following pages for symptoms and diagnoses in these areas.

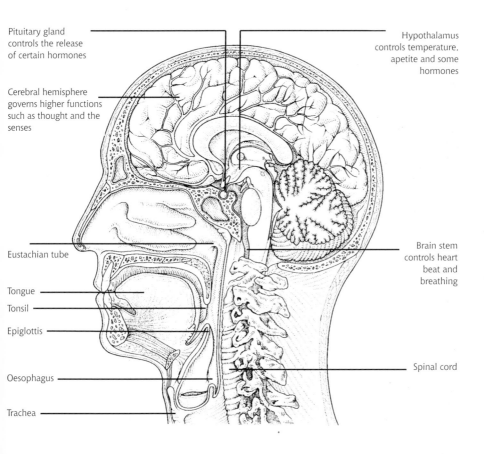

Pituitary gland controls the release of certain hormones

Cerebral hemisphere governs higher functions such as thought and the senses

Eustachian tube

Tongue

Tonsil

Epiglottis

Oesophagus

Trachea

Hypothalamus controls temperature, apetite and some hormones

Brain stem controls heart beat and breathing

Spinal cord

Bluish-purple lips

A feature of cyanosis, covered in detail on page 397. It can be caused by low body temperature. But long-term cyanosis suggests that blood oxygen levels are low.

Similar discolouration may be noticed in the ear lobes, all the mucous membranes, the tongue and anywhere that blood flows close to the surface of the skin, such as the beds of the fingernails. In general, cyanosis suggests either heart or lung disease.

Probable

◆ Low temperature

Commonly seen in shivering children on the beach. It may, however, accompany low temperature in the elderly. Consider hypothermia if there are other symptoms, such as:

- Confusion.
- Slowness of thought.
- Decreased movement

The individual should be warmed gradually: layers of blankets are best. Hot drinks, such as tea, may be given. Avoid alcohol, which increases heat loss. In all cases, seek medical help urgently – hypothermia must be dealt with in hospital.

◆ Chronic bronchitis

See page 201.

◆ Emphysema

- Shortness of breath which gets progressively worse over a period of months and years.
- The chest becomes expanded, as though permanently inhaling.
- May accompany chronic bronchitis.
- Respiratory infections.
- Cyanosis.
- Respiratory failure.

◆ Pulmonary oedema

Retention of fluid in the lungs as a result of failure of the heart to pump effectively. Heart failure may have occurred because of either poor blood supply to the heart, or because of structural abnormality such as disease of the heart's valves.

Symptoms include:

- Shortness of breath on exertion and, in severe cases, at rest.
- Shortness of breath when lying down flat.
- Night-time shortness of breath.
- Frothy sputum, sometimes pink with blood.
- Cyanosis.
- Fast or irregular heart rate.
- Swelling of ankles.

Possible

◆ Shock

Covered in detail on page 381.

Cyanosis is just one of several noticeable features. May be an emergency.

The Mouth

◆ Pneumonia

Actually, 'pneumonias' would be a better term, since there are several types. Cyanosis is a typical feature of all of them. See page 397.

Some types of pneumonia may still be fatal, particularly in the very young or the elderly: see a doctor without delay.

Rare

◆ Pulmonary embolus

Covered in detail on page 196. Bluish lips are just one of several more dramatic features, such as sudden shortness of breath, sudden onset of sharp chest pain, bloody sputum and collapse.

◆ Congenital heart disease

Cyanosis is a typical and obvious feature of new-born babies with heart abnormalities. Fallot's tetralogy and transposition of the great arteries are probably the most well known. Heart defects may also accompany abnormalities such as Down's syndrome, or those caused by the mother having Rubella during pregnancy. In addition to cyanosis:

• Shortness of breath.

• Finger clubbing.

• Toe clubbing.

• Polycythaemia – excess haemoglobin to compensate for poor oxygenation.

• Malaise.

• Poor growth.

◆ Airways obstructed by a foreign body

Any object that obstructs the free passage of air in and out of the lungs may result in cyanosis. The sudden onset of blueness, choking in someone eating, or in a child, must be considered as being possibly due to inhalation of a foreign body, perhaps a peanut, or a piece of a toy.

This is a life-threatening emergency. See *Heimlich's manoeuvre*, page 219.

◆ Laryngeal oedema

An infection (typically diphtheria or epiglottitis) or a severe allergic reaction may cause swelling of the soft tissues of the larynx, preventing air getting into the lungs.

• Blue lips.

• Stridor: a harsh and frightening noise heard as air is forced past a blockage in the airways.

• Distress.

If caused by an infection of the upper airway, all the usual features will also be noticed.

Laryngeal oedema is an emergency: get help quickly.

◆ Fibrosing alveolitis

Tends to develop in middle age and progresses gradually.

• Increasing shortness of breath.

• Dry cough.

• Clubbing.

• Cyanosis.

◆ Pneumoconiosis

A term used for a number of occupationally related chest diseases, typically associated with work in dusty environments.

- Slow onset.
- Increasing shortness of breath on exertion, and then at rest.
- Intermittent cough.
- Onset of bronchitis.
- Cyanosis.
- Respiratory failure.
- Heart failure.

◆ Extrinsic allergic alveolitis

A disease that develops because of recurrent allergic reactions to dusts from animals or plants.

Quite common in farm workers.

- Recurrent brief attacks, up to a couple of days, of shortness of breath, malaise, fever and cough, when exposed to the dust.

After repeated exposure over the years a chronic condition develops, with:

- Shortness of breath.
- Finger and toe clubbing.
- Cyanosis.
- Respiratory failure.
- Heart failure.

Cracking at corners of mouth

The medical terms are angular stomatitis or cheilosis. In isolation, this is normally of no great significance.

Probable

◆ Childhood cracking

If the corners of your child's mouth are constantly wet, they will be at increased risk of cracking. Children taking bottles or who suck their thumbs may develop inflammation at the corner(s) of the mouth. This may also occur in older children, with no very obvious cause.

- Redness.
- Cracking.
- Pain.
- Clears up of its own accord.
- May develop on one side only.

◆ Age

As individuals age, they can develop a crease running downwards from the angle of the mouth, along which saliva flows, causing skin irritation and:

- Redness.
- Cracking.
- Pain.
- May be on one or both sides. Clears up of its own accord.

Possible

◆ Brain injury

Anyone who has suffered brain injury (stroke, accident) or with chronic neurological disease may have facial weakness or swallowing problems that allow saliva to pool in the mouth and dribble out.

The Mouth

* Redness.
* Cracking.
* Pain.
* Clears up of its own accord.
* May be on one side only (after stroke) or on both sides if there is a swallowing problem.

Rare

◆ Scurvy and zinc deficiency

See pages 399 and 79 respectively. Riboflavine is a water-soluble vitamin present in many foods. Deficiency is likely to be a feature only of severe, general malnutrition. Glossitis, page 116, may be present.

Hare lip

Colloquial term for cleft lip.
See *Cleft lip and palate*, page 80

Lips – cracked, sores or patches

Sore, inflamed lips are common in adults and children: the lips look red and are often cracked. The usual cause is intermittent exposure to heat and cold. The skin of the lips loses its natural oil, becoming dry and uncomfortable or 'chapped'.

Other common causes are lip-licking and lip-chewing. The first is typical of children with colds who develop running noses and continually lick or wipe their upper lips, causing inflammation. The second is a comfort habit adopted at times of stress.

The lips and the surrounding skin are possible sites of sores or lesions for many diseases. Some are local and some are general; some are permanent and some temporary, some need treatment and some don't. The following list cannot be exhaustive, but it does highlight examples of all these types.

Probable

◆ Aphthous ulcer

May develop after injury, when the individual is run-down (physically or mentally) or more commonly for no clear reason.

* Exquisitely painful.
* After 24 hours mucous membrane breaks down to form an ulcer.
* Often a greyish/white appearance.
* Ulcer is normally about 3-4 mm in diameter and oval shaped.
* Pain can make, eating, talking or brushing teeth difficult.
* May be multiple.
* Tend to be on inner aspect of lips.
* Healing occurs between five days and two weeks.

The Mouth

◆ **Herpes simplex**

Also known as a cold sore. A virus which infects the skin.

• Often precipitated by upper respiratory tract infection when the individual is run down.

• Also precipitated by weather extremes (heat or cold).

• Initially a slightly irritating patch on the lip or local skin.

• Little fluid filled vesicles develop.

• These become crusted and a scab develops.

• The disease runs its course in ten to 14 days.

• If severe, and recognized at an early stage, can be helped by antiviral medication.

◆ **Mucocoele or retention cyst**

Blockage of one of the small glands on the inner aspect of the lips causes:

• Sudden appearance of a lump, a few millimetres in diameter.

• Painless.

• Translucent/bluish colour.

• Suddenly empties.

• Rarely lasts for more than a couple of days.

◆ **Burn**

Local areas of pain and ulceration on one lip (particularly in the middle of the lower lip) are often caused by smokers under the influence of alcohol placing the cigarette the wrong way round in their mouth. Often, the individual cannot recall the incident. The patch will heal in about five days.

◆ **Impetigo**

A nasty and highly infectious skin infection, which can occur anywhere, but commonly on the face and lips and other exposed parts. Commonest in children.

• Starts with redness.

• Vesicles and bullae (fluid filled sacs) develop on the skin surface.

• These burst and crusting occurs.

• May spread over a large area of the face.

• Asymmetrical: does not spread evenly over both sides of face.

• Needs antibiotic treatment.

Possible

◆ **Candidiasis**

A 'thrush' infection of the lips, typical of the elderly, those with dentures, those who are 'rundown' or with diets deficient in vitamins or iron. Treatment is anti-fungal creams or lozenges.

• Redness.

• Soreness.

• Slight swelling.

• Occasional cracking and bleeding.

• White plaques or patches may be seen.

◆ **Leukoplakia**

• White patches on the tongue or lining of the mouth.

• Cannot be scraped off.

The Mouth

- Occasionally disappear leaving a red base.
- Localized hardening under the patch may occur.

It is associated with smoking, spirits, spices, sepsis, sharp teeth, and syphilis.

Leukoplakia may also be an early warning sign of cancer, so long-standing firm white patches on the tongue or in the mouth must not be ignored.

Rare

◆ Zinc deficiency

Any elderly person on a poor diet or with malabsorption or malnutrition problems who develops intermittent sores on around the mouth may be zinc-deficient. A blood test may be needed to confirm this, and zinc supplements can be given.

◆ AIDS

Can give rise to multiple mouth ulcers, as well as:

- General malaise.
- Weight loss.
- Skin rashes.
- Blood tests confirm the diagnosis.

◆ Cancer

Any long-standing ulcer or growth on the lip, particularly in elderly smokers with poor oral hygiene, may be cancerous.

- Persistent ulcer or irregular lump.
- Persistent painless, but enlarged lymph nodes.
- Bleeding from lesion.

- Loss of weight.
- Malaise.

◆ Hereditary haemorrhagic telangiectasia

Also known as Osler-Weber-Rendu syndrome. A hereditary condition.

- Small red vascular lesions on lips and in mouth.
- Similar lesions throughout gastro-intestinal tract.
- The gastro-intestinal lesions may cause internal bleeding.
- Rarely seen before the age of 40.

◆ Chancre

The first sign of infection with syphilis. May occur on the lips or in the mouth after oral sex.

- Appears three to four weeks after contact.
- Initially, a hardened, elevated solitary lesion.
- Becomes a shallow ulcer.
- Painless.
- Does not bleed.
- Raised, red edges.
- Local, painless lymph node enlargement.

If suspected must be seen and treated by a doctor.

◆ Dermatitis

Any area of skin may develop sensitivity to some irritant. Habitual sucking or chewing of pens or application of some lipsticks or lip balms are examples of agents to which some may react.

The Mouth

- Redness.
- Itchiness.
- Soreness.
- Sometime crusting and weeping.
- Normal lips when the irritant is not being used

◆ Behçet's syndrome

Commonest in men from the teens to the early thirties.

- Painful ulceration of the mouth.
- Genital ulceration a few weeks after the oral lesions.
- Eye inflammation (uveitis) with the genital ulceration.

The condition repeats and relapses. Treatment is aimed at relieving the symptoms. This condition is commonest in the Middle East.

◆ Erythema multiforme

Associated with reaction to drugs or infection. Commonest in young males.

- Extensive painful ulcers inside the mouth.

- lesions can also be found on the skin.
- Gum inflammation.
- Crusting, bloodstained lesions on lips.

Treatment consists of identifying and removing or treating the cause.

◆ Lichen planus

In the over-30s.

- Multiple, fine white lines on lips, tongue and the cheek
- Tiny white spots in the same region.
- Sometimes ulcers between the spots and lines.
- Occasionally fluid-filled sacs form which then burst, causing painful ulcers.

◆ Poisons

A number of drugs, such as arsenic, bismuth, lead and mercury, will cause pigmentation of the mouth and lips, in addition to their other symptoms and signs. In the absence of other definite causes for mouth pigmentation, accidental or deliberate taking of such drugs should be considered.

Chapped lips

Essentially the same as *Sore lips*, page 77.

Cleft lip and palate

These terms cover a fairly wide range of abnormalities that occur during development in the womb.

They are quite common – one in 750

births. For some reason, generally unknown, areas of tissue fail to 'join', and the resulting gap is seen at birth, sometimes on one side, or in severe cases as a cleft lip and palate on both sides beneath the nose.

- Distortion of the nostril on the affected side.
- In more than half the cases, there is also a defect in the hard palate.

- Speech problems, typically nasal speech, will develop if left untreated.

The trend at present is to repair these deformities by plastic surgery as soon as reasonable after birth so that breast feeding and speech development are affected as little as possible.

Skin around the mouth looks pale

This is a very specific symptom, otherwise known as circumoral pallor, associated with scarlet fever. It should not be confused with more general pallor of skin, mucous membranes and nails associated with anaemia or blood loss. See page 390. The symptoms of scarlet fever are:

- Tonsillitis and pharyngitis.
- Red rash, predominantly on trunk.
- Sore and coated tongue.
- Circumoral pallor.
- Otitis media may develop; see page 58.

Bleeding gums

This is almost always due to over-vigorous brushing of the teeth, and can be a normal daily occurrence for some people.

If bleeding is persistent, or the gums are painful, some degree of gum disease (also known as gingivitis or periodontal

disease) may be present; see page 82. This may settle without treatment but if there is infection too, antibiotics may be necessary. The care of a dental hygienist may be beneficial.

A very rare cause of bleeding gums is scurvy, caused by Vitamin C deficiency.

Foul-smelling breath

Halitosis. Most dentists and doctors would attribute bad breath to poor oral hygiene. This is by far the commonest cause of bad breath.

There are, however, other causes, related to a variety of abnormalities of the mouth, the sinuses, and the lungs, as

well as disease elsewhere in the body.

Probable

◆ Poor oral hygiene

The surest way to develop bad breath is to fail to clean your teeth. Even regular

The Mouth

tooth brushing may not be enough to prevent the accumulation of food debris, which collects in the cracks between teeth and generates odours as it decays. Dental flossing (passing a special thread between teeth) clears these crevices and helps prevent bad breath.

- Staining between teeth.
- Irregular colour to teeth.
- Breath worse in the morning, on waking.

In addition to brushing and flossing your teeth, regular descaling by a dentist or an oral hygienist can help prevent bad breath.

◆ Food and drink

Individual has recently eaten spiced foods or drunk alcohol.

- No other evidence of disease in mouth or elsewhere.
- Not present if diet is confined to non-spicy food, or if alcoholic drink is stopped.

◆ Smoking

- Halitosis.
- Stained teeth.

◆ Dental caries

Caries means tooth decay. The enamel covering of the tooth is damaged by bacteria. Regular brushing and avoidance of sugary foods may help, as may fluoride – ask your dentist's advice.

- 'Sensitive teeth'.
- Painful tooth or teeth.
- Halitosis.

- Worse on drinking and eating very hot or cold foods and drinks.

◆ Mouth breathing

Any condition which makes you breath through your mouth rather than your nose may result in halitosis because of drying up of the salivary secretions which act as a rinsing agent. Thus nasal polyps, a broken nose, hay fever or even snoring may cause halitosis, because they make it difficult to breathe through the nose.

◆ Mouth or throat infection

Any mouth or throat infection may cause bad breath; all may be associated with:

- Pain.
- Fever.
- Malaise.
- Halitosis.
- Unpleasant taste in the mouth.

◆ Gum disease

Disease of the gums and tooth sockets, with inflammation of the gums (also known as gingivitis). Caused mainly by poor oral hygiene.

- Bleeding gums particularly after brushing teeth.
- Sensitive gums.
- Halitosis.
- Often associated with dental caries.

◆ Dentures

If not cleaned regularly and adequately, food debris or saliva may accumulate on dentures, giving off an offensive smell, even when in the mouth.

◆ Post nasal drip

May be present for some weeks after flu/colds.

- Mucus drips back into throat causing reflex coughing.
- Worse at night.
- General health otherwise good.
- Halitosis may be present.

See also *Phlegm in the throat*, page 120.

Possible

◆ Sinusitis

Infection of any of the sinuses may cause:

- Persistent nasal discharge (out through the nose or back into the throat).
- May be green or yellow.
- Possibly headache.
- Occasionally pyrexia.
- Malaise.
- Halitosis.

◆ Catarrh

A term with many different meanings: some use it to describe a blocked nose (because of nasal inflammation); some use it for large amounts of infected mucus. It often results in bad breath, either because of accompanying infection in the mouth or nose, or because a blocked nose is making you breath through your mouth.

◆ Chronic lung conditions

See also *Foul-smelling breath and cough*, page 85.

Any lung condition that causes persistent production of mucus, or where the lung has a long-standing focus of infection may cause halitosis. Patients with chronic bronchitis, tuberculosis, cystic fibrosis, bronchiectasis, emphysema and other diseases may well complain of halitosis. The main symptoms of the underlying disease usually include:

- Purulent (green/yellow) mucus.
- Cough.
- Fever.
- Malaise.

◆ Pyorrhoea alveolaris

A disease of gums and tooth sockets, actually a severe, advanced form of gum disease (see opposite).

- Gum margins recede.
- Teeth loosen.
- Pus caused by infection of the tooth socket leaks out between gums and teeth.
- Pain.
- Halitosis.

◆ Diabetic ketoacidosis

Diabetics whose blood sugar is not properly controlled can develop a form of abnormal blood biochemistry known as ketoacidosis.

This is characterized by a sweetish smell on the breath (some describe it as sickly).

Rare

◆ Vincent's angina

Also known as 'trench mouth', this is a bacterial disease of the tonsils which spreads to the gums. Associated with poor hygiene.

- Fever.
- Sore throat.
- Infected gums.
- Enlarged lymph nodes in the neck.

Often only one tonsil is affected, with ulceration, and a membrane which may spread to soft and hard palate.

Highly infectious. Responds rapidly to antibiotics.

◆ Cancer of the mouth, upper respiratory tract and larynx

Halitosis may be an accompaniment to any site of cancer in the mouth, upper respiratory tract and larynx, particularly if the tumour has become infected and ulcerated. Thus persistent halitosis, in addition to some or any of the following, particularly in elderly smokers, needs close investigation:

- Persistent, painless enlarged lymph nodes.
- Other lumps developing in mouth/tongue or palate.
- Change in voice.
- Loss of weight.
- Feeling unwell.
- Persistent pain in mouth or neck.
- Dentures not fitting.
- Anaemia.

◆ Renal failure

Uraemia is present. Urea is a waste product normally excreted in the urine, produced by the kidneys.

- Browny/yellow appearance of skin.
- Bruising.
- Fast rate of breathing.
- Swollen ankles.
- Heart failure.
- Breath smells of urine/ammonia.
- Altered sensation in limbs.

◆ Liver failure

This may occur as a result of a number of diseases that damage liver tissue, such as hepatitis or cirrhosis.

It may result in a large number of symptoms, including:

- Jaundice.
- Fatigue.
- Mental deterioration.
- Reddened palms ('liver' palms: the fatty parts of the palms are flushed red).
- The appearance of tiny blood vessels in the skin – 'vascular spiders'.
- Fever.
- Halitosis – sweet and faeculent – foetor hepaticus.

◆ Drugs and poisoning

Some drugs have characteristic smells, excreted in air exhaled from the lungs. Examples are paraldehyde, now rarely used, and disulfiram, a drug prescribed for alcoholics.

The Mouth

Foul-smelling breath and cough

Probable

◆ Chronic bronchitis

Covered in detail on page 201. The typical picture is:

- Smoker's cough, especially in the early morning.
- Cough in winter.
- Wheezing.
- Sputum varying from white to yellow/green.
- Increasing breathlessness over the years.
- Cyanosis.
- Halitosis.

Possible

◆ Lung cancer

Covered in detail on page 209. Associated symptoms which may be noticeable include:

- Dry cough.
- Bloody sputum.
- Hoarse voice.
- Shortness of breath.
- Chest pain.
- Infection in the lung.
- Malaise.
- Weight loss.
- Halitosis.

◆ Bronchiectasis

The air passages are widened, preventing oxygen entering the circulation efficiently. Features include:

- History of recurrent chest infections.
- Lots of yellow/green sputum with or without blood.
- Fever.
- Looking unwell.
- Weight loss.
- Malaise.
- Severe halitosis.

◆ Cystic fibrosis

See page 137.
Later in infancy, symptoms may include

- Slow growth,
- Offensive diarrhoea and/or;
- Respiratory infections, which may be associated with halitosis.

Rare

◆ Lung abscess

A collection of pus lying within the lung tissue. It may be caused by inhaling infected material, as a complication of pneumonia, or by rare causes such as spread of a liver abscess into the chest. In general, features include:

- A pre-existing infection.
- Fever.
- Shivering.
- Sweats.
- Malaise.
- Pleurisy (pain in the chest on breathing).
- Foul sputum.
- Halitosis.

◆ **Pulmonary (lung) tuberculosis**

Most often in malnourished or immunosuppressed patients.

• Malaise.

• Fatigue.

• Weight loss.

• Cough with sputum – sometimes bloody.

• Chest pain.

• Shortness of breath

• Halitosis.

Breath smells of urine

Covered in detail under *Renal failure* in *Foul-smelling breath*, page 84.

Breath smells sweet

See *Diabetic ketoacidosis* and *Liver failure*, covered in detail under *Foul-smelling breath*, pages 83 and 84.

Abnormal teeth

Including discolouration and deformity. These following diseases and predisposing factors are worth considering:

◆ **Age**

As is well known, teeth tend to become discoloured with age. Periodontal disease such as gingivitis causes gum loss, making the teeth appear longer than normal: hence the expression 'long in the tooth'.

◆ **Smoking**

Yellowy-brown staining, even with regular brushing. It also hastens the age-related colour changes of teeth.

◆ **Betel-nut chewing**

Brownish-red discolouration of all teeth, commonly seen in Asian men and women who are habitual betel nut chewers.

◆ **Transverse ridges**

Transverse ridges on teeth may be seen in people who had scurvy or rickets while the surface enamel of their teeth was forming.

Maxillary and mandibular teeth

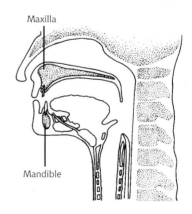

Maxilla

Mandible

The Mouth

◆ Chondro-ectodermal dysplasia

A congenital disorder. Features include:

- Short stature.
- Short fingers.
- Small teeth.
- Dry skin.
- Scanty hair.

◆ Hutchinson's teeth

Rarely seen nowadays; caused by congenital syphilis. The incisor teeth have a notch at the lower edge, are small and taper towards the notched edge. Other signs of congenital syphilis may also be present.

Grating the teeth

This is a symptom of more concern to the partner or parent of the affected person. It is observed commonly at night and may be associated with snoring. Some individuals do it habitually. The noise is caused by the opposing movement of the upper and lower teeth against each other. The symptom often disappears spontaneously. Only rarely does it cause permanent tooth damage. If the symptom persists the advice of a dentist should be sought.

'Made-to-measure' moulds which fit over the teeth can be worn at night to protect the teeth and to prevent grinding.

There is an association between tooth grinding and migraine: many people find that they have both conditions.

Damaged tooth

If possible, the broken fragment(s) should be kept, and taken with you to a dentist. If the entire tooth and root has been displaced, it may be possible to reimplant it. If there is a possibility that the jaw is fractured, get professional help quickly. The cosmetic problems of a broken or chipped tooth are less important than underlying bone damage. The bones may need to be realigned. (See *Upper and lower teeth not closing*, page 92). Cosmetic repair can be undertaken at a later date, once the bone damage has been treated.

Teething pain

The first baby teeth, normally the lower central incisors, appear at the age of six to ten months. Teeth continue to appear until about 30 months. Most infants and toddlers will have episodes of crying, fever and salivation which may be

The Mouth

attributed (not always convincingly) to teeth erupting or growing.

Fever is not a prominent symptom in a teething child: if your child has a fever, do not attribute it to teething. Pain and discomfort are the major symptoms,

leading to irritability and crying. Just as you would take a painkiller for toothache, it is reasonable to use infant paracetamol to soothe a teething child.

It is always important to exclude other causes, such as ears or throat.

Dry mouth

The probable causes are, of course, dehydration, mouth breathing and fear or anxiety.

The first two are covered on pages 444 and 60, the last on page 349.

Remove the cause, and a normal 'wet' mouth returns. If a dry mouth persists, then it might indicate underlying disease.

Anaesthetics and anti-depressants can also cause a dry mouth.

Possible

◆ Salivary gland calculus

Stones can form in the ducts of the major salivary glands, blocking saliva. They are commonest in the submandibular salivary glands but occasionally occur in the parotids.

- Swelling over the gland on one side.

- Swelling worse at meal times or in the presence of food.

- Swelling is uncomfortable.

- Sensation of dryness on the same side of the mouth.

- Swelling suddenly goes down – you may note saliva trickling into mouth.

Salivary glands

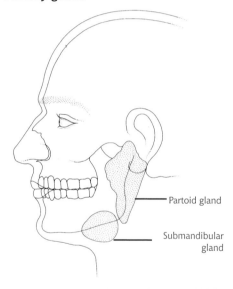

Partoid gland

Submandibular gland

Sometimes the stones are passed, sometimes they need surgical removal.

Rare

◆ Sjögren's syndrome

Probably an auto-immune disease, commonest in middle-aged women.

The Mouth

- Dry eyes, causing a painful, gritty feeling.
- Dry mouth, with halitosis.

- Salivary gland swelling.

  Other connective tissue disorders may be associated, such as rheumatoid arthritis.

Generally infected mouth

Severe generalized infection of the oral cavity, including tongue, palate and gums, is a medical emergency. It is rare, and happens if oral hygiene is extremely poor, or indeed absent.

Rare

◆ Vincent's angina and Vincent's acute ulcerative gingivitis

Named after the infecting organisms. Also known as trench mouth. These are bacterial diseases of the mouth which may originate in the gums between the teeth, or the tonsils (Vincent's angina). May spread rapidly to adjacent tissues.

Vincent's angina:

- Pyrexia.
- Local pain.
- Sore throat.

- Enlarged neck lymph nodes.
- Often only one tonsil affected which is ulcerated, with a membrane present.
- The membrane may spread to soft and hard palate.
- Excessive salivation may occur.
- Highly infectious.
- Responds rapidly to appropriate antibiotics.

  Vincent's acute ulcerative gingivitis: in addition to the preceding symptoms,

- Deep gum ulcers.

◆ Cancrum oris

A severe form of the conditions described above which occur in poorly nourished children.

Even with treatment, gross scarring of the cheek can result, also limitation of jaw movement.

Difficult to open mouth

This is usually the result of a disease affecting structures involved in opening the mouth, causing a combination of either pain or swelling. Pain gives the impression that it is difficult to open the jaw. It is, however, rarely a primary symptom.

The diseases are listed here in order of frequency, not in order of how often they give rise to difficulty in opening the mouth.

Probable

◆ Aphthous ulcer

See page 118.

◆ Dental caries

See page 82.

The Mouth

◆ Dental infection

See page 129.

◆ Upper respiratory tract infection

See page 128.

◆ Tonsillitis

See page 116.

◆ Mumps

Inflammation of the parotid glands, often mistaken for lymph glands.

- Both glands affected and markedly swollen.
- Swelling makes opening the jaw uncomfortable.
- Occasionally, pancreas and testes are affected (after puberty).

Possible

◆ Infectious mononucleosis

See page 118.

◆ Peritonsillar abscess

See page 130.

◆ Impacted wisdom tooth

Emerging wisdom teeth, especially if obstructed by existing teeth, may cause such pain, discomfort and infection at the back of the mouth that it is difficult to open your mouth. Dental opinion should be sought if suspected.

◆ Arthritis in temporo-mandibular joint

This joint is where the mandible hinges with the skull. Arthritis can develop with age, or after injury.

Temporo-mandibular joint

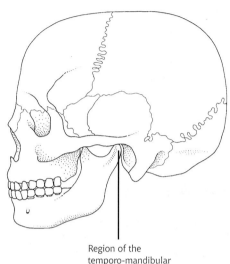

Region of the temporo-mandibular joint

- Pain localized just in front of the ear.
- Pain may extend across side of face.
- Pain worse on chewing or moving jaw.
- A grinding sensation over the joint may be noted.
- At first, only on one side.
- May eventually affect both sides.

Rare

◆ Tetanus

A disease caught by soil penetrating a trivial skin wound and contaminating it with the organism Clostridium tetani. It can be fatal.

The Mouth

- Local muscular weakness near the wound.
- Muscular spasms develop.
- Inability to open the mouth, called trismus or 'lockjaw'.
- The spasms and trismus give rise to a grinning appearance, 'risus sardonicus'.
- Fever.

    Gradually, spasms are caused by the slightest stimulus. In severe cases, the number and frequency of spasms increases until death occurs. Keeping your tetanus immunization up to date is essential.

◆ Strychnine poisoning

The symptoms of strychnine poisoning are similar to those of tetanus (see opposite), but without a history of wound contamination.

Too much saliva

In the absence of any other problems, this is rare. Any condition that causes painful swallowing or a sore throat may lead to an apparent excess of saliva, as the pain prevents the usual frequency of clearing of the saliva from mouth to stomach.

However, there are some conditions in which excessive saliva is a notable feature:

Probable

◆ Smoking

Many smokers, especially pipe and cigar smokers, notice that they salivate excessively when smoking, an effect of nicotine.

It is unclear why this is not noticed by all smokers.

◆ Nausea and vomiting

Prior to vomiting, the mouth often appears to fill with salty saliva.

◆ Tonsillitis

See page 116. Excessive saliva is a typical feature.

◆ Pharyngitis

See page 115. There may be an apparent excess of saliva because of pain on swallowing.

Possible

◆ Infectious mononucleosis

See page 118.

◆ Brain injury

See page 76.

◆ Neurological disease

See multiple sclerosis, Parkinson's disease, motor neurone disease, pseudobulbar and bulbar palsy, under *Problems with swallowing plus weight loss*, page 114.

The Mouth

◆ **Peritonsillar abscess**

See *Enlarged lymph glands in the neck*, page 345.

◆ **Cancer of the oesophagus**

See page 113.

Impacted tooth

Meaning a tooth that cannot erupt because it is blocked or otherwise prevented from emerging by other teeth. This applies most frequently in adult life to the wisdom teeth.

The unerupted tooth may be covered by a flap of gum that can become infected and painful. Extraction of the unerupted tooth is the usual – and effective – treatment. It may have to be done under general anaesthetic.

Loose teeth

See *Dental caries*, page 82; *Gum disease*, page 82; *Pyorrhoea alveolaris*, page 83.

These are associated with, or lead to, loose teeth, decaying teeth and toothache.

Upper and lower teeth not closing properly

Medical term, malocclusion. Teeth should snap shut directly opposite each other. Most people have some degree of malocclusion, typically protruding front teeth – overbite), and this needs no further treatment. Some have irregular teeth because as babies their teeth developed too slowly; because of infection, or because of an extra tooth.

Dentists can correct deformities to improve function and cosmetic appearance.

Damage to the jaw bones, into which the teeth are bedded, can also give malocclusion. If bone damage is suspected, specialized treatment is essential.

Deformity will give rise to pain around the face and ear – see *Difficult to open mouth*, page 89. Arthritis may develop.

The Mouth

Sensitive teeth

Most people suffer from sensitive teeth at some time, frequently caused by over-vigorous brushing of the teeth, leading to receding gums. This exposes the nerve fibres around the tooth, producing sometimes extreme sensitivity to heat and cold. When a tooth is damaged or infected, again the nerves will be exposed and unusually sensitive.
See *Dental caries*, page 82; *Gum disease*, page 82; *Pyorrhoea alveolaris*, page 83.

Special toothpastes for sensitive teeth coat the nerves and reduce sensitivity. They will not work in cases where there is gum disease, dental caries or infection.

Decaying teeth

See *Dental caries*, page 82;
Gum disease, page 82;
Pyorrhoea alveolaris, page 83.

Toothache

See *Dental caries*, page 82;
Gum disease, page 82;
Pyorrhoea alveolaris, page 83.

The Mouth

The face: introduction

Many symptoms of the face can also appear elsewhere on the body. This section concentrates on conditions most likely to be localized to the face.

Swollen or puffy face

Generalized swelling or puffiness of the face, as distinct from, say, swelling in the neck, is rather uncommon. Considered here is true, overall facial swelling or puffiness.

For causes of local swelling, see the sections on skin, and on the neck.

Because the tissues around the eye are so soft, relatively minor inflammation may in turn cause considerable swelling of the eyelids, which can swell and close the eye.

Probable

◆ Insect bite

- Sudden onset of swelling localized to site of bite and surrounding tissues.
- Often quite itchy.
- Subsides after a day or so.
- Occasionally becomes infected, with swelling becoming red and hot, and fever developing with malaise.

◆ Dental abscess

- Painful swelling above or below lower or upper jaw.
- Whole cheek may be swollen.
- Obvious dental pain or decay (caries).
- Swelling worsens over two to three days.

A visit to your dentist plus a course of antibiotics should provide rapid relief. Dental treatment may subsequently be required.

◆ Trauma

- Clear history of injury.

Bruising on the face can cause marked swelling, particularly when the bruise is only a day or two old and begins to change colour.

Possible

◆ Angionuerotic oedema

Often associated with urticaria (hives) – see *Skin* section.

Normally caused by an allergy, typically to a food or a drug, but often the cause is not identifiable.

Symptoms may include:

- Swelling of lips and eyes.

Can involve the tongue and cause some obstruction to breathing, in which case it is a medical emergency.

◆ Erysipelas

An infection of the skin and underlying tissues. Often, bacteria get in through a minor cut or graze.

The word literally means 'like

lightening', and it can come on remarkably quickly.

- Red, shiny, hot skin.
- Painful.
- Fever
- Malaise.

Needs antibiotic treatment (sometimes in hospital, via a drip).

◆ Cushing's syndrome

See page 251.

◆ Hypothyroidism

Weight gain and other changes associated with this condition may give the appearance of a puffy face, although there is no true swelling. See page 320.

Rare

◆ Acromegaly

In this condition, excess growth hormone is produced in adult life. Enlargement of the jaw and forehead is part of the picture of acromegaly and might be mistaken for facial puffiness. See page 258.

◆ Glomerulonephritis

One of the conditions described by *Nephritis*, page 291.

◆ Nephrotic syndrome

See page 30.

Facial nodules or bumps

A possible cause is gout, covered in detail on page 261.

A very rare cause is leprosy, page 50.

Facial blisters or ulcerations

Probable

◆ Cold sore

Common, and caused by a *Herpes* virus. They often develop with, or after, a febrile illness, or if you are generally run-down. However they can also be provoked by anything that causes a rise in skin temperature, such as direct sunlight or even the slight temperature rise that women experience before menstruation.

- Initially, irritation noted on skin, usually around mouth.

- Becomes progressively more painful.
- Skin reddens and little vesicles (fluid-filled blisters) appear.
- Vesicles burst and sometimes crusts form.
- Clears up in about two weeks.

A similar type of infection may occur in the genital region.

◆ Impetigo

A bacterial infection of the skin. Very contagious. May occur in children and adults.

- Blisters may develop in the form which

The Face

occurs in newborn babies.

- Honey coloured scabs develop rapidly.
- Large areas can be infected if untreated.

At some stages, impetigo can be difficult to distinguish from a cold sore (and impetigo can develop on cold sores).

Antibiotics are required: if the condition is mild, treatment is by ointment; but if it is severe, by tablets.

Possible

◆ Eczema

Sometimes called dermatitis.

On the face, cosmetics are a common cause, but other causes include hair dyes, nail lacquer and some plants

Features include:

- Redness (where the cosmetics were applied).
- Red, raised spots.
- Small blisters which weep.
- Crusting and scaling.

It is not uncommon for patches of eczema to appear eventually all over the body.

◆ Shingles

An infection caused by the same virus that causes chickenpox.

- Red, blistering rash.
- Can be very painful (pain preceding the rash).
- May be extensive (typically covering one side of the face).
- Localized to one side of the body's centre line.
- Crusting of the blisters.

- Heals in about two weeks, but pain may persist for months or years.

Can occur at any age, including in young people. The older the individual, the more severe it usually is.

If the side of the nose (or interior of the nostril) is affected, there is a risk that the eyeball may be involved. This demands urgent medical attention.

Rare

◆ Rodent ulcer

A small cancerous sore, which virtually never spreads to distant parts of the body. Often appears in the elderly around nose, eyes, ears or mouth.

- Starts as a small pink lump.
- After some weeks or months may become ulcerated.
- Gradually, if undiagnosed and untreated, it invades underlying tissues, for example the bones of the nose.

Once diagnosed, treatment is usually straightforward.

◆ Pemphigus vulgaris

See page 225.

◆ Dermatitis herpetiformis

See page 225.

◆ Pemphigoid

See page 224.

◆ Erythema multiforme and Stevens-Johnson syndrome

The second is a severe form of the first where the inside of the mouth is involved.

Both are reactions to provocations such as infection or medications. Features include:

- Red rash of different shapes which may be present all over the body.
- Raised red lesions and blisters may occur.
- Each episode may last two to three weeks.

Stevens-Johnson syndrome may also include:

- Fever.
- Malaise.
- Lung inflammation.
- Kidney damage.

Reddened face

The probable causes are, of course, embarrassment, heat and alcohol, all of which can make the blood vessels in the skin widen so that they carry more blood than usual. In each case, the redness may well extend across not only face and head but neck and upper trunk.

That the blood vessels can respond to a state of mind is proof, if any were needed, that mind and body are indeed not separate but complementary.

Possible

◆ Acne rosacea

Most common in the middle-aged and elderly.

- Facial reddening.
- Some inflamed pustules.
- Skin is shiny.
- May become permanent.

Hot or spicy food, alcohol, embarrassment or temperature changes can exacerbate the reddening.

◆ Epilepsy

Epileptics may be aware of facial flushing just before a fit, and observers will often notice it afterwards.

◆ Medication

Several drugs can cause flushing, especially calcium antagonists, which are commonly used to treat blood pressure.

A possibility if flushing follows a change of medication.

◆ Menopause

Flushing is one of the commonest symptoms women experience as they approach the 'change of life'.

Symptoms can persist for years.

Rare

◆ Mitral valve disease

- Shortness of breath.
- Lung congestion.
- Coughing blood.
- Bronchitis.
- Heart failure.
- Facial flush, very marked below the eyes.

◆ Carcinoid syndrome

A tumour that may occur in many parts of the body.

Most of its symptoms are caused by chemicals it secretes, and may include:

The Face

- Facial flushing, extending over body.
- Diarrhoea, abdominal pain.
- Enlarged liver.
- Wheezy chest.
- Heart problems.

◆ **Phaeochromocytoma**

Another tumour whose symptoms are caused by the chemicals it secretes.

It is very rare.

- High blood pressure.
- Diarrhoea.
- Nausea.
- Abdominal pain.
- Facial flushing.

◆ **Systemic lupus erythematosus**

See page 417.

Adenoidal face

A term used for individuals who tend to mouth-breathe, rather than breathe through the nose. They tend to walk, move about and even sit with their mouths permanently open. This is because their enlarged adenoids prevent them from breathing through their nose. Their voice may also be affected and is often described as 'adenoidal'. Symptoms may include:

- Breathing through the mouth.
- Snoring.
- Open mouth – the jaw hangs down.
- Nasal speech.

Grinning

One of the several symptoms of tetanus (see page 90) is spasms which contort the face in to the so-called 'sardonic grin'. There is nothing funny about this, or the other potentially fatal symptoms, which is why immunization – and keeping your protection up to date – is essential. Gardeners are particularly at risk from skin wounds being contaminated by soil containing the tetanus organism.

Expressionless face

Parkinson's disease is the classic reason for an expressionless, immobile face. However, a number of conditions can give rise to a similar appearance as a result of damage to the part of the brain that controls facial, and other, movement.

Probable

◆ **Parkinson's disease**

A slowly progressive disease of the middle-aged and elderly.

- Tremor.

- Rigidity and some muscle pain.
- Slow movement.
- Immobile, mask-like face.
- Difficulty in writing.
- Occasional swallowing disorders.
  Can be controlled with medication.

◆ Depression

A depressed person may progressively lose the expression from his or her face. A dull, saddened, flat face is characteristic of depression.
See also page 363.

Possible

◆ Drugs

Drugs that may cause some (but not necessarily all) of the symptoms of Parkinson's disease include phenothiazines and butyrophenones.
Both of these groups of drugs are sometimes used as tranquillizers.

◆ Scleroderma

A multi-system disease, affecting women more than men, which is likely to have been diagnosed already; See page 242

- Stiffness of hands leading to rigidity.
- Smooth, hard, shiny skin.
- Difficulty in opening mouth.
- Immobile face with loss of expression.
- Alimentary tract, heart and kidneys may become involved.

Rare

◆ Hepatolenticular degeneration

Wilson's disease. An inherited disorder, usually showing itself during the teens.

- Parkinson's disease symptoms, plus:
- Liver damage leading to jaundice in some cases.
- Yellow-brown rings on the eyes.

Part of the face paralysed

Excluded here is immobility of the entire face, covered under *Expressionless face*, page 98.

Probable

◆ Bell's palsy

The cause is unknown, but the facial nerve is damaged on one side. The affected individual may note the symptoms on waking up one morning, or after having been out in cold weather, or in a draught:

- May be a dull ache on the affected side.
- Cannot close eye.
- Mouth drawn to the side, away from the damaged nerve
- Saliva may dribble from the affected side.
- Cannot smile properly or bare the teeth.
- Occasionally, taste sensation to one side of the tongue is affected.

  With luck, recovery commences within seven to ten days, but may take several weeks.

The Face

If you suspect Bell's palsy, see a doctor as soon as possible.

Recent evidence has confirmed that many cases are caused by the *Herpes simplex* virus. Early antiviral treatment, together with steroids, can improve the outcome significantly. Rare causes include a late stage of Lyme disease and Guillain-Barré syndrome.

Some doctors believe that high doses of steroids, given early enough, may improve the chances of recovery.

◆ Stroke

Any stroke may damage part of the brain that controls the nerve that makes the facial muscles work.

Different types of stroke may affect the face in slightly different ways so that a number of symptoms can be present to a greater or lesser degree. These include:

- Difficulty or inability to wrinkle the forehead.
- Difficulty or inability to blink or close the eye.
- Difficulty or inability to smile symmetrically.
- Difficulty or inability to bare the teeth.
- Difficulty or inability to whistle.
- Saliva may leak out of the affected side of the mouth.

The body is usually affected on the same side as the face: for example, weakened left hand and face paralysed on left-hand side. When the dominant side of the body (right side in right-handed people) is affected, speech is often affected. Paralysis of the face is unlikely to occur in the absence of other symptoms – which may help to determine the diagnosis.

Possible

◆ Injury

All or part of the facial nerve, which controls movement of the facial muscles, may be damaged – sometimes permanently. The symptoms are the same as for Bell's palsy (see page 99). Knife wounds to the face may be a cause (including surgery, especially on the parotid gland). The facial nerve travels through the ear, just behind the ear drum, and is easily injured at this site too.

◆ Poliomyelitis

'Polio' can also affect the facial nerve, with similar results to *Bell's palsy*, page 99.

Rare

◆ Tumours

Primary or secondary cancerous tumours developing in the part of the brain that controls facial movement or that involve or press on the facial nerve, may cause a mixture of symptoms similar to those of *Stroke* or *Bell's palsy*, page 99.

◆ Herpes varicella zoster

A herpes infection of the mouth, palate or ear can damage the nerve supply to the face causing symptoms similar to *Bell's palsy*, page 99.

This is known as Ramsay-Hunt syndrome.

◆ Guillain-Barré syndrome

A disease of the neurological system with many different symptoms, ranging from mild to severe.

Most cases recover, but this may take many months.

- Altered sensation in the arms and legs.
- Shoulder and back pain.
- Facial palsies.

- Muscles of respiration may be so weakened that artificial ventilation is required.
- Swallowing may be affected and tube-feeding may be needed while recovery progresses.

◆ Motor neurone disease

See page 253.

Facial pain

Covered here are causes of pain that have no visible symptoms, so, for example, shingles is excluded.

Probable

◆ Dental disease

Check teeth and gums first if local face pain develops with no obvious cause. Is it an abscess? If in doubt, always check with your dentist.

◆ Sinusitis

See page 423.

◆ Referred pain

Because the body's 'wiring'– its nervous system – is interconnected, pain arising in one place can travel onwards or be 'referred' to another. If the teeth and gums appear normal, then pain in the face may arise from elsewhere in the head, for instance the facial sinuses.

◆ Temporo-mandibular joint dysfunction

A common cause of pain, particularly if there is any problem with biting. The

Trigeminal neuralgia

Trigeminal nerve

patient's partner often complains that he or she grinds their teeth at night.

Possible

◆ Migraine

See page 105, for full details. Facial pain can be felt as part of a migraine attack.

- The pain will usually be severe and piercing.
- In classic migraine, only one side of the face will be affected. But can be

The Face

bilateral in common migraine: the word 'migraine' come from the French meaning 'half face'.

◆ Cluster headache

• Intensely severe pain in or behind one eye.

The eye often looks bloodshot during an episode, and there may be some stuffiness in the nostril on the affected side.

Typically, episodes of pain occur at precisely the same time each day (often in the middle of the night) and clusters continue for a few weeks before remitting.

◆ Post-herpetic neuralgia

Persistent burning pain at the site of a previous attack of shingles; see page 34.

• Normally in elderly patients.

• Pain is so severe that suicide may be considered.

• Even touching the site may start an attack of pain.

◆ Trigeminal neuralgia

Also called tic douloureux. Pain in the face in an area supplied by the trigeminal nerve (see diagram on previous page).

• Stabbing, intermittent facial pain.

• Can be triggered by touch, or for no reason.

• Attacks come in bouts.

Many different treatments have been tried, some with more success than others. A specialist opinion is usually recommended, as the symptoms can be incapacitating.

Rare

◆ Malignant disease

A doctor will consider the possibility of a cancerous tumour of the nose, mouth, sinuses or pharynx, particularly if the individual is an elderly smoker.

◆ Eagle's syndrome

Sharp localized pain to side of the jaw, below the ear. Pain can be felt inside the mouth.

Caused by an overgrowth of a bony spike from the underside of the skull. (called the styloid process because it looks like the tip of a pen)

◆ Paget's disease

This disease (see also page 107) can cause local pain in the bones affected, including those of the face.

◆ Psychological or atypical

In a few individuals no cause of pain is ever found, despite full investigation and assessment. This pain is described as 'atypical'. Recent research by dental experts and pain specialists has found that tricyclics, a group of drugs generally used to treat depression, can be helpful to patients with 'atypical facial pain'.

It is certainly worth trying these drugs before accepting that 'only psychotherapy will help'.

Oversized head

There are two possibilities: hydrocephalus and Paget's disease. For details of the latter, see page 407.

Hydrocephalus, literally 'water in the head', is a problem of new-born and very young babies. Within the brain, large quantities of clear fluid are constantly being produced. This fluid normally circulates through cavities within the brain and down the spinal cord. It goes out through tiny holes on to the outer surface of the brain, where it is reabsorbed. Occasionally damage to this circulation results in a backlog of fluid in the cavities of the brain, causing increased pressure and swelling. The result is increased pressure in the skull, with:

• Progressive enlargement of the head.

• Bulging fontanelles (soft spots on the top of a baby's head).

The increased pressure damages the brain and can cause:

• Intellectual impairment.

• Epilepsy.

• Physical impairment.

• Vulnerability to infection.

Hydrocephalus needs specialist treatment: the fluid can be drained away, bypassing the blockage, to the stomach (abdomen) by a tube set permanently below the skin on the scalp.

Bulging or sunken places on the head

Several causes of bulges in the head are worth considering in their own right, separately from lumps, bumps and swellings that can occur anywhere on the body, and which are covered in detail in other major sections of this book.

One somewhat specialized area should also be mentioned in this context: the fontanelles. These are the soft 'gaps' that can be felt in babies' heads at the points where the skull bones have not yet fused into a consistent bony covering. The smaller, posterior fontanelle closes soon after birth, while the larger one, the anterior fontanelle, usually closes by one and a half years of age.

The size of the fontanelles varies enormously from child to child. Your doctor will often feel the fontanelle if your child is unwell. A bulging fontanelle can indicate raised pressure in the head – as in meningitis. It can also mean only that your baby is screaming the house down. It is best to check any changes or concerns regarding the fontanelle with your doctor.

Probable

◆ Dehydration

A baby who is short of fluid, typically after a bout of diarrhoea, will show:

• Sunken eyes.

- Sunken fontanelle.
- Loss of skin elasticity.
- Listless, apathetic behaviour.
- Dry lips and mouth.

Dehydration is a serious condition in any baby or child; if you suspect it, see a doctor urgently. It can be effectively treated, but time is of the essence.

Possible

◆ Paget's disease

See page 407.

Rare

◆ Hydrocephalus

See under *Oversized head*, page 103.

◆ Raised intracranial pressure

A tumour or infection raises the pressure inside the skull. It is normal for the fontanelles to bulge outwards when a baby cries or strains, say when coughing. But if intracranial pressure is raised, the fontanelle bulges permanently.

There may well be other symptoms such as vomiting and headache. See a doctor.

When the fontanelle is closed, after around 18 months, it cannot bulge. After this time the main features of raised intracranial pressure will be vomiting and headache.

Blood vessels stand out in head

An obvious feature of temporal arteritis; see page 106.

Head twisting to one side

Stiff neck? See *Stiffness or pain in neck*, page 126.

A common cause is torticollis, also considered in detail on page 126.

Headaches and fits or convulsions

See *Convulsions*, page 356.

Headache

It is so rare for headache to be the symptom of grave underlying disease, such as a brain tumour, that worrying about it – though understandable – is

usually a waste of time: better to worry about other aspects of your health which really might be significant, such as smoking or excess alcohol or cholesterol intake. As a rough rule of thumb, even the most vicious, throbbing headache is in all likelihood 'innocent': the headache that signifies a brain tumour is something else entirely, and will almost always be accompanied by other symptoms. Ninety-eight per cent of all headaches that doctors treat are caused by tension or sinus trouble.

Probable

◆ Tension headache

Often develops in people with work or family problems. May also arise if an individual finds him- or herself under pressure, whatever the circumstances. The source of tension is not always obvious.

* May be intermittent for weeks and months in a previously fit individual.
* Normal periods in between.
* Band-like, crushing pain around head.
* No other physical abnormalities present.
* Disappears after a variable length of time.

◆ Sinusitis

See page 423.

Any inflammation of the sinuses (air-spaces in the facial bones) can cause headache. This can be due to infection, catarrh and even hay fever.

* Tends to be a remorseless, low-grade, throbbing pain.

◆ Menstruation or menopause-related

Alterations of body hormone production, either naturally, during,

before or after a period, can cause variable headaches.

Your doctor may be able to advise you on treatments or check-ups from which you might benefit.

◆ Infection

Viral infections of any kind are notorious for producing multiple symptoms of which headache, often dull and persistent is but one. Other features are:

* Fever.
* Muscle and joint pain.
* Malaise.
* These are in addition to other, more specific, symptoms, typically sore throat.

Possible

◆ Migraine

Recurrent, severe headaches, often but not always accompanied by visual disturbance. Often starts in adolescence. Many different symptoms are described, including:

* Vision affected before the headache starts.
* Occasionally numbness or weakness of one limb before the headache starts.
* Pain starts on one side of the head, but may spread.
* The pain throbs.
* A wish to avoid light.
* Vomiting may occur.
* May last for a couple of days, but normally four to 12 hours.

The cause is not fully understood but probably related to abnormal blood flow in the fine vessels of the scalp. Some relief is available from modern medications – see your doctor.

◆ Cluster headache

- Commonest in men.
- Tends to be one-sided.
- Often severe.
- May occur at night.
- Occurs several times within a period of a few weeks, then disappears, returning some months later.
- Is harmless.

◆ Temporal arteritis

Inflammation of the temporal artery, which runs along the side of the face. Commonest in the elderly.

- Severe pain on the side of the face.
- Skin over the artery is inflamed.
- Artery is thickened and painful to touch.
- There may be fever and malaise.

If suspected, urgent medical treatment is needed, as the eye may become involved.

◆ Eye, ear, nose, throat or dental disease

See those sections for full detail.

All these organs can produce pain that is referred to the head. The pain may be dull and persistent. These possibilities should therefore be excluded if a headache persists for longer than expected.

◆ Drugs

Including cigarettes and alcohol. The system is poisoned by the body's inability to eliminate the broken-down by-products.

Some prescription drugs can cause headache, too. You must reasonably suspect this if the headache is noted after taking the drug. One such drug is the anti-angina medication, glyceryl trinitrate, which gives some people a throbbing headache. Overuse of painkillers containing codeine, found in many over the counter remedies, is now a well recognized cause of chronic headache.

If headaches coincide with taking a prescribed drug, always report it to your doctor – there may well be an alternative to try instead.

◆ Toxic fumes

Dry-cleaning agents, tar and diesel fumes are among regular culprits. Some people suddenly develop a sensitivity to fumes, even having worked with them for years.

Low-grade poisoning with carbon monoxide, for example from a faulty central heating boiler, can cause headaches. Other features include drowsiness and an abnormally pink complexion. Everyone should be alert for situations in which carbon monoxide poisoning might arise – thy are common.

Rare

◆ Meningitis

An infection of the membranes that enclose the brain and spinal cord. If you suspect it, see a doctor immediately

- Severe headache.

- Stiff neck; bending the neck worsens the pain.
- Reduced level of consciousness.
- Photophobia – fear of light.
- Vomiting.
- Fever.
- Very ill.
- A rash may appear.

◆ Subarachnoid haemorrhage

A leakage of blood from a vessel into the liquid that bathes the spinal cord and brain. The following may occur:

- Sudden onset of severe headache, sometimes after a period of exertion – often described as being like a blow on the back of the head. However:
- The headache may have a slower, more insidious, onset.
- Vomiting.
- Stiff neck.
- Mental confusion.
- Speech difficulties.
- Limb weakness.
- Visual disturbances.
- Convulsions.

  If suspected, see a doctor urgently.

◆ Brain tumour

Because the adult skull is rigid, a growth within it can increase the internal pressure, giving rise to headache. However, not every brain tumour has this effect.

Brain tumours can be primary – a pituitary tumour is an example – or secondary, that is, having spread from elsewhere in the body, for example from a primary breast cancer. There will almost always be a range of symptoms:

- Gradually increasing, dull headache.
- Vomiting.
- Impaired consciousness.
- Pulse becomes slower.
- Respiration rate becomes slower.
- Convulsions may occur.
- Vision may be affected.
- Headache often present when you wake in the morning.

  If the first three symptoms develop in an individual, along with other signs of neurological damage, say weakness or numbness of a limb, urgent medical assessment is needed.

  The symptoms can be relieved, even if the tumour itself cannot be removed.

◆ Subdural haemorrhage

Blood collects between the layers of tissue covering the brain. When this blood breaks down into a bruise, it draws more fluid to it, causing raised pressure. May happen in the elderly after an (apparently) insignificant bump on the head. Symptoms may develop some weeks later and include:

- Headache, often minor.
- Periods of sleepiness and unconsciousness.
- Increased confusion and incontinence.
- Possibly speech difficulties.
- Possibly convulsions.

  May often be mistaken for 'getting

old' – so not to be discounted if someone has recently received a blow to the head.

◆ **Brain abscess**

Infection enters the brain in one of several ways: a broken skull-bone with overlying skin damage; from ear, throat, sinus and lung infection; or occasionally from facial infection.

- Symptoms of the initial infection, for example, earache.
- Progressive headache.
- Progressive drowsiness.
- Fever.
- Vomiting.
- Malaise.
- Anorexia.
- Convulsions.

Headache with high fever

The commonest illnesses which give fever combined with headache are common viral infections such as influenza and glandular fever. There are, however, several rare but dangerous infections which may also be responsible for similar symptoms. Don't read this summary without also reading the sections on fever, page 410.

Headache plus chills and fever

See *Fever*, page 410.

Headache: babies and children

Babies and children can get headaches for the same reasons as adults. But in seeking the cause, you should consider two other factors: First, babies and young children, say up to the age of five or even six, are notoriously inexact about where pain is coming from. 'Head pain' often turns out to be earache or sore throat. So, explore every possibility before settling for headache.Second, complaining of recurrent headaches can be characteristic of a child who is unhappy or under stress: typically he or she is going through a bad patch at school. You can detect no other symptoms; and if illness or disease can really be ruled out, then you should find out what is causing the problems.

Removing the cause can make the headaches vanish overnight.

Recurring headache

See *Headache with high fever*, page 108.

Slurred or unclear speech

Hoarseness is covered separately on page 110.

Listed here are the main causes of impaired speech; but bear in mind that impaired speech is not always a feature of these conditions, and that their other symptoms usually predominate.

Look up specific entries elsewhere in the book for further details.

Probable

◆ Alcohol and drugs

- Temporary slowness and slurring.
- Deafness.

If an individual is unable to hear their own voice, he or she is unable to create the precise intended sound.

◆ Septal deviation

- Muffled or nasal quality to speech. See page 56.

◆ Nasal injury

- Muffled or nasal quality to speech.
- Mouth ulcer.
- Anaethesia, for example from recent dental treatment. See page 50.

◆ Common cold

- Muffled or nasal quality to speech. See page 423.

◆ Adenoids

- Muffled or nasal quality to speech. See page 56.

◆ Stuttering

Tends to begin as a child begins to learn to talk, from two years onwards.

◆ Lisping and rolling Rs

Not necessarily a speech impairment, but a variation of normal. Common when children first learn to speak, and tends to disappear by the age of six. If marked or persistent, speech therapy may be appropriate. Indeed, early attention from a speech therapist can prevent speech disorders becoming permanent.

Possible

◆ Cleft palate

See page 80.

◆ Neurological disease

Any disease that can affect control of the tongue, soft palate and related structures will give slurred and unclear speech. A stroke, motor neurone disease, multiple sclerosis and Parkinson's disease are examples. Cerebellar disease, in particular, can give rise to a speech impediment.

◆ Chronic sinusitis

May give a muffled or nasal quality to speech. See page 53.

◆ Benign tumours

Including nasal polyps, may give a muffled or nasal quality to speech. See page 52.

Rare

◆ Malignant tumours of nose or mouth

See *Cancer of the nose*, page 54.

The Throat

The Throat

Hoarse voice or no voice

Severe cases of hoarseness may suffer complete loss of voice; mild cases merely a temporary thickening or roughening.

The causes can be divided into three main categories: those affecting the vocal cords themselves; those affecting the nerves supplying them; and those caused by other disease of the larynx. All cases of hoarseness lasting more than 10 days should be reported to a doctor. See also *Problems wth swallowing plus hoarse voice*, page 113.

Probable

◆ **Smoking, drinking, excessive talking or shouting**

Obvious and familiar when combined, but also capable of inflaming the vocal cords in isolation.

• Hoarseness.

• Sore throat.

• Settles with resting the voice in three to four days.

If you keep up these insults to your vocal cords, recovery may be slow, indeed you may suffer total loss of voice. Rest (not talking) is the only answer.

Excessive coughing can also damage the vocal cords.

◆ **Laryngitis**

See page 116.

◆ **Common cold**

May occasionally involve the larynx, resulting in hoarseness.

Throat and larynx

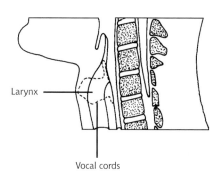

Larynx

Vocal cords

Possible

◆ **Vocal nodules**

Also called singer's nodes. Typically in singers pitching their voice higher than their natural range.

• Progressive hoarseness.

• The nodules often need to be removed by surgery.

◆ **Surgery**

Surgery to the neck, particularly to the thyroid gland, may damage the recurrent laryngeal nerve. Recovery takes a few weeks but the hoarseness can be permanent. If so, there are methods of improving the speech.

After any operation where a breathing tube has been passed down the throat, slight hoarseness and a sore throat is usual.

◆ **Myxoedema**

Swelling around eyes and feet as a result of an underactive thyroid gland, plus highly distinctive, deep, gruff voice.

◆ **Epiglottitis**

See page 211.

◆ **Cancer of the larynx**

See page 84.

◆ **Inhalation**

Of smoke or chemicals can cause temporary hoarseness.

Rare

◆ **Foreign bodies**

See page 53.

◆ **Thoracic aortic aneurysm**

The aorta is the main artery in the chest. An aneurysm is a swelling due to weakness of the wall. This can cause hoarseness by local pressure on the recurrent laryngeal nerve.

◆ **Cancer**

Any malignant tumour in the chest, but especially on the oesophagus or lung, may press on or invade the recurrent laryngeal nerve causing hoarseness. However, this symptom is usually one of the last to occur.

See *Noticeable blood vessels in the neck*, page 123; *Swollen lymph nodes in neck*, page 128; and *Problems with swallowing*, this page.

◆ **After radiotherapy**

Radiotherapy is sometimes used to treat cancer of the larynx, leaving the patient hoarse.

◆ **Sarcoidosis**

A disease (cause unknown) giving enlarged lymph nodes and deposits in various tissues, including larynx, hence hoarseness.

◆ **Myasthenia gravis**

See page 27.

The Throat

Clearing the throat

See *Phlegm in the throat*, page 120.

Problems with swallowing

Probable

◆ **Tonsillitis and pharyngitis**

See pages 116 and 115.

Possible

◆ **Globus hystericus**

Often seen in young women with a history of anxiety-related illness: a certain belief that there is something stuck in the throat; sensation of choking. Requires full medical examination and often intensive investigation to exclude other causes. If all is normal, strong reassurance is all that is needed.

◆ **Oesophagitis**

See below.

Rare

◆ **Achalasia**

A narrowing of the gullet at the lower end. Appears in young adults.

• Difficulty in swallowing.
• Regurgitation of undigested food into the mouth.
• Vomiting.
• Loss of weight.
• Occasionally, chest infections with fever.

◆ **Congenital atresia of the oesophagus**

At birth:

• All feeds regurgitated.
• Frothy saliva from mouth.
• Difficulty breathing while being fed.
• Episodes of cyanosis (blueness).
• Recurrent pneumonia, either from overspill into the lungs or a fistula (communication) between the oesophagus and main windpipe.

◆ **Cancer of the oesophagus and cancer of the stomach**

See pages 113 and 438.

◆ **Epiglottitis**

See page 211.

◆ **Neurological disease**

Typically MND/Myasthenia gravis – see page 27.

Problems with swallowing plus regurgitation or vomiting

Probable

◆ **Oesophagitis**

Caused by stomach acid flowing back up into the gullet.

• Burning pain on swallowing.
• Food and fluid regurgitated.
• Bitter taste in mouth.
• Heartburn.
• Pain in middle of chest, at front or at back, or down arms.
• Food 'sticks' behind breast bone.
• Aggravated by spicy foods and alcohol.
• Relieved by antacids.

Possible

◆ **Peptic stricture**

A narrowing of the gullet caused by long-standing reflux oesophagitis.

• Food regurgitated with fluid.
• Heartburn.
• Associated with weight loss after prolonged period.

The Throat

- Chest infections associated with regurgitation.
- May be associated with hiatus hernia; see page 217.

◆ **Pharyngeal pouch**

See page 125.

Rare

◆ **Cancer of the oesophagus**

Commonest in 50-plus age group.

- Difficulty in swallowing.
- Liquids swallowed more easily than solids.
- Some regurgitation of food.
- Rarely pain.
- Weight loss.
- Poor appetite.
- Fatigue.
- Anaemia (particularly in women).
- Hoarse voice.
- Occasional chest infection with fever – due to regurgitation.

◆ **Stomach cancer**

Similar symptoms to oesophageal cancer, but there may also be:

- Abdominal pain.
- Poor appetite, developing earlier.
- A feeling of fullness soon after eating very little.
- Symptoms of indigestion which persist, do not respond to usual treatment, or become more severe.
- Feeling bloated.
- A previous ulcer.
- Anaemia.
- In later stages, occasional difficulty in swallowing.

◆ **Other cancers**

Secondary tumours or large primary tumours outside the oesophagus, but within the chest, can compress the oesophagus giving rise to:

- Difficulty in swallowing.
- Weight loss.
- Poor appetite.
- Weakness.
- All in addition to the symptoms of the primary tumour.

◆ **Thoracic aortic aneurysm**

See page 111.

Problems with swallowing plus hoarse voice

Probable

◆ **Laryngitis**

See page 116.

Possible

◆ **Foreign body (such as a bone) in gullet**

- Pain and discomfort on swallowing.
- Hoarseness.
- Feeling of 'something in the throat'.

Rare

◆ Myasthenia gravis

A disorder causing weakness and tiring of the muscles.

- Weakness of muscles.
- Drooping eyelids.
- Double vision.
- Hoarse, weak voice.
- Difficulty in swallowing.
- Possibly weight loss.

> Hoarseness which persists in the absence of other symptoms can be a sign either of laryngeal polyps or of cancer. Early treatment will significantly affect the outcome for the better. Seek your doctor's advice as early as possible.

◆ Cancer of the oesophagus

See page 113.

Problems with swallowing plus weight loss

This combination of symptoms is likely to be an indication of serious illness. Seek help soon, since early intervention will significantly improve your chances of recovery. Smoking and drinking to excess will increase the risk of oesophageal problems and cancer of the stomach.

Probable

◆ Oesophageal stricture

See *Peptic stricture*, page 112. The symptoms are the same, but can be caused by, for instance, accidental or deliberate swallowing of toxic chemicals.

◆ Cancer of the oesophagus

See page 113.

Possible

◆ Benign tumour of the oesophagus

Such as a fibroma, leiomyoma or haemangioma.

- Intermittent difficulty in swallowing.
- Sensation of 'something' in the gullet.
- Health otherwise good.
- Minimal weight loss, unless tumour is large.

◆ Multiple sclerosis

In addition to motor and sensory changes (see page 298):

- Difficulty in swallowing.
- Some risk of regurgitation of food into chest.
- Gradual weight loss.

◆ Motor neurone disease

Progressive muscle weakness with:

- Difficulty in starting to swallow because of poor tongue muscle control.
- Risk of inhaling food or fluids.
- Gradual weight loss.

  See also page 379.

◆ Parkinson's disease

In addition to the tremor, mask face and slowness of movement:

- Difficulty in starting to swallow.
- Occasional choking.
- Weight loss.

◆ Pseudobulbar and bulbar palsy

These conditions are usually set off by a stroke (pseudobulbar palsy) or motor neurone disease (bulbar palsy). They cause:

- Difficulty in speech.
- Difficulty in swallowing.
- Regurgitation of food into nose.
- If prolonged, weight loss.

Rare

◆ Chagas' disease

Common in South America. Caused by infection with *Trypanosoma cruzi*.

Symptoms are similar to those of *Achalasia*; see page 112.

◆ Myasthenia gravis

See page 38.

◆ Scleroderma

A disease which can affect many organs and which will usually have been diagnosed already. Typically affects women in their 30s and 40s.

- Associated with pain because of oesophagitis; see page 112.
- Slow weight loss.

◆ Systemic lupus erythematosus

See page 417.

◆ Cancer of the stomach

See page 113.

Problems with swallowing plus pain

Probable

◆ Tonsillitis

See page 116.

◆ Pharyngitis

The pharynx lies behind the tonsils at the back of the mouth, above the voice box and gullet.

- Pain on swallowing.
- Back of throat is noticeably red.
- Possibly enlarged lymph nodes – similar to tonsillitis, but tonsils not inflamed.

If you have had your tonsils removed, pharyngitis may develop in response to an infection which would otherwise have caused tonsillitis.

◆ Laryngitis

See page 116.

Possible

◆ Candidiasis (thrush)

- Discomfort making swallowing difficult.
- White patches seen at the back of the throat and sides of mouth.

Most often nowadays caused by overuse of inhaled steroids. Common in the immuno-suppressed (including those with HIV) and the elderly.

The Throat

The Throat

◆ **Oesophagitis**

Similar to reflux oesophagitis, but the main symptom is:

• Burning pain behind the breast bone within a few seconds of swallowing, plus:

• Spread of pain to the arms.

• Heartburn.

• Aggravated by spicy foods or alcohol.

◆ **Oesophageal spasm**

Spasm of the muscles of the gullet.

• Chest pain initiated by eating or emotional stress (if severe can be mistaken for a heart attack).

• The condition can be mild or severe.

• Pain varies in intensity during an attack.

• Can be painless.

• Intermittent difficulty in swallowing, often at the same time as the pain.

◆ **Ulcers of the tongue and mouth**

See pages 77.

◆ **Glossitis**

Swollen, painful tongue, occasional fever, sometimes associated with riboflavine deficiency.

◆ **Herpes simplex**

A viral infection causing pain and formation of fluid-filled spots or ulcers. May be present in mouth, throat or oesophagus.

• Severe pain associated with the herpes sore.

• Vesicles and intensely painful ulcers seen in mouth.

• Feeling very unwell.

• Fever.

Rare

◆ **Cancer of the oesophagus**

See page 113.

◆ **Cancer of the larynx**

• Persistent hoarseness.

• Occasionally pain on swallowing because of spread or ulceration.

Problems with swallowing plus fever

Probable

◆ **Tonsillitis**

Tonsils at the back of the mouth, either side of the throat, become inflamed.

• Enlarged tonsils.

• Occasional white spots on tonsils.

• Reddening in the throat.

• Pain on swallowing.

• Occasionally, associated cough.

• Fever.

• Enlarged lymph glands in neck may be tender.

◆ **Laryngitis**

Infection involving the larynx – the 'voice box' in the neck.

• Hoarse voice, or difficulty in speaking at all.

- Fever.
- Pain on swallowing, but less severe than with tonsillitis.

Rare

◆ Ludwig's angina

Severe infection of the floor of the mouth.

- Severe pain.

- Can cause breathing difficulty – because of swollen upper airways.
- Pain on swallowing.

The condition is usually associated with poor oral hygiene, and problems with infected teeth or gums.

◆ Cancer of the oesophagus

See page 113.

The Throat

Swollen throat

See *Swollen lymph nodes in neck*, page 128.

Lump in throat

See *Problems with swallowing*, pages 111.

Sore throat

Common reasons for a sore throat are covered under *Problems with swallowing plus pain*, page 115.

If you think you have this symptom in isolation, see *Swollen lymph nodes in the neck*, page 128; *Isolated lumps and swellings in or on the neck*, page 124; *Stiffness or pain in the neck*, page 126; *Problems with swallowing plus pain*, page 115 and *Ulcers in the mouth*, page 77.

It is however most likely to occur along with fever. See below.

Sore throat with fever

Probable

◆ Common cold

See page 423.

◆ Tonsillitis

See opposite.

◆ Laryngitis

See opposite.

Smoking

Smokers are likely to suffer from exaggerated symptoms if they have any of the conditions listed here. They are also likely to take longer to recover than non-smokers; and are at greater risk of developing complications, such as secondary infections of the ears or chest.

◆ **Phayrngitis**

See page 115.

Possible

◆ **Infectious mononucleosis**

'Glandular fever'. See page 129.

◆ **Dental infections**

See page 129.

Rare

◆ **Glossitis**

See page 116.

◆ **Ludwig's angina**

See page 117.

◆ **Adverse drug reaction**

Sore throat, inflammation of the mucous membranes of the mouth and fever are all possible symptoms of adverse drug reactions, especially if accompanied by a rash.

Ulcers in the mouth

Probable

◆ **Aphthous ulcer**

- Small and multiple (or larger and solitary).

- Anywhere in mouth or on tongue, typically behind lower lip at the front.

- Extremely painful; aggravated by acid fruits.

- May be aggravated by sharp dentures or other dental problems.

- Often appears at times of stress.

   Most heal after a few days, but larger ones take longer, though rarely more than eight to ten days. Treatments for aphthous ulcers are often unsatisfactory. Pain-relieving gel or tablets may be bought from a chemist. Most brands of toothpaste contain sodium laryl suphate (SLS) and sensitivity to this is sometimes the cause.

◆ **Drugs**

The commonest drug cause is nicorandil (an anti-angina treatment).

◆ **Herpes simplex**

See page 116.

Possible

◆ **Erythema multiforme**

Irregular red marks. May be associated with a reaction to drugs or an infection. Commonest in children and young women.

- Itchy rash anywhere on body; not unlike measles rash.

- Pale-centred wheals, sometimes called 'target lesions'.

- Sore throat.
- Headache.
- Fever.
- Ulceration in the mouth and throat.

There is a severe form of the condition, called Stevens-Johnson syndrome.

Rare

◆ Cancer of the mouth or throat

May occur anywhere in mouth or throat. Tobacco users at risk, especially pipe-smokers, tobacco-chewers.

Suspicion is aroused by:

- Long-standing, large ulcers (more than two weeks).
- Ulcer with irregular shape.
- Ulcers on surfaces of polyps.
- Ulcers with raised edges.
- Feeling unwell.
- Bad breath.
- Enlarged lymph nodes in neck.

◆ Syphilis

Ulcers in the throat can mean primary, secondary or tertiary syphilis. Ulcers are likely to be:

- Single.
- Shallow.
- Hard at the base.
- Painless.
- Non-bleeding.

And they have:

- A raised, reddened margin.
- Enlarged lymph nodes may be present.

◆ Pemphigus

A skin disease in which fluid-filled sacs appear on the skin at sites of pressure and trauma.

- Fluid-filled sacs in the mouth.

These burst, forming:

- Ulcers which may remain for weeks.

◆ Crohn's disease

The following symptoms always accompany other signs of gut disease.

- Aphthous-type ulcers. See opposite.

Recurrent diarrhoea, with or without weight loss, in an otherwise fit person who has aphthous ulcers suggests the possibility of Crohn's disease.

◆ Coeliac disease

See page 137.

◆ Behçet's syndrome

Most common, though still rare, in some Middle Eastern countries.

- Recurrent major ulceration in mouth and throat.

Followed by:

- Ulcers on the genitals.
- Eye inflammation and arthritis.

◆ Leukaemias/Myeloma

- Ulceration in the mouth.
- Persistent sore throats.
- Infections.
- Feeling unwell.
- Bruise easily.

See also page 450.

The Throat

◆ **Tuberculosis**
- Small ulcers.
- Sore throat.
- Difficulty in swallowing.

- Excessive salivation.
  See also page 208.

◆ **Heamatological i.e. blood disorders**
Any cause of marrow suppression.

Phlegm in the throat

Which, typically, you are always trying to clear.

Probable

◆ **Vasomotor rhinitis**
- More or less constant production of mucus in the nasal passages.
- Clear discharge from front of nose. The mucus also dribbles into the throat from the back of the nose (the two are connected). This last is known as post-nasal drip.
- Brought on by a change of environment or atmosphere.
- Difficulty in breathing through nostrils.
- Not associated with other symptoms of *Allergic rhinitis*; see below.

◆ **Allergic rhinitis**
You are likely to have a known allergy, typically to pollen, dust or animals.
- Clear discharge from front of nose and into throat.
- Difficulty in breathing through the nostrils.
- Watery eyes.
- Sneezing.
- Wheezing.

A family history of asthma, eczema or hay fever is often found in those with this condition.

There is some evidence that modern living, with its double glazing, central heating and indoor life, has increased the volume of house dust generally, and that rhinitis is, as a consequence, much more common.

◆ **Chest infection/chronic lung sepsis**
Particularly in patients with chronic chest conditions, for example, bronchitis, cystic fibrosis, bronchiectasis. Smokers are also a high-risk group.
- Persistent coughing up of green or yellow phlegm.
- Fever.
- Feeling unwell.
- Sometimes, difficulty in breathing.
- Normally requires antibiotics.

Possible

◆ **Sinusitis**
Any of the nasal sinuses may become infected causing local pain/discomfort.

- Persistent nasal discharge (green or yellow).
- Headache.
- Pain over affected sinus.
- Fever.
- Bad breath.

◆ Nasal polyps

Polyps are fleshy growths or tumours, almost never malignant. Often multiple.

- Can sometimes be seen by looking into nose.
- Obstruction in nose.
- Clear discharge occasionally.
- Loss of sense of smell.
- Often associated with allergies.

Rare

◆ Cancer of the nasal fossa or nasopharynx

Most common in the elderly.

- Foul smelling and tasting nasal discharge.
- Persistent pain.
- Bad breath.
- A lump may be seen in the mouth or nose; or a facial swelling may develop.
- Toothache may develop.
- Bloodstained nasal discharge or sputum.

White spots visible in mouth and throat

Probable

◆ Milk – especially in babies.

Can easily be wiped off, leaving a healthy oral surfaceh.

◆ Candidiasis

Otherwise known as thrush or monilia. Most commonly seen in new-born babies or infants. (It has been known for parents to mistake thrush for milk on the inside of a baby's cheek; but the white patches are hard to remove and doing so will cause the baby some discomfort.)

- White patches in mouth (which, unlike milk, are hard to remove and cause discomfort).
- Associated reddening.
- Lips, tongue and cheek may be painful.
- Patches may be dislodged, but not always easily.

    Often associated with antibiotic therapy, general ill-health and (more rarely) immunosuppression.

◆ Tonsillitis

See page 116.

Possible

◆ Koplik's spots

A sure sign of measles (see page 415).

- White spots inside the mouth opposite the molar teeth.

The Throat

Persistent, white patches in the mouth can be a sign of serious illness, and should not be ignored.
    Consult your doctor if:

- Patches persist.
- They cannot be removed easily.

- Spots are about the size of a grain of salt with surrounding reddening.

    Other symptoms of measles are:

- A red rash starting by the ears spreading over seven days to the body and limbs.
- Runny nose.
- Reddened eyes.
- Cough.

◆ **Lichen planus**

Irregular, small, shiny purplish lesions on the skin. Can occur all over the body, including the genital area. Very itchy.

Commonest in the middle-aged.

- Multiple fine white lines on lips, tongue and cheek.
- White spots in the same region.
- Sometimes ulcers between the spots and lines.

A small risk of progression to mouth cancer.

◆ **Leukoplakia**

- White patches on the tongue or lining of the mouth.
- Cannot be scraped off.
- Occasionally disappear leaving a red base.
- Possibly localized hardening under the patch.

A not insignificant risk of progression to mouth cancer, so persistent white patches should never be ignored.

Associated with smoking (particularly pipe-smoking), and rubbing dentures. Also, it is increasingly found in people with AIDS.

Noticeable blood vessels on the neck

Newly developed, visible blood vessels are a sign of underlying disease that need careful investigation, and probably tests, before treatment can be started.

Probable

◆ Heart failure

The pump fails to pump blood adequately, typically after a heart attack. May be associated with one or more of the following:

- Prominent symmetrical veins on each side of the neck, that distend more as the patient lies flat.
- The prominence varies with respiration and heart beat.
- Shortness of breath worse on lying flat.
- Shortness of breath on walking.
- Bluish discolouration of face.
- Swelling of ankles and legs.

Possible

◆ Malignant tumour within the chest

Malignant tumours (primary or secondary) within the chest can compress the great veins inside the chest giving rise to:

- Symmetrical prominent veins on head, neck and upper chest unaffected by bodily position.
- Face may appear congested and reddened.
- The face, neck and upper chest may be swollen.

- Breathing may be normal.

In addition, there may well be the following general symptoms of:

- Weight loss.
- Poor appetite.
- Weakness.
- Feeling unwell.

◆ Pericardial effusion

Fluid distends the sac around the heart. May be caused by infection, auto-immune disease, tumour or after a heart attack and can cause:

- Shortness of breath when lying flat.
- Prominent neck veins (symmetrical).
- Tightness in the chest, varying with movement.
- Fever (with infection).
- Feeling unwell.

Rare

◆ Benign tumour within the chest

Large benign tumours within the chest can compress the great veins inside the chest giving rise to the same symptoms as malignant tumours – see above.

◆ Constrictive pericarditis

Increasing rigidity of the sac round the heart. Caused by tuberculosis, or other infection or injury, often many years previously.

- Rapid pulse (sometimes irregular).
- Low blood pressure.
- Tiredness.

The Neck

- Prominent neck veins – more prominent on breathing in.
- Fluid in the abdomen.
- Liver enlargement.

Isolated lumps may be associated with a number of structures in the neck in addition to the lymph nodes (see page 128: read with this).

These include the skin, and the salivary or thyroid glands. A few are present from birth.

Isolated lumps or swellings in or on the neck

Probable

◆ Boil

A skin infection commonly originating in a hair follicle or follicles.

- Painful.
- Localized reddening.
- Skin warm to the touch.
- Localized swelling.
- A yellow centre that may discharge pus.

◆ Sebaceous cyst

- Superficial.
- Painless (unless infected).
- Present for many years.
- Slowly increases in size.
- Has a central 'punctum' – the opening to the blocked sweat gland that causes the cyst.

◆ Lipoma

A benign fatty tumour which can be superficial or extend under the skin.

Same characteristics as a sebaceous cyst except:

- No punctum.

Possible

◆ Diffuse thyroid gland enlargement

The thyroid gland lies on both sides of the neck below the Adam's apple.

- Movement of swelling up and down on swallowing.
- Diffuse swelling – no separate lumps.
- No other symptoms.

Other causes of diffuse thyroid swelling can be divided into those causing excess thyroid hormone secretion, and those causing an underactive thyroid. Both require professional attention.

Further details, pages 319 and 320.

◆ Isolated thyroid nodule – benign

A localized lump within the thyroid, which can be benign or malignant – see opposite.

- Can be felt either side of the neck below the Adam's apple.
- Moves up and down on swallowing.

May be associated with signs of overactive or underactive thyroid. See above.

◆ Submandibular duct stone

Beneath the jaw, each side of the tongue, are two salivary glands, the submandibular glands. Stones may form in the ducts of the glands, or the body of the gland, causing:

• Painful swelling (normally on one side).

• The swelling increases when eating and reduces between meals.

• Swelling can sometimes be felt in the mouth, under the tongue.

Rare

◆ Cervical rib

See page 127.

◆ Diffuse thyroid gland enlargement – malignant tumour

Features of thyroid enlargement plus:

• Irregular symmetric enlargement.

• Movement of swelling up and down on swallowing may be lost.

• Trachea (wind pipe) may be compressed, causing difficulty in breathing.

◆ Isolated thyroid nodule – malignant

A localized lump within the thyroid gland.

• Moves up and down on swallowing.

• May have no other symptoms, but can cause:

• Hoarseness.

• Pain.

• Drooping of one eyelid (Horner's syndrome).

Thyroid gland

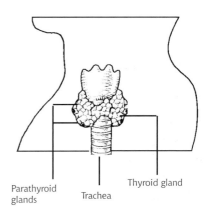

Parathyroid glands

Trachea

Thyroid gland

◆ Thyroglossal cyst

Lies in the middle of the neck at the front.

• Near the surface.

• Moves up if the tongue is stuck out.

• Painless.

◆ Pharyngeal pouch

A swelling on one side of the neck caused by a defect in the upper gullet.

• Varies in size.

• Causes variable difficulty in swallowing.

• Enlarges while eating or drinking.

• May 'gurgle' as fluid empties from it.

• Old food may regurgitated.

• Can be emptied by direct pressure on it.

• Not painful, but can be uncomfortable as it increases in size.

The Neck

◆ **Sternomastoid tumour**

Present from birth – not a true tumour:

- Lump sited in the middle of the muscle at the side of the neck.
- The face is turned away from the side of the lesion.

◆ **Submandibular tumour**

May be benign or malignant.

- One-sided enlargement of gland.
- Progressive.
- May become painful.
- Lymph nodes may be involved.

Stiffness or pain in neck

Probable

◆ **Acute stiff neck**

Associated with sleeping in awkward position; also with exposure to cold.

- Pain on movement localized to neck.
- Neck movements limited by pain and muscle spasm.

◆ **Acute neck sprain**

Associated with sudden twisting/turning or bending.

- Extreme pain on any movement.
- Pain in upper back and head.
- Marked muscle spasm limiting neck movement.

◆ **Whiplash injury**

Typically present after a car crash (hit from behind or from the front).

- Pain in neck and upper back.
- Neck held stiffly.
- Pain may have taken a few hours to develop after injury.
- Pain and stiffness may persist for weeks.
- May have pain and weakness in arms.
- Reduced range of neck movement.

◆ **Wry neck (Torticollis)**

- Head pulled down on affected side.
- Chin points towards the opposite shoulder.
- The affected muscle is a solid band.
- Neck movements are considerably restricted.
- Typically the condition occurs on waking: suddenly you cannot move your neck freely. Wears off in a day or two.

Possible

◆ **Cervical spondylosis**

Caused by degeneration of the lower cervical intervertebral discs.

- Sufferer is typically middle-aged.
- Pain in neck and back.
- Painful over neck.
- Worse on waking.
- Slight limitation of movement. Occasionally:
- Pain in arms.
- Numbness in arms.
- Weakness in arms.

A scan of the neck might show a prolapsed lower cervical intervertebral disc.

◆ Cervical rib

Some people are born with an extra rib, or with fibrous band which constricts nerves and arteries in the neck. Symptoms may appear in the late twenties.

- May be a palpable lump in the neck.
- Neck is rarely painful.
- Pain behind collar bone.
- Pain on the inner side of the arm after or when carrying shopping.
- Intermittent coldness and blueness of fingers.

◆ Rheumatoid arthritis

Patients with known rheumatoid arthritis may get degenerative changes in the neck.

- Pain is common.
- Range of movement is reduced.
- Weakness and sensory changes may be present in upper and occasionally lower limbs.

Rare

◆ Cervical spine infection

Tuberculous infection still occasionally occurs.

- Mild neck pain.
- Pain on any movement.
- Head may be held in hands.
- Stiffness, with reduced movement.
- Occasionally there may be sudden paralysis as the spinal cord gets involved.

Prolapsed lower cervical invertebral disk

Prolapse

Spinal cord

◆ Meningitis

Infection of the lining of the brain and spinal cord. Usually other marked symptoms, such as fever, will be present.

- Neck stiffness – inability to bend the neck forward because of pain and muscle spasm.
- Headache.
- Feeling unwell.
- Fever.
- Fine purple rash which does not blanch under pressure from a glass tumbler.

If meningitis is suspected, call a doctor immediately.

◆ Prolapsed cervical disk

May be caused by sudden movements, and degeneration of the intervertebral discs. There is a sudden onset of symptoms which may include:

The Neck

- Neck pain and stiffness.
- Pain and altered sensation in the arms.
- Muscular spasm of the neck and upper back.
- Symptoms may resolve and then return.

◆ **Spinal cord tumours**

Progressive onset of symptoms may include:

- Altered sensation in arms and legs.
- Areas of numbness.
- Weakness in arms and legs.
- Wasting of muscles.
- Ability to pass urine may be affected.

Swollen lymph nodes in neck

Most people have temporarily enlarged lymph nodes (also known simply as glands) in the neck at some time.

This is generally associated with infection or inflammation, either locally or of the whole body. Sometimes just one is enlarged, giving a single swelling. Occasionally, recurring or persistent enlargement may indicate more serious underlying disorders.

Enlarged lymph nodes need to be distinguished from other lumps in the neck, such as enlarged salivary glands – see *Isolated lumps or swellings in or on the neck*, page 124.

Probable

◆ **Common cold or upper respiratory tract infection (URTI).**

These can occur alone or in combination:

- Tender lymph nodes enlarged symmetrically below ears and under jaw.
- Fever.
- Malaise.
- Sore throat.
- Cough.

Lymph nodes of the neck

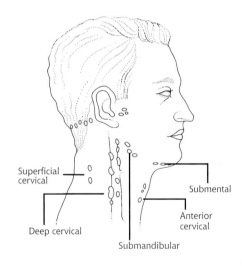

Superficial cervical

Deep cervical

Submandibular

Submental

Anterior cervical

- Runny nose.
- Earache.
- Usually cures itself.

◆ **Tonsillitis**

- Tonsils enlarged
- Throat looks red.
- Tender lymph nodes enlarged below and behind jaw.

- Often enlarged more on one side than the other.
- White spots often apparent on tonsil surface (pus emerging from tonsil).
- Fever.
- Feeling unwell.

Requires antibiotics. Your doctor may take swabs from the tonsils, particularly if the surface is purulent. Frequent attacks may necessitate referral to a specialist throat surgeon.

◆ Local infection or inflammation (e.g. acne, impetigo, sebaceous cyst)

- Nearest lymph nodes will be enlarged and may be painful.
- Pain and tenderness in scalp (look in hair).
- If a lump is present it may be an infected sebaceous cyst.

If an area is scaly/reddened/weeping /itchy consider impetigo, dermatitis, eczema/psoriasis – see your doctor to distinguish which.

◆ Dental infection

Diseases of the gums or teeth may be associated with lymph node enlargement.

- Enlarged tender nodes which tend to be those nearest the affected tooth.
- Toothache.
- Bleeding gums (gingivitis).
- Teeth with loose fillings.
- Dental abscess (painful tooth/gums and local swelling).

Possible

◆ Glandular fever – infectious mononucleosis

Caused by infection with the Epstein-Barr virus and sometimes known as 'kissing disease'. A disease of children and young adults.

- Generalized lymph node enlargement and tenderness, but neck nodes, including those at the back of the head, may be worst affected.
- Fever.
- Sore throat.
- Feeling unwell.
- Symptoms may last for a few days to a few weeks.
- Characteristic changes in the blood: your doctor may confirm the diagnosis with a blood test.
- Spleen may become enlarged in up to 50 per cent of cases.

◆ Toxoplasmosis

A parasite which infects 50 per cent of us. Mostly cures itself in one to three weeks.

Acquired by eating infected, raw or lightly cooked meat (or through contact with cat faeces).

Only about 20 percent of people affected actually have symptoms.

- Fever.
- Enlarged lymph nodes – neck nodes predominant – which may also be tender.
- Feeling unwell.

Diagnosis is confirmed by blood test

The Neck

or by removing a lymph node and examining it under a microscope.

If a pregnant mother develops toxoplasmosis there is a risk of the baby being damaged. Brain and eyes are primarily affected.

In many countries there is routine screening for toxoplasmosis, but not in the U.K.

Avoiding toxoplasmosis in pregnancy:

- Never eat raw or uncooked meat.
- Wash all fruit, vegetables and salads well.
- Do not empty cat litter trays. (If you must do so, wear protective gloves.)
- Wear gloves for gardening.

◆ **Peritonsillar abscess**

Similar signs to tonsillitis, but:

- Pain on opening mouth also present because abscess or 'quinsy' has developed.
  Requires surgical drainage.

◆ **Epiglottitis**

- Very painful throat.
- Pain on swallowing.
- Breathing changes.
- Breathing through an open mouth.
- Lymph nodes may be enlarged.
- High Fever.

  Get medical help urgently.

Rare

◆ **German measles**

Rubella. Commonest in children.

- Runny nose.
- Red rash, mainly on body.
- Enlarged, tender neck lymph nodes, particularly over the back of the scalp, just above the neck.
- In teenage and adult females there may be pains in the joints of the hands.

The use of the MMR vaccine can erradicate this illness.

◆ **Tuberculosis**

Isolated non-tender lymph node enlargement, commonest in immigrants.

- Redness.
- Skin overlying node(s) breaks down.
- Intermittent fever.

Skin tests and blood tests, or biopsy of the node, confirms the diagnosis. Drug treatment required.

◆ **Cancer of the mouth or upper respiratory passages (including larynx)**

All these cancers can cause enlarged lymph nodes, often as a result of the cancer spreading.

These are diseases especially of smokers in the 50-plus age range.

- Persistently enlarged but painless lymph nodes.
- Other lump developing in mouth/tongue or palate.

- Change in voice.
- Weight loss.
- Feeling unwell.
- Persistent pain in mouth or neck.
- Dentures not fitting.
- Anaemia.

◆ Cancer elsewhere in the body

Enlarged painless lymph nodes above the collar bone may suggest spread of a tumour from within the chest or abdomen, but would normally be accompanied by other symptoms from those areas.

◆ Leukaemias

Some or all of the following in combination:

- Enlarged painless lymph nodes in the neck or elsewhere.
- Persistently feeling unwell.
- Pallor, due to anaemia.
- Shortness of breath.
- Fatigue.
- Bruising.

◆ Lymphomas

May have no symptoms apart from:

- Painless, generalized enlargement of lymph nodes.

Later stages include:

- Fever.
- Weight loss.
- Anaemia.

◆ HIV/ARC/AIDS

HIV stands for the *Human immunodeficiency virus*, which tends to infect people for years without making them ill. Eventually, however, it causes ARC – an AIDS-related complex, and finally, full-blown AIDS.

The symptoms listed below cover the whole range from ARC to AIDS.

- Enlarged lymph nodes.
- Fever.
- Feeling unwell.

Anyone in a high-risk group for HIV infection should report persistently enlarged lymph nodes to their doctor. Effectiveness of treatment depends on early diagnosis.

The Neck

> **Persistent symptoms**
>
> If enlarged lymph nodes persist in the neck for more than two weeks, and particularly if other symptoms are present, you must see your doctor.

The abdomen – digestive and urinary systems

The abdominal cavity: introduction

It lies below the rib cage and above the pelvic bones. The terms tummy, stomach and gut are often used, the latter two incorrectly since they are organs that lie within the abdominal cavity.

The abdomen contains the organs of digestion and absorption; part of the oesophagus; the stomach, then the small intestine (including the duodenum, jejunum and ileum); and finally, the large bowel (including the appendix, colon and rectum). It also contains organs connected to the gut which supply the chemicals necessary for digestion: liver, pancreas, gall bladder and biliary tract.

The abdomen also contains organs covered in other sections of this book, including the kidneys, ureters and bladder, which are concerned with excreting urine; and the adrenal glands, which are responsible for secreting hormones that control many of the body's functions. The spleen, which is essentially like a very large lymph gland, is under the rib cage on the left side.

In men, there are also the prostate gland and the seminal vesicles, part of the reproductive system; and likewise in women, the uterus or womb, the Fallopian tubes and the ovaries.

There are also many important blood vessels and nerves.

Vomiting

Vomiting can be forceful or it can be passive, as when one regurgitates food into the mouth.

Sometimes bitter gastric or duodenal juices are vomited, sometimes undigested food, and sometimes blood (either fresh or old – sometimes called 'coffee grounds' because of its appearance). In order to diagnose the underlying cause, you have to take precise note, however disagreeable, of the nature of the vomit. Excluded from this section are the all-too-familiar and obvious causes of vomiting: too much to drink, too much rich food to eat; and travel sickness.

Terminology:

- 'Gastric contents' means typical vomit: partially digested and undigested food, pinkish-yellow, frothy, foul-smelling.

- 'Duodenal contents' means bile-stained (green), thin fluid, mixed with slime and clear secretions.

- 'Faecal vomit' is exactly as the name suggests. It is associated with more severe or chronic forms of vomiting in which partially digested bowel contents are returned to the stomach and vomited.

Probable

◆ Gastroenteritis/food poisoning

Gastric or duodenal contents. Likely to be viral or can occur as part of food poisoning. Abdominal pain may be a feature.

Vomit is likely to contain partially-digested and undigested food, and will look like 'typical vomit' at first. After several vomits, clear, greeny-yellow liquid and slime.

See page 157.

◆ Acute gastritis

Gastric and duodenal contents with old blood, which appears as streaks of brown staining or looking like coffee granules. This is likely after a very heavy drinking bout. Abdominal pain might be a feature. See page 161.

◆ Pregnancy

Gastric and duodenal contents. Other symptoms of pregnancy will be pronounced:

- Nausea, usually most marked on waking.

- Tendency to acid stomach and heartburn.

  See also page 139.

◆ Migraine

Gastric and duodenal contents. See page 105. Other migraine symptoms will be present.

Possible

◆ Peptic ulcer

Gastric and duodenal contents.
  See page 159.

◆ Hiatus hernia and Oesophagitis

A feeling akin to regurgitation.

- A feeling of acid in the lower throat; bilious taste.

- Symptoms of heartburn.
- If severe, vomiting undigested food; also,
- Vomiting old blood, sometimes fresh.

◆ Cancer of the stomach

Vomiting can be a late feature of stomach cancer and may be present with other signs of cancer, such as malaise, marked weight loss and anaemia. Gastric and bowel contents. Likely to follow a progressive feeling of fullness after eating small quantities.

See also *Stomach disease*, page 154.

◆ Intestinal obstruction

- Pain in abdomen that comes and goes.
- No wind or faeces passed rectally.
- Abdomen becomes distended.
- Bloated feeling.
- Gastric and bowel contents, occasionally like diarrhoea.

See also page 162.

◆ Post-gastrectomy syndrome

See page 158. Duodenal contents.

◆ Pyloric stenosis

The pylorus (the word comes from the Greek for a 'gate-keeper') is a muscular narrowing at the outlet of the stomach. Rarely, in newborn babies (invariably less than six weeks old), there is some over-development of this muscle which then blocks emptying of the stomach. Effortless and sometimes projectile vomiting of undigested milk develops within a few minutes of a feed. A very simple operation remedies the problem.

In adults, the gastric outlet can be narrowed by chronic scarring from an ulcer or from a cancer in this area. The vomit will be gastric contents (never bile stained) and can be quite spectacular as the stomach attempts to empty against the blockage.

◆ Drugs

Many drugs have nausea and vomiting as side effects, including opiates and drugs used as chemotherapy agents for cancer.

◆ Radiotherapy

Exposure to irradiation is a potent cause of nausea and vomiting. It typically comes on about four to eight hours after exposure, and can limit a patient's ability to tolerate their treatment.

◆ Diabetes

Uncontrolled diabetes, particularly insulin-dependent diabetes, can cause a dangerous situation with vomiting and rapid onset of dehydration. Sometimes this can be the first presentation of diabetes.

◆ Inner ear disease

Vertigo from vestibular neuronitis or BPPV (Benign paroxysmal positional vertigo) can cause severe nausea and vomiting.

Rare

◆ Chronic pancreatitis

See *Pain in the abdomen and diarrhoea*, page 157.

- Gastric contents.

◆ **Brain tumours**

See *Brain* section,
page 368.

• Gastric contents.

◆ **Brain-stem stroke**

A stroke in the brain stem can cause very
severe vomiting, but other features are
usually over-whelming.

◆ **Renal failure**

• Acute or chronic.

• Mental confusion.

• Headache.

• Breath smelling of urine.

• Vomiting gastric contents.

• Coma.

◆ **Bulimia**

See *Anorexia nervosa*,
page 396.

◆ **Botulism**

A dangerous but extremely rare form of
food poisoning.

• Malaise.

• Nausea.

• Dizziness.

• Vomiting gastric and duodenal contents.

• Abdominal cramp and diarrhoea.

• Breathing problems.

• Pupils wide open.

• Collapse leading to coma.

◆ **Cholera**

See page 147.

◆ **Bezoas**

A fur ball can develop inside the stomach
from constantly chewing on the hair. This
gradually fills the stomach cavity.

Any food consumed then results in
discomfort and sometimes in vomiting.

**Abdomen:
Digestive System**

Vomiting blood

See *Abdominal pain plus vomiting blood*,
page 161.

Vomiting and headache

See especially *Migraine*, page 105; also
other causes of headache and headache
with fever, pages 104.

Regurgitation

See *Vomiting*, page 133.

Prominent blood vessels on the abdomen

Unusually large surface veins sometimes develop on the skin of the abdomen. They are may be a sign of an abnormality of underlying blood vessels, and can be caused by blockage of vessels; pressure from some types of abdominal distension; or local pressure on veins, from growths.

Other symptoms that may be present if any of these causes apply are:

- Leg swelling, sometimes one-sided.
- Lower abdominal wall veins most prominent.

- Caput medusae (literally the 'head of Medusa', one of the Gorgons in Greek mythology whose beautiful hair was changed into a head of serpents by the god Athena) – distended veins radiating out from the umbilicus.

Some conditions (all rare) that can cause these symptoms are:

- *Acute pancreatitis* – page 140.
- *Cirrhosis of the liver* – page 141.
- *Malignant ascites* – page 141.
- *Ovarian cyst* – page 160.

Generalized swelling of the abdomen in babies and children

Probable

◆ **Normal variant**

The pot-bellied child is simply made that way and because the tummy naturally bulges in childhood, it will not necessarily do so in adulthood.

◆ **Constipation**

In some toddlers and children there is a strong psychological element to constipation. It may well develop at potty-training, when the child resists parental exhortation to pass stools; and it can develop into a life-long habit.

Clothes may get soiled with faeces – 'apparent diarrhoea' – The underlying problem is a hard, constipated stool blocking the rectum. This causes irritation and a constant urge to defecate. The irritation causes 'hurry' in

the colon, resulting in a rather liquid stool reaching the rectum before the fluid content has been reduced. This fluid stool then leaks past the the blockage and escapes without conscious control.

See also *Constipation*, page 152.

Whatever you do, don't allow potty training to become a battleground between you and your child. A relaxed approach is usually best. All children will learn in time to control their bowels and bladder. Most problems are caused by over-zealous carers pushing a child to be 'clean' before he or she is ready. If you are in any doubt, take advice from your GP or health visitor.

Possible

◆ Cystic fibrosis

Most symptoms of this hereditary disease are caused by abnormal body secretions.

- Failure to thrive, but healthy appetite.
- Thin, with distended abdomen.
- Recurrent chest infections.
- Large amounts of smelly faeces.
- Finger clubbing.
- Occasionally the rectum may slip out through the anus (rectal prolapse).

◆ Coeliac disease

Caused by an allergy to gluten, a component of wheat (in cereals, for example). Normally, the child will be underweight and will not grow as expected.

- Often, the child has a fair complexion.
- Child is unhappy.
- Appetite is poor.
- Muscles are wasted.
- Abdomen is distended.
- Occasional diarrhoea and vomiting.

  Treatment is a gluten-free diet for life, and a complete recovery can be expected.

◆ Pre-term

Babies born preterm may become constipated with bowel distension due to the presence of meconium, the greenish bowel contents present at birth. This stage usually passes quickly.

Prematurity is a measure of birth weight – i.e less than 2500g.

Rare

◆ Hirschsprung's disease

Part of the bowel fails to develop proper nervous tissue and fails to work correctly, resulting in the progressive distension of the large bowel by faeces. Large quantities may be retained. The abdomen may become massively swollen. Symptoms of constipation appear soon after birth, but the diagnosis is sometimes not made for years.

◆ Kwashiorkor

Malnutrition caused by insufficient protein. All too common in underdeveloped countries, especially in poor, rural areas in the tropics.

- Unhappy child.
- Distended abdomen.
- Swelling of face and limbs.
- Dry, thin hair.
- Pigmented areas of skin.
- Occasional diarrhoea.

**Abdomen:
Digestive System**

Generalized swelling of the abdomen

Described by doctors as distension. The common causes are fat, wind, faeces, fluid or, in a woman, pregnancy. Doctors often find it difficult to decide whether there really is distension.

This section does not deal with isolated lumps or bumps felt in the abdomen and it excludes pregnancy.

These aside, there are many causes of abdominal swelling: some, as one would expect, are harmless, and some suggest serious underlying disease.

It is important to consider whether symptoms associated with abdominal swelling are new and uncomfortable (such as pain and indigestion) or have built up slowly, possibly during a period when your personal circumstances altered (for example, reduced exercise, 'comfort eating', family crisis or bereavement).

Usually it will be clear to you whether your symptoms are part of a long, even lifelong, history of abdominal discomfort, or are new and therefore more likely to suggest an illness.

Probable

◆ Obesity

An obvious, and extremely common diagnosis, but worth considering in its own right. Fat does not just accumulate below the skin, it accumulates in the body cavities. Work out your correct weight for height and age, or ask your doctor what it should be. Then compare every stone you are overweight with the bulk created by 28 half-pounds of butter. It all has to be stored somewhere.

◆ Wind

Doctors call it flatus. Produced by the fermentation of food in the gut. Most of us are aware of those foods that cause most wind.

◆ Poor muscle tone

Many women develop protruding abdomens after childbirth. Often, intensive exercise is needed to get the abdominal wall muscles to revert to

their original tone, and sometimes they never do.

Men can also find that they acquire a 'pot belly', either when they stop exercising or when they indulge in the steady consumption of beer.

◆ Constipation

Most people have one bowel movement a day for most of their lives. Constipation is a term individuals may use if they believe they are not passing stools either easily or frequently enough. In fact, constipation should be divided into three types.

First, that in which hard, pellet-like or rock-like stools are passed, a common condition caused by change in diet and / or lifestyle, often in younger people and in children.

Second, there are people who have bowel movements at long intervals – say every week or fortnight. This has been their pattern for a long time, but they describe themselves as constipated. In fact, there is nothing essentially wrong: they are a variant of normal.

The third type is constipation of sudden onset, often in the elderly.

Most people have regular bowel movements (even though they may be preoccupied, perhaps even obsessed, by variations). Often, bowel movements occur at about the same time every day. However, it is not necessarily abnormal not to have such a regular habit. What is always important is a change from your usual pattern. It is this that should be reported to your doctor.

Sometimes it is impossible even to pass wind. This may suggest an underlying disorder: report it to a doctor – it must be investigated.

Possible

◆ Pregnancy

Again, an apparently obvious diagnosis, but some women are taken unawares by pregnancy. Enough to say that an enlarging abdomen, missed periods, heartburn, fullness and discomfort of the breasts, with or without morning sickness in a sexually active woman in the reproductive years are sound reasons for doing a home pregnancy test.

◆ Irritable bowel syndrome

This is a remarkably common condition in Western society, affecting most people to some extent from time to time.

Sometimes the symptoms are quite severe and unpleasant and cause considerable concern to the patient, even though investigations are all normal. It is probably caused by abnormal motility of the gut. It tends to come and go, and to be related to anything that affects the gut's activity: for example, stress, change of diet, unusual food.

The typical picture is:

• Intermittent abdominal pain relieved by opening the bowels.

• Variable bowel habit fluctuating from loose, frequent stools to constipation.

• Passage of mucus.

• Abdominal distension.

• Wind.

◆ Diverticular disease

A diverticulum is a small pouch on the wall of the large bowel. Along the length of the large bowel are three longitudinal muscles. Between these, the wall of the bowel is relatively weak. Chronic, low-grade constipation results in the bowel having to squeeze harder to move the stool down, and this increased pressure causes small pouches to develop in these weaker areas. Most people develop them as they get older, but only a few will get symptoms. These usually arise if one of the diverticula becomes inflamed.

• Change of bowel habit.

• Steady or colicky abdominal pain, often on the left side.

• Abdominal distension.

• Pellet-like stools.

• Occasional passage of dark to bright red blood from the rectum.

If the inflammation becomes severe, with:

• Fever.

• Intense pain.

• A tender lump in the abdomen.

This condition is then called diverticulitis. It usually settles down with antibiotic treatment.

Decreasing the amount of food you eat allows the gut to rest and will also help.

It is important to maintain a high-fibre diet to enable the large bowel to function at reduced pressure, as the stools become softer.

Abdomen: Digestive System

◆ **Heart failure**

Severe untreated heart failure can result in the accumulation of fluid in the abdominal cavity in addition to several other symptoms. See page 198.

◆ **Perforated viscus (hollow internal organ)**

The major symptom of this condition is pain, which will dominate any discomfort or swelling of the abdomen.

Any of the hollow organs within the abdominal cavity can become inflamed or damaged. If the inflammation or damage is severe enough, the wall of the organ – typically the stomach, small bowel, colon or appendix – bursts. Gut contents leak into the abdominal cavity. This material contains organisms that can cause peritonitis – inflammation of the abdominal cavity – if treatment is delayed. This can be fatal.

The symptoms are similar whichever organ perforates, although initially the site of pain may be different. An inflamed appendix, a peptic ulcer and a diverticulum may all burst.

• Sudden onset of severe pain.

• Fever.

• Very tender abdomen (muscles of the abdominal wall appear rigid).

• Pale, sweating face, sunken eyes.

• Eventually, distension of the abdomen caused by leakage of gas and contents from the gut.

• Shock may develop. See page 381.

◆ **Bowel cancer**

Includes cancer of colon and rectum.

This can block the intestine, either gradually or suddenly. Though a common symptom is a change in bowel habit (type or frequency of stool), swelling (distension) of the abdomen may be caused by a build-up of food, fluid, faeces or wind. Other possible symptoms may include:

• Colicky, abdominal pain.

• Possibly intermittent symptoms.

• Slime or mucus in stool.

• Abnormal stools.

• Blood in stools.

Rare

◆ **Acute pancreatitis**

Abdominal pain will be a major and primary symptom of this condition. It is inflammation of the pancreas, which lies at the back of the abdominal cavity and produces chemicals, known as enzymes, which help with digestion of food. If inflamed, the pancreas can actually start digesting your own innards. There are mild or very severe, and some times fatal forms.

People who drink excessive amounts of alcohol, or who have a history of gall bladder disease are at increased risk. Features include:

• Continuous, central abdominal pain.

• Pain may radiate to the back.

• Vomiting.

• Malaise.

• Slight jaundice may appear a couple of days after the initial attack.

• Bruising/discoloration around the

umbilicus or flanks after two to three days.

Some individuals who collapse for no apparent reason are later found to have pancreatitis.

◆ Cirrhosis of the liver

An irreversible degeneration of the liver that has many causes. Perhaps the most well known is alcohol abuse.

Features of advanced cirrhosis are:

- Malaise, weakness.
- Weight loss.
- Anorexia.
- Swelling of the ankles.
- Abdominal distension due to fluid in the abdominal cavity – ascites.
- Vomiting, sickness.
- Vomiting blood, blood in stools.
- Jaundice.
- Mental deterioration.
- Easy bruising.
- Red vascular marks on skin (spider naevi).
- Clubbing of the nails. See page 276.

In men:

- Enlargement of the breasts.
- Shrinkage of the testes.

Other causes of cirrhosis, of which there are several different types, include:

- Active chronic hepatitis.
- Haemochromatosis.
- Wilson's disease.
- Primary biliary cirrhosis.
- Budd-Chiari syndrome.

- Chronic cardiac failure.

In most cases the individual is aware of the primary diagnosis before cirrhosis develops.

◆ Malignant ascites

Cancer of any organ within the abdominal cavity may lead to the formation of fluid in the abdominal cavity, or ascites. In addition to the symptoms of the original cancer individuals may develop:

- Tense, distended abdomen.
- Swelling of the ankles.
- Shortness of breath (due to pressure on the diaphragm).

◆ Ovarian cyst

Very occasionally, an enormous cyst may develop on an ovary, causing abdominal distension. It requires surgery.

◆ Intestinal obstruction

The intestine is a term for the stomach, the small and the large bowel. Blockage can occur for many reasons. The features are similar:

- Colicky often central abdominal pain (site dependent on cause).
- Abdominal distension: if low, ileum or colon/rectum obstruction is likely.
- Vomiting may be an early feature of stomach or jejunal obstruction, later involving the ileum. It tends to be a late feature of colon obstruction.
- Constipation – no stools and often no wind.
- Loops of bowel may be seen undulating

Abdomen: Digestive System

under the skin surface as they try to overcome the obstruction.

- Perforation may ultimately occur (see *Perforated viscus*, page 140).

Urgent medical attention is needed. Causes include:

Strangulated hernia

- Hernia (rupture) in groin may become painful and not be able to be pushed back.

Cancer

- Other features of cancer may have been present before, for example, altered bowel habit (constipation/diarrhoea), weight loss, anorexia, anaemia.

Inflammation

- For example, with Crohn's disease, diverticular disease.
- A fibrous internal band, sometimes referred to as adhesions, common after abdominal surgery.
- Bowel gets twisted internally around fibrous tissue present from, or after, birth.

Volvulus

- Bowel twists on itself, causing a blockage.

Gall-stone

Occasionally a gall-stone passes into the bowel and gets jammed in the narrowest part (the end of the ileum).

◆ Ulcerative colitis

Chronic disease of the colon.
Main features:

- Diarrhoea.
- In acute attacks, blood, mucus and pus are passed.
- Abdominal pain and fever in acute cases.
- As a complication of some cases, abdominal swelling.

Overall swelling of the abdomen plus diarrhoea

Probable

◆ Obesity

◆ Wind

See page 138.

Possible

◆ Constipation

Occasionally someone, especially an elderly person, can become so constipated that other gut contents leak out of the rectum past the impacted mass of faeces. This gives the impression of diarrhoea.

◆ Irritable bowel syndrome

◆ Diverticular disease

See page 139.

◆ Factitious diarrhoea

Some people take laxative medicine as a matter of habit and yet complain of diarrhoea. They may be doing so in order to lose weight, but sometimes doctors are faced with people who cannot explain why they take laxatives so often, or they may deny it altogether. So, this is worth considering for any individual who complains of diarrhoea, yet is otherwise well.

Some laxatives cause associated abdominal distension and discomfort.

◆ Crohn's disease

- Tends to occur in young adults.
- Intermittent, colicky pain with or without diarrhoea.
- With or without weight loss.
- Spontaneously resolves and relapses.
- Sometimes taken for a 'grumbling appendix'.

- Occasionally intestinal obstruction due to narrowing of bowel.

Drug treatment and/or surgery may be needed.

See also page 119.

Rare

◆ Bowel cancer

See page 140.

◆ Ulcerative colitis

See page 416.

Overall swelling of the abdomen plus constipation

Probable

◆ Wind

◆ Constipation

See pages 138 and 152.

Possible

◆ Irritable bowel syndrome

◆ Diverticular disease

See page 139.

Rare

◆ Bowel cancer

Most bowel cancer originates in the rectum, colon or caecum. It may present in many ways, or be found incidentally on routine examination.

It is possible to divide symptoms into right colon + caecum and left colon + rectum. See also *Intestinal obstruction*, page 141.

Right colon plus caecum:

- Vague lower abdominal pain.
- Pain may localize to right side.
- Mass in right side of abdomen.
- Change in bowel habit: often diarrhoea; occasionally constipation.
- Anaemia and associated symptoms (see page 390) due to slow blood loss.

Left colon plus rectum:

- Increasing constipation.
- Intermittent diarrhoea.
- Colicky abdominal pain and distension.
- Blood present when passing stools.
- Mass in left side of abdomen.

Any persistent change in bowel habit in someone over 50 must be assessed by a doctor.

Quickly feeling full on eating

◆ Post-gastric surgery

If surgery to remove a diseased stomach leaves only a small part behind, relatively small meals make you feel replete.

◆ Stomach cancer

See *Stomach disease*, page 154.

◆ Bezoa

• General malaise (see page 135).

Worms

There are four types of worm that most commonly affect humans.

In developed countries, the only type of worm normally seen is the threadworm.

Probable

◆ Threadworm

• Anal irritation.

Threadworms are an extremely common infestation among schoolchildren. Most children will have them at some time. Typically, a child wakes with an itchy anus at night: the female worm typically comes out on to the anus at night in order to lay her eggs. Small, white, thread-like worms can be seen on the skin of the anus, and, less easily, in the stools. Treatment is simple, with medicine which should normally be taken by all family members. The commonest source of threadworm infestation is another child, but the eggs can live in garden soil. Washing hands and scrubbing nails helps prevent infection or re-infection.

• May prevent sleep.
• Worms observed in stools.

Possible

◆ Roundworms – ascaris lumbricoides

• May be no symptoms.
• Worm observed in stools.
• Occasionally abdominal pain.
• Occasionally the lungs become inflamed.
• Occasionally an urticarial skin reaction develops; see page 242.

◆ Hookworms

• May cause chronic bleeding from small intestine.
• Anaemia.
• Malaise.
• Diarrhoea.

◆ Tapeworms

• Abdominal discomfort.
• Increased appetite.
• Segments of worms seen in stools.

All types of worm infestation should be assessed and treated by a doctor.

Abdomen:
Digestive System

Tar-like stools

See *Blood from the back passage*, page 148.

Pale-coloured faeces

Faeces are normally coloured brown by a mixture of the body's bile pigments and bacteria. Certain conditions hinder this pigmentation; and sometimes bile is excreted instead via urine, which then appears dark brown or orange. There may also be jaundice and sometimes itching.

Jaundice occurs when pigments which are normally excreted in bowel or urine waste products build up in the body to such an extent that they colour the eyes and skin with a yellow tinge.

Probable

◆ **Gall stones**

See *Cholecystitis*, page 162.

◆ **Hepatitis**

Several different types of virus cause hepatitis. Some are more significant than others and so suspected hepatitis needs professional attention. In some cases, the disease is so mild it is assumed to be a cold or flu.

- Lethargy.
- Loss of appetite.
- Loss of desire for cigarettes and alcohol.
- Nausea.
- Joint pains.
- Variable rash.

Gall stones

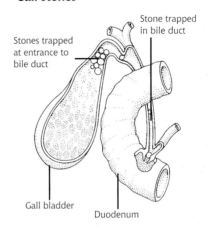

Stones trapped at entrance to bile duct

Stone trapped in bile duct

Gall bladder

Duodenum

- Right-sided upper abdominal pain.
- Fever.
- Diarrhoea.

The pale stools, dark urine and jaundice appear (if, indeed, they are going to) after a few days. In mild cases, jaundice may not be a feature.

Possible

◆ **Cancer of the pancreas**

See *Diseased pancreas*, page 169.

◆ **Chronic pancreatitis**

See page 157.

◆ **Cirrhosis of the liver**

See page 141.

◆ **Liver tumours**

See *Liver disease*, page 401.

◆ **Drugs**

Certain drugs can cause damage and swelling of the tiny bile ducts in the liver. This gives a picture similar to blockage of the main bile duct, with pale stools and jaundice.

Rare

◆ **Jaundice of pregnancy**

Occurs in a small proportion of women. Normally harmless and appears in the final three months.

◆ **Biliary atresia**

Failure of the biliary tract to develop properly in a foetus.

• Jaundice a few days after birth.
• Itching.
• Retarded growth.
• Cirrhosis develops.
• Malabsorption.
• Liver transplants offer hope.

◆ **Sclerosing cholangitis (adult)**

For some unknown reason the bile ducts grow fibrous and shrink.

• Progressive jaundice.
• Itching.
• Liver failure after a few years.

◆ **Cancer of the bile ducts**

Very rare. Causes jaundice with pale faeces and dark urine associated with other signs of cancer, such as weight loss.

Diarrhoea

Can be difficult to define: perhaps the most useful criterion is whether the passage of stools is loose enough or frequent enough to be inconvenient.

Diarrhoea may be watery; green-yellow; bloody (bright red, dark or tarry); a normal colour; or mixed with mucus and pus.

Strictly speaking, blood passed via the anus is not diarrhoea, but as it is often difficult to tell it from liquid stools, it is also included under this heading.

Probable

◆ **Gastroenteritis**

• Loose, runny, watery.
  See page 157.

◆ **Irritable bowel syndrome**

• Slightly loose normal stool.
  See page 139.

◆ **Diverticular disease**

• Normal stool, but may be blood-streaked, or with dark blood mixed in.
  See page 139.

Possible

◆ Factitious diarrhoea

- Loose, but normal.
  See page 142.

◆ Crohn's disease

- Loose, but normal.
  See page 119.

◆ Ulcerative colitis

- Loose stools with blood, mucus and pus. See page 416.

◆ Bowel cancer

- Loose, but normal, and may be blood-streaked. See page 140.

◆ Coeliac disease

- Loose, pale and bulky. See page 137.

◆ Chronic pancreatitis

- Loose pale, bulky, smelly. See page 157.

◆ Bacillary dysentery

- Loose, bloody, pus and mucus. See page 158.

◆ Sprue

Malabsorption that starts with an initial attack of diarrhoea.

- Persistent diarrhoea.
- Stools are bulky, pale and fatty.
- Progressive weight loss.
- Anorexia.
- Anaemia.
- Oedema.
- Inflamed tongue.
  Requires antibiotics.

◆ Traveller's diarrhoea

Diarrhoea after travelling in countries with poor standards of hygiene.

Needs investigation if bloody or persistent, or the sufferer feels very unwell.

◆ AIDS-related diarrhoea

AIDS patients commonly have diarrhoea and abdominal pain as symptoms. Investigations are needed to decide whether these symptoms are related to AIDS alone or to bacterial infection.

◆ Hyperthyroidism

- Loose, but normal. See page 319.

◆ Kwashiorkor

- Loose, but normal. See page 137.

◆ Post-gastrectomy syndrome

After the removal of part of the stomach (a gastrectomy), diarrhoea is a common complaint. Fortunately, since the introduction of modern ulcer-curing drugs, gastrectomy is no longer as common an operation as it once was.

◆ Drugs (such as metformin)

Many drugs cause diarrhoea as a side effect. Discuss with your doctor.

Rare

◆ Carcinoid syndrome

See page 159.

◆ Cholera

- Profuse, watery. See page 135.

◆ Typhoid

- Loose, watery. See page 158.

Abdomen:
Digestive System

Blood from the back passage

This can appear in several forms: fresh, bright red; darkish, coming from the colon; or 'tarry,' coming from even higher up the gut, say the duodenum. In general, any disease that can cause bleeding in the gut can produce either vomited blood, and/or blood passed in stools.

Probable

◆ Piles

Medical term, haemorrhoids. These lumps are engorged veins from the lining of the rectum which get pushed out from the anal canal: a very common complaint.

- Bright red bleeding after defaecation, seen in the lavatory pan and on the paper.
- Pain is not a symptom of uncomplicated haemorrhoids.
- Fleshy lumps felt protruding intermittently from the anus after defaecation, which can and should be encouraged back above the anal sphincter. However, some piles remain permanently protruding.

Piles are normally caused by a diet which is abnormally low in roughage; stress, leading to changes in diet; or pregnancy, which puts pressure on the veins around the rectum. You can usually cure 90 per cent of piles by increasing the amount of roughage in your diet, ideally by adding bran.

Severe cases may need injection or, rarely, surgical treatment.

Intussusception

◆ Anal fissure

See opposite page.

Possible

◆ Polyps

Intestinal polyps (growths of the tissue lining the ileum), which are initially benign growths, may cause anaemia, or episodes of rectal bleeding. As they grow, the risk of cancerous change increases. See also *Bowel cancer*, page 140.

◆ Diverticular disease

See page 139.

◆ Bowel cancer

See page 140.

◆ Bleeding peptic ulcer

This can cause a black, tarry motion, in association with other symptoms. Sometimes a black stool is the first and only sign of a significant episode of internal bleeding from the gut. The stool is black because the blood is altered by its passage through the gut. The stool is shiny black and has a distinctive, unpleasant smell. The black stool that occurs with iron therapy does not have the same smell and is matt black.

◆ Drug-induced

Certain drugs (particularly steroids and non-steroidal anti-inflammatory drugs, including aspirin) may cause gastric bleeding. Initial symptoms may include vomiting blood or tarry stools.

Rare

◆ Oesophageal varices

Delicate, distended veins in the lower end of the oesophagus. They may be present with cirrhosis of the liver (see page 141). They may cause massive vomiting of blood and also bleeding from the back passage or the appearance of black stools. This condition can be fatal because of sudden blood loss.

◆ Intussusception

See diagram opposite. This condition is extremely painful and a medical emergency. It is a bowel abnormality which tends to occur when the body tries to expel unwanted tissue, such as polyps.

In children it is the commonest form of bowel obstruction. Often no underlying cause is found, but sometimes it can be caused by inflamed lymph nodes in the wall of the intestine, or a condition known as a Meckel's diverticulum.

- Severe, colicky, abdominal pain.
- Thighs and knees drawn up because of pain.
- Blood-stained stools and mucus are passed (though this is usually a late sign).
- Vomiting.
- Abdominal distension.

◆ Jejunal diverticula

Like the colon, the jejunum may develop multiple diverticula. See *Diverticular disease*, page 139.

- Tarry stools.
- Often pain-free.
- Sometimes diarrhoea due to altered digestion and absorption.

◆ Meckel's diverticulum

This is like an extra appendix but originates in the ileum.

Very rarely, it can cause bleeding or an intussusception. See page 160.

Pain around anus or in rectum

Probable

◆ External piles

See opposite page.

◆ Anal fissure

A small tear in the surface tissue of the anal canal, usually caused by the passage of hard faeces. Sometimes this can be a feature of Crohn's disease, though it may have been caused by injury (perhaps during anal intercourse).

- Local pain, worse after passing a stool.
- Pain stops the individual wanting to open their bowels, and they can become constipated.
- Occasional bleeding (bright red) may be noted (in lavatory pan or on paper).
- Pain-relieving creams or GTN cream which allows anal muscle relaxation may help healing, which will often occur spontaneously.

◆ Proctalgia fugax

This odd condition is probably due to cramp of the muscles that internally support the anus. Brief episodes of intense deep anal pain can occur without warning. Often relieved by reducing stress levels and ensuring a high fibre diet.

Possible

◆ Anal abscess

The anus or anal canal and rectum are common sites for infection, because of the moist environment and the many organisms present in faeces.

- All abscesses need surgical assessment and treatment.
- Localized throbbing pain (either around the anus or in the rectum).
- Local tender swelling.
- Reddening of the skin if near the surface.
- Often fever.
- Often malaise.
- Often a fast pulse rate.

Possible underlying diseases that cause severe or recurrent abscesses are diabetes mellitus (see page 168) and Crohn's disease (see page 119).

Rare

◆ Fistula-in-ano

May be the final result of an abscess which has burst through skin and bowel creating a false passage.

- Persistent faecal discharge on skin near anus.

Itching anus

Itching is usually a sign of inflammation, infection or infestation of the skin's surface. It can occur as a result of an underlying illness in the rest of the body, which makes the skin more vulnerable to this sensation in one particular area.

Probable

◆ Occupational hazard

The term is a euphemism for the fact that, by its nature, the anal area, moist and subject to infective organisms, is prone to infection and irritation. People who sit all day (particularly in well-contoured car seats) and who have stressful jobs, are perhaps especially prone to this problem.

Regular washing and proper drying will reduce itching. (See below) On the other hand, over-zealous washing and wiping can damage the skin surface, also causing minor irritation and itching.

A mild steroid cream can be helpful; get a doctor's advice.

◆ Threadworm

See pages 144.

◆ Piles

See page 148.

◆ Yeast infection

Because this area is continuously moist and damp, it is vulnerable to yeast and fungal infections such as thrush, which is caused by the yeast candida. Simple anti-fungal creams can cure the condition. However, it may recur.

In children especially, a low-grade infection with a bowel organism (*Strep. faecalis*) can cause a chronic anal irritation. This merits a swab and appropriate antibiotic treatment.

Possible

◆ Pruritis ani

Some people scratch the anal region as a matter of habit, or when tense. Constant scratching causes inflammation, cracking, itching and discomfort.

◆ Lichen sclerosis et atrophicus

This condition is not rare, but is often missed. See *Dermatology* section.

◆ Anal fissure

See page 149. Individuals with anal fissures occasionally complain of local itching or irritation.

◆ Fistula-in-ano

See opposite page. Those with anal fistulas occasionally complain of local irritation and itching.

◆ Pilonidal sinus

A small hole underneath the skin between the buttocks, thought to be created by a hair growing into and under the skin. It can cause recurrent infection and itching.

Rare

◆ Diabetes mellitus

See page 168. Some diabetics complain of an itching perianal region, for which no other local cause is apparent.

◆ Shingles

Can occur in the anal region. Pain and itching can precede the onset of this unpleasant, blistering condition. A medical priority.

Abdomen: Digestive System

Change in bowel habit

See *Constipation*, page 152 and *Diarrhoea*, page 146. Any change in bowel habit which does not have a simple explanation, such as a sudden change in diet, should be reported to your doctor.

Constipation

A diagnosis as well as a symptom. For details on constipation as a diagnosis, see page 152.

Probable

◆ **Inadequate diet**

A diet too low in fluids and/or too low in roughage will cause constipation.

◆ **Pregnancy**

There are two main causes for constipation in pregnancy.

- Decreased movement of the gut.
- The pressure of the growing womb on the colon.

See page 133.

◆ **Anal fissure**

See page 148.

◆ **Drug side effect**

Many painkillers, in particular codeine and morphine, contain substances which may cause constipation. Many other drugs also cause constipation as a side-effect.

Possible

◆ **Diverticular disease**

See page 139.

◆ **Intestinal obstruction**

See page 141.

◆ **Bowel cancer**

See page 140.

◆ **Pre-term**

See page 137.

◆ **Immobility**

Anyone relatively immobile or bedridden (for example, the elderly, or anyone who has had a head injury, stroke or progressive neurological disease) is prone to constipation.

Rare

◆ **Crohn's disease**

See page 119.

◆ **Hirschsprung's disease**

See page 137.

A swelling felt within the abdomen

Any organ inside the abdomen can, if diseased, appear as a swelling, a lump or a mass. You might notice this yourself, or your doctor may do so at a routine examination.

This is such a general symptom that it makes sense to list only the principal possible causes.

You must a see a doctor if you suspect any of these problems. Pregnancy is excluded from the possibilities.

Probable

◆ **Inguinal and femoral hernias**

Hernias are protrusions of bowel through weak spots in the muscular wall of the

Abdomen: Digestive System

abdomen. Although not, strictly-speaking, in the abdomen, they may be noticed as lumps in the groin. Inguinal hernias are very much more common than femoral hernias.

- May make a gurgling sound.
- Can be pushed back into the abdomen.
- May disappear at night, reappearing once you are up and about.
- In men, hernias may extend down into the scrotum.
- Hernias gradually enlarge.

Sometimes the bowel gets trapped in the hernia, causing intestinal obstruction (see page 141). If this happens, the following may be noticed:

- The hernia becomes painful.
- It cannot be pushed back.
- Intermittent abdominal pain.
- Possibly vomiting.
- Surgery may be needed.

◆ Umbilical hernia

Symptoms are the same as for inguinal and femoral hernias, above, but are less likely to obstruct the gut. They are commonest in babies and infants, particularly if they are black. They sometimes disappear as the abdominal muscles develop.

Possible

◆ Enlarged bladder

Usually caused by *Enlarged prostate*, page 172.

- Mid-line swelling in the lower abdomen above the pubic bone.

- Constant pain.
- Inability to pass urine.
- Possibly dribbling of urine.

◆ Aortic aneurysm

Swelling of the body's main artery. It may burst without warning.

- Abdominal pain.
- A swelling in middle of abdomen which pulsates in time with the heart beat.
- Back pain.
- Sometimes, sudden collapse.

Often the individual is unaware of the aneurysm until the sudden onset of severe pain.

◆ Cancer of the colon or rectum

See *Bowel cancer*, page 140.

◆ Gall bladder

The gall bladder may become enlarged for two main reasons. If it is caused by infection:

- Upper right abdominal pain.
- May be a tender mass jut below the right rib margin.
- Pain may be made worse by breathing in.
- Fever.
- Malaise.

If it is a tumour (of the pancreas, bile ducts or gall bladder):

- Jaundice.
- Non-tender mass in right upper abdomen.
- Pale stools.

Abdomen:
Digestive System

- Dark urine.
- Other signs of malignant disease may be present.

◆ Problems of the ovaries

Ovarian cysts (page 141) and cancer of the ovaries can produce abdominal swelling which can be extreme.

◆ Stomach disease

Virtually the only reason for a palpably enlarged stomach in an adult is tumour, although even in established cases, for example stomach cancers, the enlarged stomach can only be felt in a minority of individuals. The pylorus may be felt occasionally in babies with hypertrophic pyloric stenosis (see below).

Other features of stomach cancer (rare under the age of 45) include:

- Anorexia.
- Indigestion and abdominal pain.
- Weight loss.
- Anaemia.
- Upper abdominal midline mass.
- Occasionally vomiting, if the pylorus in blocked.
- Even more occasionally, vomiting blood.

Sometimes the individual goes to a doctor complaining of jaundice and ascites (see page 233) both the result of the tumour having already spread.

◆ Hypertrophic pyloric stenosis

Mostly in baby boys. The stomach outlet is blocked by thickened intestinal muscle.

Rare

◆ Appendicitis

Inflammation of the appendix. A lump is rarely a noticeable feature of appendicitis; however, if appendicitis is not diagnosed at an early stage, a lump may subsequently appear a few days later which can be felt in the right side of the abdomen, called an appendix mass.

- Right-sided lower abdominal pain – often starts over the 'belly button' or umbilicus, and then moves down and to the right.
- Pain worse on pressing over appendix.
- There may be fever.
- Anorexia.
- Nausea and sometimes vomiting.
- Malaise.

◆ Kidney disease

Kidney enlargement may be noticed on the right or left sides of the abdomen and in the loin, and may be felt as a mass.

Enlargement is caused by tumour, polycystic disease or urinary obstruction (see relevant entries in *Abdomen: urinary system*). Enlargement is one, not often very noticeable, symptom of these conditions.

◆ Liver disease

The liver lies under the right rib cage but extends across the midline. The individual may feel or see the enlargement as a mass moving in and out with respiration.

The main reasons for enlargement are:

Cirrhosis

See page 141.

Cancer

Several types of cancer can spread to the liver, including breast and lung. But they do not automatically do so; and in most cases, the cancer is already diagnosed and being treated. Occasionally, the liver is the original site of the tumour, known as a hepatoma; can be treated surgically.

Infection

The liver may become infected by a number of organisms and liver abscesses may develop.

- Swinging fever.
- Sweating.
- Right upper abdominal pain.
- Enlarged, tender liver.
- Sometimes jaundice.
- Malaise.

Hydatid disease

Infection from a tapeworm: causes cysts to form in the liver.

- Often, no symptoms.
- Occasionally the liver is enlarged because of a big cyst.

◆ Diseased pancreas

The pancreas lies at the back of the abdomen and may enlarge through inflammation or malignant disease.

Cancer of the pancreas

- Abdominal pain.
- Wasting.

- Nausea.
- Jaundice.
- Pale stools.
- Dark urine.
- Occasional vomiting.

Pancreatitis

See page 140. Acute pancreatitis sometimes develops a complication called a pseudocyst: a large cyst which may be felt as a mass in the middle of the abdomen.

◆ Diseased spleen

The spleen may be felt as a mass in the abdomen when enlarged two to three times its normal size. Its tip can be felt under the left rib margins. It may be enlarged by any viral infection (typically glandular fever), but if it is noticed as a mass; the main causes would be:

Malaria

See page 422.

Kala-azar

An infection spread by sandflies.

- Fever.
- Sweating.
- Massive splenic enlargement.
- Liver enlargement.
- Lymph gland enlargement.
- Anaemia.

Chronic myeloid leukaemia

- Anaemia.
- Discomfort in abdomen due to large spleen.
- Night sweats.

- Fever.
- Loss of weight.
- Occasional generalized itchiness.

Myelofibrosis

Often in association with other illnesses such as cancer.

- Anaemia.
- Weakness.
- Enlarged spleen.
- Gout.

◆ **Diseased uterus**

See *Cancer of the womb*, page 311.

Rigid abdomen

See *Perforated viscus*, page 140.

Tender abdomen

See all symptoms involving abdominal pain: this page. and pages 159-60, 161, 162, 163, 433-5.

Constant very severe pain in the abdomen

As a main symptom this will quite rightly send you straight to a doctor. Don't delay the visit. The causes listed here are not common, but they need immediate attention.

Possible

◆ **Perforated viscus**

See page 140.

◆ **Mesenteric vascular occlusion**

The blood supply to the gut is interrupted because of blockage in the gut's main blood vessels.

- Severe pain, starting suddenly.
- Bloody stools.
- Vomiting.
- Shock.
- Occasionally, abdominal distension.

Rare

◆ **Acute pancreatitis**

Occasionally, pancreatitis starts suddenly with very severe upper abdominal pain; see page 140.

◆ **Ruptured aortic aneurysm**

See *Aortic aneurysm*, page 153.

Severe but intermittent abdominal pain

This suggests a different set of causes to those of constant severe pain, above.

Probable

◆ **Kidney stones**

See page 171.

◆ Early appendicitis

See page 154.

Possible

◆ Intestinal obstruction

See page 141.

◆ Biliary colic

Caused by gall stones temporarily blocking a bile duct.

- Intense pain lasting from minutes to hours.
- Pain is in upper abdomen, and may pass to shoulder tip.
- Vomiting.
- Individual is pale and clammy.

- Possibly jaundice.
- Possibly fever or shivering.

◆ Heart attack

Very rarely the pain from a heart attack can be present as abdominal colic.

◆ Uterine cramps (period pains)

◆ Ectopic pregnancy

◆ Torsion of an ovarian cyst

◆ Torsion of the testicle

Torsion of the testicle can present with abdominal pain as the nerve supply to the testicle is dragged down into the scrotum, and therefore pain is referred to the central abdomen.

Diarrhoea plus abdominal pain

Probable

◆ Gastroenteritis

Otherwise known as food poisoning. Often caused by viral infections but certain bacterial causes (such as *Campylobacter*) characteristically cause painful and sometimes bloody diarrhoea. Very common. Episodes rarely last more than 24 to 36 hours, and cure themselves.

- Abdominal pain.
- Vomiting.
- Watery diarrhoea.
- Muscle/joint pains.
- Headache.
- Occasional fever.

◆ Irritable bowel syndrome

See page 139.

Possible

◆ Bowel cancer

◆ Crohn's disease

◆ Ulcerative colitis

See pages 140, 119 and 416.

◆ Chronic pancreatitis

Inflammation of the pancreas resulting in permanent and irreversible damage. Alcohol is commonly implicated: if you have the condition, you will have to stop drinking.

- Pain worsened by food and alcohol. Often very persistent.

Abdomen:
Digestive System

- Malabsorption, due to lack of digestive enzymes, causes fatty diarrhoea.
- Weight loss.
- Diabetes develops; see page 168.
- Occasionally associated with jaundice, pale stools and dark urine.

◆ **Bacillary dysentery**

Caused by person-to-person spread of a bacterium.

- Fever.
- Abdominal pain.
- Watery diarrhoea.
- After one to three days, bloody diarrhoea with mucus.
- Most cases cure themselves, although antibiotics may help.

Rare

◆ **Pernicious anaemia**

The lining of the stomach stops producing acid and other essential substances. Occurs in people over 30 years of age.

- Anaemia, slow onset.
- Sore tongue.
- Tingling and/or numbness of extremities (peripheral neuropathy)
- Fever.
- Abdominal pain.
- Diarrhoea.
- Mild jaundice.

◆ **Cholera**

Common in India and some other underdeveloped countries. Caused by an organism present in water. A major problem when water supplies are contaminated.

- Initially, mild diarrhoea.
- Then large volumes of diarrhoea.
- Vomiting.
- Abdominal pain.
- Thirst.
- Muscle cramps.
- Slight fever.

Treatment aimed at minimizing dehydration.

◆ **Typhoid fever**

Caused by one of the salmonella organisms. In the first week:

- Increasing fever.
- Abdominal pain.
- Headache.
- Cough.

In the second week:

- General malaise.
- Apathy.
- Fever.
- Abdominal distension.
- Diarrhoea.
- 'Rose' spots on abdomen.

Fatal in some cases, but antibiotics can change the course of the disease.

◆ **Post-gastrectomy syndrome**

Gastrectomy is surgical removal of the stomach.

After a meal, within two or three hours, there may be:

- Upper abdominal distension.
- Faintness.

- Weakness.
- Palpitations.
- Sweating.
- Diarrhoea.

◆ Carcinoid syndrome

Carcinoid tumours may appear in any part of the gut. They cause many symptoms, due to the chemicals they secrete, including:

- Facial flushing.
- Explosive, watery diarrhoea.
- Abdominal pain.
- Asthmatic wheeze.
- Pain in the abdomen and weight loss.
- Sweating.

Abdominal pain and progressive loss of weight

This combination needs to be taken seriously. Your doctor will consider the following possibilities. They are not listed in order of probability: diagnosis depends upon accompanying symptoms.

◆ **Crohn's disease** page 119.

◆ **Ulcerative colitis** page 416.

◆ **Chronic pancreatitis** page 157.

◆ **Cancer of the pancreas** page 169.

◆ **Cancer of the stomach** page 154.

◆ **Cancer of the bowel** page 143.

◆ **Spread of cancer to the liver** page 405.

Abdominal pain plus vomiting

Probable

◆ Gastroenteritis

See page 157.

◆ Mesenteric adenitis

Often mistaken for appendicitis in children; see page 154. This condition is caused by enlargement of lymph glands in the abdomen, usually caused by a viral infection with an adenovirus. Typically, there are common cold symptoms, plus:

- Pain and tenderness in the right lower abdomen; pain may also be present throughout the abdomen.
- Fever.
- Nausea and vomiting.
- The adenitis settles of its own accord.

Possible

◆ Peptic ulcer

The term covers ulcers of the stomach and duodenum. There is a wide range of symptoms which vary considerably from person to person:

- Pain in the epigastrium (upper middle part of the abdomen).

- Pain is recurrent.
- Heartburn may be present.
- Pain may radiate to the back.
- Pain may be present for a few weeks at a time.
- Night waking because of pain is common.
- Possibly nausea and vomiting.
- Food can either improve or worsen the pain.

Ulcers can bleed, causing anaemia and tarry stools or haematemesis. See *Blood from the back passage*, page 148 and *Abdominal pain plus vomiting blood*, page 161.

They can also perforate – see *Perforated viscus*, page 140.

◆ Appendicitis

See page 154.

◆ Kidney stones

See page 171.

◆ Ovarian cyst

Ovarian cysts may be attached to the ovary on a stalk. If the cyst rotates, it will tighten the stalk, causing severe pain.

- Sudden onset of lower abdominal pain.
- Vomiting.
- Cyst may bleed, causing pain and irritating the inside of the abdominal cavity.
- May mimic appendicitis if on the right ovary.

Meckel's diverticulum

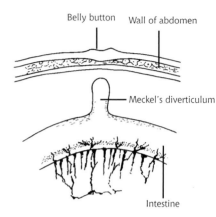

Belly button   Wall of abdomen

Meckel's diverticulum

Intestine

◆ Salpingitis (pyosalpinx)

Abscess on a fallopian tube – one possibility in the wider picture of *Pelvic infection*, page 304.

◆ Biliary colic

See page 157.

◆ Stomach cancer

See *Stomach disease*, page 154

Rare

◆ Meckel's diverticulum

A diverticulum (see diagram) is an out-pouching – a little sac; this type occurs in the ileum. Symptoms mimic appendicitis if it becomes inflamed (see page 154) and may also cause:

- Anaemia.
- Intestinal obstruction.
- Rectal bleeding.

- ◆ **Acute pancreatitis**

- ◆ **Intestinal obstruction**

  See pages 140 and 141.

- ◆ **Porphyria**

  A group of metabolic diseases. The following are the commonest features:

  - Intermittent abdominal pain.
  - Vomiting.
  - Constipation.
  - Fever.
  - Fast pulse.
  - Neurological abnormalities.

- ◆ **Toxins**

  Poisoning from various toxins, for example arsenic, can cause abdominal pain plus vomiting.

Abdominal pain plus vomiting blood

A rare combination, but if you have both these symptoms, you must consult your doctor.

Bleeding may continue even without vomiting, putting you in danger until the source is detected and the bleeding stopped.

Probable

- ◆ **Mallory-Weiss tear**

First noticed in studies of alcoholics. Any case of severe, repeated retching or vomiting can cause a small tear in the lining of the upper stomach or lower oesophagus (gullet).

- Vomiting, often recurrent.
- Fresh blood may be vomited (medical term, haematemesis).
- Tarry stools.

Normally self-healing without further treatment, but admission to hospital is usually recommended in order to control any further vomiting and to stabilize any consequence of potentially severe blood loss.

- ◆ **Acute gastritis**

Inflammation of the lining of the stomach caused by food, drugs, alcohol or infection.

- Indigestion.
- Occasionally blood is vomited.
- This usually looks like coffee grounds; the blood is altered by the gastric juices.

- ◆ **Peptic ulcer**

See page 159.

- ◆ **Drug-induced**

Some drugs, particularly steroids and non-steroidal anti-inflammatory drugs, including aspirin, can cause gastric bleeding.

This may be experienced as vomiting up blood or passing tarry stools (melaena).

Possible

- ◆ **Hiatus hernia and oesophagitis**

Inflammation of the gullet caused by

reflux of stomach contents.

- Heartburn.
- Difficulty in swallowing.
- Bitter fluid comes into mouth ('waterbrash' or 'repeating').
- Vomiting.
- Nausea.

- Occasional anaemia.
- Occasionally, if very severe, may cause melaena or haematemesis.

Rare

◆ **Cancer of the stomach**

See *Stomach disease*, page 154.

Abdominal pain plus vomiting and fever

Probable

◆ **Gastroenteritis**

See page 157.

◆ **Urinary tract infection**

See page 171.

Possible

◆ **Acute pyelonephritis**

See *Kidney infection*, page 171.

◆ **Pelvic inflammatory disease**

See page 304.

◆ **Appendicitis**

See page 154.

◆ **Cholecystitis**

The gall bladder may become inflamed and infected because of gall stones, which form from fats, calcium and pigment.

Many people have them, but they often remain unnoticed unless the individual develops cholecystitis.

- Upper right abdominal pain.
- Tenderness just below the right rib margin.
- Pain may be made worse by breathing in.
- Fever.
- Malaise.
- Vomiting.
- Jaundice may develop if stones block biliary tract.

  See a doctor without delay.

Rare

◆ **Intestinal obstruction**

See page 141.

◆ **Acute pancreatitis**

See page 140.

◆ **Meckel's diverticulum**

See page 160.

◆ **Porphyria**

See page 161.

Abdominal pain, vomiting and jaundice

Probable

◆ **Cholecystitis**

◆ **Biliary colic**
See opposite page, and 157.

Possible

◆ **Acute pancreatitis**
See page 140.

Rare

◆ **Cancer of the pancreas**
See page 169.

◆ **Cancer of the stomach**
See *Stomach disease*, page 154.

Apparent constipation alternating with diarrhoea

This is a possible combination, but it is best to explore the possibilities in detail by separately reading *Constipation*, page 152 and *Diarrhoea*, page 146 and *Change in bowel habit*, page 151.

Constipation and abdominal pain

Explore the full possibilities by reading *Constipation*, page 152 and *Abdominal pain*, pages 156-163. and pages 433-5.

Indigestion

Indigestion, heartburn, dyspepsia – these terms tend to be used interchangeably for a variety of symptoms of upper abdominal pain, flatulence, belching, acid in the mouth (waterbrash), and nausea. Occasional, mild indigestion, which settles with simple, over-the-counter remedies, is of little significance. It becomes an important symptom when it recurs frequently, or becomes more persistent than usual. It is a sign of change in your normal pattern of tolerance to food and carries a clear message: seek medical advice.

Probable

◆ **Non-ulcer dyspepsia**
A term used to describe groups of symptoms such as:

• Upper abdominal pain.

• Nausea.

Abdomen:
Digestive System

- Flatulence and belching when there is no evidence of an ulcer after special tests.

◆ Oesophagitis and hiatus hernia

See page 133.

◆ Peptic ulcer

See page 159.

◆ Pregnancy

See page 133.

Possible

◆ Gall stones

See page 145.

◆ Ischaemic heart disease

Sometimes angina ('heart pain') is misinterpreted by the patient as indigestion.

If the pain is not immediately relieved by an antacid, or is aggravated by exertion, this possibility must be considered.

Rare

◆ Cancer of the stomach

See *Stomach disease*, page 154.

◆ Cancer of the oesophagus

See page 113.

◆ Achalasia

See page 112.

◆ Chronic pancreatitis

See page 157.

Cramping pains in the abdomen

See all combinations of symptoms involving *Abdominal pain*, pages 156-163, and pages 433-5.

Loss of appetite

See page 437.

Flatulence and belching

See *Indigestion*, page 441.

Diarrhoea, bloody

See *Diarrhoea*, page 146 and *Blood from the back passage*, page 148.

Abdomen: Digestive System

Diarrhoea plus vomiting

See *Diarrhoea*, page 146 and *Vomiting*,
page 133; also *Gastroenteritis*, page 157.

'Stomach ache'

See all combinations of symptoms
involving *Abdominal pain*, pages 156-163,
and pages 433-5.

Nausea

See *Vomiting*, page 133.

Dyspepsia

See *Indigestion*, page 163.

Heartburn

See *Indigestion*, page 163.

Abdomen:
Digestive System

Incontinence

Lack of control over the act of urination so that accidental or unplanned leakage occurs. Any irritation or inflammation may predispose to some degree of leakage. Age often worsens these problems. It is estimated that over 3,000,000 people in the UK have some degree of incontinence of faeces and urine.

Probable

◆ Enlarged prostate

See page 172.

◆ Bladder neck obstruction

See page 176.

◆ Urinary tract infection

See page 171. Especially in the elderly.

◆ Irritable bladder

See page 176.

◆ Stress incontinence

• Often in women after a pregnancy.
• Leakage of urine when coughing, laughing, sneezing and on exercise.
• Leakage when straining.

Possible

◆ Cystocele and rectocele

These two conditions are common in women who also suffer from stress incontinence – above.

They are caused by weakness of the vaginal wall, which allows the bladder (cystocele) or rectum (rectocele) to bulge into the vagina. This distortion of anatomy (often felt as a lump) can cause leakage of urine.

◆ Prolapse

The structures that keep the womb in place deteriorate after childbirth and with age. In some women this allows the womb to prolapse – to drop down into the vagina – where it may often be seen or felt.

• Red lump at vagina.
• Sometimes bleeds.
• Discharge may be present.
• Associated with urinary leakage.
• May be pushed back internally.
• Comes back out on straining/coughing/sneezing.

◆ Stroke

Anyone who has suffered a stroke may develop incontinence or difficulty in urination. Sometimes the bladder distends with urine, but because of lack of sensation no pain is felt, although the individual may appear restless and sweaty. Some overflow incontinence may develop.

◆ Epilepsy

In major epileptic fits (see page 409), symptoms include:

• Jerking movements.
• Tongue biting.
• Urinary incontinence (the entire bladder empties spontaneously during the fit).

◆ Multiple sclerosis

See page 378.

Early symptoms reported to a doctor can include:

- Weakness, numbness and pins and needles in a limb(s).
- Heaviness in a limb(s).
- 'Jumping' legs.
- Muscular spasms.
- Blurred vision.
- Hesitancy, frequency, incontinence and retention of urine may all be present.
- Altered sensation in limbs and trunk.

Rare

These diseases can be associated with very sudden loss of bladder control – together with other symptoms.

◆ Spinal cord injury

- Weakness of the limbs below the level of damage.
- Sensory loss below the level of damage.
- Loss of bladder control – usually resulting in retention of urine.
- Urgent medical attention is required.

◆ Cauda equina syndrome

Meaning damage to the lowest part of the spinal cord. Can be caused by bone damage, tumour or a 'slipped disc'.

- Back pain.
- Loss of sensation at the lower back and around the buttocks and anus.
- Leg weakness.
- Loss of bladder control.
- Urgent medical attention is required.

Need to urinate urgently or often

This symptom usually suggests that the bladder itself is irritated. The commonest cause is urine infection – cystitis.

See page 171; also *Problems with urinating*, page 175.

Urinating too much or too often

The obvious cause is drinking too much tea, coffee or alcohol. These all stimulate the production of urine and can make you want to urinate during the night.

Probable

◆ Urinary tract infection

See page 171. Causes frequent urination and discomfort on urination, rather than excessive volume.

Possible

◆ Enlarged prostate

See page 172. Again, causes frequent urination, rather than excessive volume.

◆ Diuretics

A range of drugs given to reduce high blood pressure or to treat heart failure. Their intended effect is to increase the amount of urine passed, in order to reduce the amount of fluid in the system and so lessen tension in the blood vessels.

Some people taking these drugs find that they need to get up at night in order to urinate.

◆ Diabetes mellitus

See page 151.

New cases may suddenly experience:

- Increased volume of urine (polyuria).
- Increased thirst (polydipsia).
- Rapid weight loss.
- Malaise.
- Other symptoms such as vomiting, muscle cramps, abdominal pain.

If untreated, coma and death may follow.

In older people diabetes may cause few other symptoms and is often discovered simply on routine testing of urine or blood for sugar.

Rare

◆ Diabetes insipidus

See page 446. Don't confuse it with diabetes mellitus, above. It may arise spontaneously or after injury to the head (typically after surgery or an accident); because of brain tumours; or because of infection.

The main symptom is:

- Enormous volumes of urine – about 9 pints/5 litres passed daily.

◆ Chronic kidney failure

Any disease resulting in kidney failure (see *Inability to urinate*, page 178) can cause excess urine at some stage.

◆ Aldosteronism

You may hear this described as Conn's Syndrome, which is one form of the disease. Caused by a tumour of the adrenal gland. The blood chemistry becomes abnormal, leading to:

- Muscle weakness.
- Excessive urination.
- Excessive thirst.
- High blood pressure.

◆ Hypercalcaemia

High levels of calcium in the blood may be caused by a number of conditions and diseases including:

- Abnormalities of the parathyroid glands (see diagram page 125).
- Excess Vitamin D.
- Sarcoidosis: a rare illness of body tissues leading to the deposit of material, described as sarcoid, in various sites in the body.
- Malignant bone tumours (primary or secondary).
- Thyrotoxicosis: an illness caused by having too much thyroid hormone.

The symptoms of excess calcium in the blood are:

- Anorexia.
- Nausea.
- Vomiting.
- Thirst.
- Polyuria (passing urine more often than normal).
- Constipation.
- Muscle fatigue.

Urine looks dark

Probable

◆ Concentrated urine

If you have spent a long time in a hot atmosphere, or if you have been physically very active, without also increasing your fluid intake, you may notice that your urine is a dark yellow colour, and that it is passed in small amounts. In the absence of other symptoms, this is normal.

By increasing your fluid intake, or by avoiding the heat or exercise, urine will be back to normal within 24 hours.

Possible

◆ Hepatitis

Inflammation of the liver. There are several different types, some, particularly hepatitis B and C, are more serious than the others.

If you suspect hepatitis, you must see a doctor. General symptoms may include:

* Fever.
* Malaise.
* Anorexia.
* Muscle and joint pains.
* Jaundice.
* Dark urine: it can be dark yellow, orange or brown.
* Stools may become pale.

◆ Food or drug

Several foods and drugs can cause discolouration of different hues.

Examples are:

* Orange – rhubarb, senna.
* Red – beetroot, blackberries.
* Green/blue – methylene blue dye.
* Some drugs used in the treatment of TB (tuberculosis)
* After stopping the food or drug, urine should be back to normal within about 24 hours.

Rare

◆ Cancer of the pancreas

A malignant tumour of the pancreas which blocks the bile ducts.

This means that yellow bile is passed out in the urine.

* Jaundice.
* Dark yellow/orange/brown urine.
* Pale stools.
* Abdominal and back pain.
* Weight loss, anorexia.

◆ Haemaglobinuria

In contrast to haematuria (which is the medical term for blood in urine, see the following page) haemoglobinuria means broken down red blood cells in the urine. It is caused by several different diseases or conditions and the urine is often more brown than red. It appears in association with illnesses and diseases such as: haemolytic anaemias; thrombocytopaenia purpuras; cardiac disease (for example, after valve replacement); malaria; septicaemias.

Abdomen:
Urinary system

Discoloured urine is unlikely to be the first or only symptom of these conditions, and in most cases the individual will already be under a doctor's care.

◆ 'Crush' syndrome

See page 179.

◆ Melanoma

A melanoma is a skin cancer (see page 317). In some advanced cases, the pigment melanin gets into the urine and colours it dark brown or black.

◆ Alkaptonuria

This is an example of 'inborn errors of metabolism': in other words, the body fails to deal correctly with certain chemicals in the blood, which are then excreted in urine, which becomes progressively darker if left standing.

Blood in urine

The significance of blood in the urine varies greatly from the simple and easily treated to the severe and life-threatening. It should never be ignored as a symptom. If recurring, its significance increases. Again, do not ignore. Red blood cells in the urine (the medical term is haematuria) may come from any part of the urinary tract – the kidneys, the ureters (which connect the kidneys to the bladder), the bladder and the urethra (see illustration, page 173). Blood may also appear in urine because of generalized disease.

It may become apparent in several ways. The urine may appear the colour of blood (frank haematuria), or in smaller quantities it may only colour it pinkish, or give it a smoky or cloudy appearance. Occasionally clots of blood are passed with minimal colouring of the rest of the urine. Also, blood may appear only at the beginning or end of urination.

The male and female urinary tracts differ in that the male has a prostate gland and two seminal vesicles (see illustration, page 172). In females of child-bearing age, menstrual loss of blood may some-times be mistaken for blood in the urine. In these cases, the bloody discolouration disappears as the period ends.

Some foods, particularly beetroot, can discolour the urine.

Children

Blood in the urine should always be taken seriously. Investigation will be required. While an adult may commonly suffer an infection causing blood to appear in the urine, this is not acceptable in children. Any urine infection in a child is an unusual event. It may be the first sign of an abnormality in the structure of the urinary tract. Rarely, accompanying swelling in the abdomen may be due to a Wilm's tumour – a malignant tumour of the kidney seen in children usually up to the age of three.

Probable

◆ Cystitis

Inflammation of the bladder lining, giving symptoms of urine infection.

- Frequent passing of urine.
- Burning or scalding as you urinate.
- Bursting to go but little result.
- Having to rush to pass urine with urgency.
- Dull ache in lower abdomen; may persist or worsen after urination.
- Fever; backache.
- Dark, cloudy or blood-stained urine.

Mild cases may clear without the use of antibiotics.

◆ Urinary tract infection

Symptoms as for cystitis; in addition, there may be more severe symptoms such as:

- High fever.
- Pain in the back, loin, groin, front of abdomen.
- Vomiting, nausea.
- Sweating.

Will require antibiotics.

◆ Kidney infection

Medical term: pyelonephritis. In this instance, the urine reveals infection but in addition the kidney itself is affected.

- Symptoms as for cystitis, plus:
- Severe fever.
- Loin pain.
- Tenderness and sensitivity in the loin and side of abdomen.

- General feeling of being unwell.

Cystitis symptoms may not be marked, particularly in the early stages, when the symptoms may be confined largely to the upper abdomen; for example:

- Pain, vomiting, nausea.
- Rigors – a medical term for shivering.

Severe and advanced cases (also termed acute nephritis) will show diminished urine output, swelling of face and ankles, headache and other symptoms as above.

Treatment is with antibiotics, sometime intravenously.

Resistance to infection

Increasingly, the bacteria causing urinary infections (and cystitis) do not respond to commonly prescribed antibiotics. This is known as bacterial resistance. Hence the importance, where possible, of sending a urine culture test to the laboratory before treatment starts.

Possible

◆ Kidney stones

Extremely severe pain, coming and going in unbearable waves, localized to one side over kidney area (loin and extreme side of abdomen).

- Vomiting.
- Sweating.
- Typically, pain spreads from the back,

Abdomen: Urinary system

Persistent symptoms

If you find symptoms persist after, or during, treatment with antibiotics, seek the result of your urine culture test. It will reveal which antibiotics can kill the bacteria. You will hear this referred to as a test to reveal bacterial sensitivity.

---

around the side to the front of the abdomen and from there to the scrotum/groin area.

◆ Prostatitis

- Men only.
- Fever.
- Pain in the rectal area behind scrotum.
- Difficulty in passing urine.
- Sensation of passing hot urine.

◆ Benign tumours of bladder/kidney

Benign tumours of the urinary tract may cause bleeding. Symptoms may include:

- Painless haematuria (blood in urine), sometimes copious.
- General health is otherwise sound.
- Occasional obstruction of the passage of urine, due to blood clot.
- Anaemia (if there has been unrecognized bleeding for some time).

Urological assessment is required.

◆ Enlarged prostate (men)

Difficulty in:

- Passing urine.

- Starting/stopping stream.
- Holding on to pass urine later.
- Preventing dribbling.

Inability to pass urine (retention of urine) requires medical intervention and catheterization.

◆ Cancer of prostate

As for enlarged prostate. Diagnosis is frequently made only during operative intervention for enlarged prostate symptoms. Some authorities now suggest screening for cancer of the prostate by means of a blood test for PSA (prostate specific antigen). Consult your doctor.

After about 80 years, nearly every male has cancer of the prostate. It lies

Male bladder

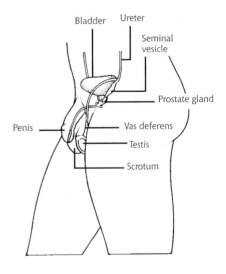

Bladder
Ureter
Seminal vesicle
Prostate gland
Penis
Vas deferens
Testis
Scrotum

dormant in the gland, seldom causing severe problems at that age.

◆ Chronic nephritis

- Nocturnal passage of large quantities of urine.
- Anaemia.
- Swelling.
- Shortness of breath.

◆ Injury

Injuries to the lower chest or pelvis (such as a blow or a stab wound) may damage underlying structures. If you have any blood in your urine after such an injury, whether in large or small quantities, you will need a full medical assessment in order to rule out serious damage to the urinary, or any other, system.

◆ Exercise

It is now widely recognized that certain types of prolonged, repeated exercise – in particular, marathon running – may cause transient appearances of blood in the urine.

Rare

◆ Cancer of the bladder/kidney

Simple tests such as urine cytology, to examine the cell content of urine, can reveal the presence of malignant cells.

- Commonest in adults over 50.
- Painless haematuria – blood in urine.
- Pain in the loin.
- Swelling in loin or abdomen.

Female bladder

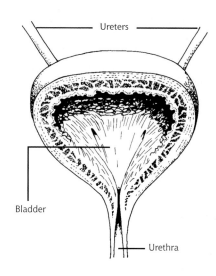

Ureters

Bladder

Urethra

- Occasionally bone pain, due to spread of the tumour.
- Fever.
- Loss of weight.
- Anaemia.

◆ Wilm's tumour (children)

The child has:

- One-sided, abdominal swelling.
- Painless blood in urine.
- Loss of appetite.
- Anaemia.
- Pain in late stages only.

Modern drugs and medical techniques have revolutionized the treatment of this condition.

Early diagnosis is important.

◆ **Endocarditis**

Multiple symptoms appear. The affected individual will be very ill.
Symptoms include:

• Rash.

• Joint pains.

• Finger clubbing (see page 276).

• Fever.

• Chest pain.

◆ **Anticoagulant therapy**

Individuals who are taking anticoagulants (blood-thinning medication) may notice blood in their urine.

They should consult their doctor, who will probably recommend reducing the dose of the drug.

◆ **Bilharzia**

Or schistosomiasis. Caused by an organism that inhabits water.
    Common in Africa, the West Indies, South America and Japan.

• Blood in urine.

• Pain on passing urine.

• Frequent passing of urine.

• Cancer of the bladder can develop, as well as liver damage.

Blood in urine plus pain when urinating

The probable causes are: urinary tract infection; cystitis; kidney stone.
    The possible causes are: acute pyelonephritis; prostatitis.
    The rare cause is: bilharzia, above. All covered under *Blood in urine*, page 170.

Kidney pain

The kidneys are situated at the side of the abdomen, towards the back. This area is known as the kidney or loin area.The most likely cause of pain in this area is infection.

There are a number of other possible causes all of which are covered in *Blood in urine*, page 170 and *Blood in urine plus pain when urinating*, page 174.

Pain when urinating

Pain when passing urine is almost always a sign of cystitis or urine infection. Rarely, it can be one of the symptoms caused by a kidney stone or venereal infection such as NSU; see *Non-specific urethritis*, page 176.

Also, the conditions listed under *Blood in urine*, page 170, may all cause pain on passing urine as an early symptom, prior to the appearance of blood in the urine.

**Abdomen:
Urinary system**

Urine looks cloudy

A number of body products, but mainly blood, pus cells and microrganisms, can have this effect. Other symptoms may well be noticed at the same time. Urine which is concentrated but normal often goes cloudy if left standing. Cloudy appearance does not always signify illness.

Probable

◆ **Urinary tract infection**

◆ **Cystitis**

◆ **Kidney stones**

See *Blood in urine*, page 170.

Possible

◆ **Acute pyelonephritis**

◆ **Prostatitis**

See *Blood in urine*, page 170.

◆ **Gonorrhea**

A sexually transmitted disease. Often has no symptoms in women, although vaginal discharge, pelvic inflammatory disease and pain on passing urine may be experienced.

If a man has genital symptoms (and he may not) there will be:

• Urethral discharge.

• Discomfort on passing urine.

• Cloudy urine.

• Reddening and pain around the glans of the penis and urethra.

• Enlarged lymph nodes in the groin.

Rare

◆ **Bilharzia**

See page 174.

Problems with urinating

These include such symptoms as hesitancy or difficulty in starting to urinate; poor urine stream; and dribbling. The underlying causes tend to be either obstruction to the passage of urine; or structural abnormalities of the urinary tract; pain on urinating due to other causes such as infection; neurological defects may also affect urination.

Probable

◆ **Enlarged prostate (men)**

The gland can be enlarged as a result of

benign or malignant growth. Symptoms may be similar in both cases:

• Difficulty or hesitancy when starting to urinate.

• Poor stream.

• Terminal dribbling.

• Feeling as though the bladder has not emptied.

• Need to urinate in the night (nocturia).

• Sudden desire to pass urine.

• Some blood in the urine.

- Sometimes, leakage of urine: overflow incontinence.

Later in the disease, acute obstruction occurs with inability to pass urine at all. Severe abdominal pain develops because of the distended bladder.

In some cases, the obstruction develops so slowly that the bladder compensates by enlarging over a period of weeks or months. There is minimal discomfort and the urine frequently leaks out, without the individual being able to control it. The bladder does not empty properly, remaining distended, which is often seen as abdominal swelling. This type of urine loss is called overflow incontinence.

Medical assessment is always needed. Cancer of the prostate may also cause:

- Back pain.
- Bone pain.

◆ Bladder neck obstruction

Symptoms similar to an enlarged prostate, but occurring in a younger age group and, occasionally, in women. Caused by overgrowth of the bladder muscle at its outlet to the urethra.

◆ Urinary tract infection

See page 171.

◆ Gonorrhea

See page 175.

◆ Non-specific urethritis

A common sexually transmitted disease caused by an organism called Chlamydia. Often there are no symptoms.

If there are symptoms, men will have:

- Discomfort or itch on passing urine – making it difficult to urinate.
- Discharge (white, yellow) from penis.

Women will have:

- Pain/burning on passing urine.
- Occasional vaginal discharge.
- The womb and fallopian tubes can be infected; see also *Pelvic inflammatory disease*, page 162.

Possible

◆ Irritable bladder

A term encompassing different symptoms caused by irritation of sensory or motor nerves to the bladder. Other causes (such as infection) must be excluded first. Special tests are needed to confirm the diagnosis.

Symptoms can be one or more of:

- Frequent desire to pass urine (for example every 30 minutes).
- Pain over the bladder.
- Difficulty in passing urine (small volumes) and the bladder still feels full.
- Sometimes retention of urine occurs.
- Occasionally leakage of urine.

NSU or non-specific urethritis

It is very important to have this disease treated. Both partners must receive treatment, since, even with a total absence of symptoms, Chlamydia may be present. Untreated chlamydial infections can cause infertility.

◆ Urethral stricture

Urethral stricture is a narrowing of the outflow passage from the bladder. It is commoner in men than women and may be caused by previous infection (perhaps gonorrhoea), surgery, damage by an instrument or a catheter (typically during delivery of a baby). Symptoms are progressive:

- Poor stream.
- The urine sprays.
- Needing to strain hard to empty bladder.

◆ Prostatitis

See page 172.

◆ Kidney stones

See page 171.

◆ Drugs

See page 178.

Rare

◆ Urethral tumours

Benign or malignant tumours may cause progressive obstruction of the urethra in men and women, leading to:

- Need to strain harder than usual, to pass urine.

◆ Spinal cord damage

◆ Neurological disease

◆ Stroke

See *Incontinence*, page 166.

Urine dribbles

Meaning either a poor stream, or dripping when trying to stop the flow of urine. Can be a form of incontinence. The following, all dealt with in detail under *Problems with urinating*, page 175, can all be occasional causes of dribbling:

Probable

◆ Enlarged prostate

◆ Bladder neck obstruction

◆ Urinary tract infection

Possible

◆ Urethral stricture

◆ Prostatitis

Rare

◆ Urethral tumours

Urinating at night

You may often have had to get up during the night to pass urine, especially if you have had anything to drink within a few hours of going to bed. It is only abnormal

if it develops as a new symptom, or if the number of times you get up increases significantly.

The commonest causes are an enlarged

prostate gland (in men) and bladder irritability (in women). Drugs are another important cause. Diuretics can often be taken once daily, in the morning, to minimize this difficulty.

See also *Problems with urinating*, page 175, and *Urinating too much, or too often*, page 167.

Inability to urinate

The medical term is anuria, and it is a serious problem.

Don't confuse it with passing small volumes of concentrated urine infrequently, as in hot atmospheres or after strenuous exercise.

Urination can be arrested for three main reasons: first obstruction in the urethra (see illustration page 173); second, failure of the bladder muscle to contract; and third, both kidneys may stop producing urine, because they are diseased or are affected by disease elsewhere.

The first two cases are described as retention of urine. In all three cases, but particularly in the last, there may be a period of hours or days when the volume of urine gradually diminishes.

In the case of obstruction, there will be severe pain because of an increasingly distended bladder. Failure to excrete urine results in a build-up of toxic chemicals in the blood – and so it is, of course, a medical emergency.

Probable

◆ Enlarged prostate

Much the most common reason (in men only) for a sudden inability to pass urine is an enlarged prostate gland causing an obstruction to the outlet from the bladder.

You will feel pain as the bladder distends. See page 172. All the other causes in this section are much less common.

◆ Kidney stone

See page 171. If a stone lodges in the urethra or at the neck of the bladder it will block the passage of urine. In addition to urine failure:

• Pain because of distended bladder.

• Inability to pass urine.

• In men, pain may radiate to the tip of the penis.

◆ Urethral stricture

See page 177.

Possible

◆ Surgery or injury

Any event that causes uncontrolled blood loss, and thus low blood pressure, can damage the kidneys and prevent them from working. The elderly, and those with chronically raised blood pressure, are vulnerable to this type of kidney damage.

◆ Drugs

A number of drugs may unexpectedly cause retention of urine, particularly in patients with prostatic disease. Examples of are amitryptiline and imipramine.

Abdomen: Urinary system

◆ Pyelonephritis

See *Kidney infection*, page 171.

In severe, untreated cases, the kidneys may be so badly damaged that they stop working. No urine is produced and the patient gets more and more sick, with:

- Weak pulse.
- Fever.
- Rigors.
- Vomiting.

◆ Malignant tumours

Any malignant tumour of organs in or near the pelvis can involve parts of the urinary tract, blocking the urethra, ureters, bladder or kidneys. Cancers of the colon, uterus, ovaries, bladder and prostate can all have this effect. But it is very rare for anuria to be the first symptom, and the diagnosis has usually been made long before.

◆ Shock

See also page 381. If shock is untreated or untreatable, the kidneys fail to produce urine and gradually urine output tails off to nothing. A grave condition, as is:

◆ Septicaemia

Infection of the bloodstream and whole body from any cause. It can lead to shock (see page 381), which, if untreated or severe, results in acute kidney failure. Possibly fatal.

Rare

◆ Injury

Direct injury to the urethra (particularly in men) occurs typically in car accidents where the pelvis has been fractured. Because of the damage, urine cannot pass: a medical emergency which in most cases is promptly treated because the patient is already in hospital.

Very occasionally, a kick to the male scrotum, or crotch, may damage the urethra, or indeed the spinal cord.

◆ Spinal cord damage

◆ Neurological disease

See page 430.

◆ Poisoning

A number of drugs may directly damage the kidneys, causing kidney failure. These include mercury, arsenic and bismuth.

◆ Blood transfusion

If a patient is given blood which is incompatible with his or her own, the result may damage the kidneys and cause kidney failure.

This is one reason why such care is taken when giving blood, and why it is only given when needed.

◆ 'Crush' syndrome

Damaged leg muscles, sustained in a crushing injury to the lower limbs, causes toxins to enter the blood stream, resutling in direct damage to the kidneys.

- Discoloured urine may be a symptom.

The longer the limb is crushed, the greater the risk.

Abdomen:
Urinary system

The heart, chest, lungs and breathing

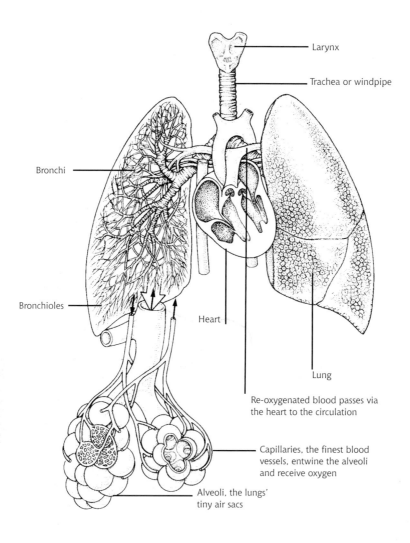

Larynx

Trachea or windpipe

Bronchi

Bronchioles

Heart

Lung

Re-oxygenated blood passes via the heart to the circulation

Capillaries, the finest blood vessels, entwine the alveoli and receive oxygen

Alveoli, the lungs' tiny air sacs

The heart: introduction

The heart is a superb pump: it gives years of service, responding automatically to all the varied demands of growth, activity and stress, so that we are rarely aware of its action.

How does the heart work? Two major systems, both electrical, control the heart's activity; there is also an in-built mechanism that increases the heart's muscular effort in response to high demand.

Emotion and stress are communicated to the heart by a branch of the nervous system called the autonomic system. It is this system that, for example, sets the heart beating faster when you notice a bull in the next meadow, and continues to increase both its speed and power when you realize there is no fence between you and the bull.

Next, within the heart itself there are two electrical pacemakers that control the rate of heartbeat. The main one, the sino-atrial node, normally sets the rate, transmitting a regular firing signal down an electrical pathway to the second pacemaker, a relay station called the atrio-ventricular node. From there, the signal to beat is transmitted to the rest of the heart by other electrical tracts. The atrioventricular node may also act as a pacemaker should the sino-atrial node fail for some reason.

Clearly there are many opportunities for malfunction in this system. If there is a problem, heart-rhythms may be too fast, too slow or irregular. These irregularities are felt in various ways: perhaps a thumping in the chest or a fluttering sensation; sometimes only skilled examination can detect a problem. This section analyses the possibilities.

It is important to realize that occasional rhythm disorders are common and are not necessarily a sign of disease. It is remarkable that there are not more of them, considering that an average heart will be making some three thousand million heart beats during a 70-year lifetime. Where irregularities decrease the pumping efficiency of the heart significantly, faintness, dizzy turns or, at worst, collapse may follow.

It is worth remembering that the diagnosis of heart irregularities, palpitations and similar disorders can be a highly technical matter; tremendous advances in research have been made in recent years. The sources of electrical malfunction can now be traced to individual sections of wiring in the heart, in some cases allowing precise surgery to control the fault.

The journey from seeing the heart as something that can break, to thinking of it as a mechanism that would do credit to a Grand Prix Formula 1 computerized fuel management system, has been long. As with so many other systems in our bodies, with a more precise understanding has come admiration of the sophistication of an activity we take for granted.

The Heart

Heart makes extra beats

This is a common symptom with an interesting explanation. What happens is that the heart beats twice in rapid succession. The extra beat goes unnoticed.

However, the next beat of the heart is delayed by a fraction of a second and it is this slight delay that you may be aware of. During the delay, blood continues to fill the heart, bringing into play an automatic mechanism that makes the heart beat more forcefully the fuller it gets. The next beat after the delay is, therefore, extra-powerful, and is felt as a thump in the chest.

Probable

◆ Unexplained

- In the young or early middle-aged.
- Happens occasionally.
- Otherwise sound health.
- The extra beat causes no other symptoms: no faintness or chest pain.

◆ Too much coffee or tea

The small amounts of caffeine in these drinks is responsible for the 'lift' they provide.

Taken in excess – and what constitutes excess is an individual matter – the caffeine will cause:

- Rapid heart rate.
- Extra beats.
- Tremor.
- Anxiety.

- Increased output of urine.

  Treatment is simply to reduce intake.

◆ Alcohol

Alcohol has a direct effect on the heart. This increases with time and excessive use and can lead, in rare cases, to heart failure.

◆ Cigarette smoking

Nicotine has a stimulant effect on the heart, increasing its rate and output. Extra beats are one reflection of this.

◆ Fever

Heart rate rises by about ten beats per 0.5 degree centigrade rise in temperature and increases the chance of extra beats. Some infections, as well as causing fever, can irritate the heart.

Possible

◆ Anxiety

Has its effect via the autonomic nervous system (see *The heart: introduction*, page 181), increasing the resting rate of the heart and the chances of extra beats. Other well-known features include:

- Tension in neck, shoulders.
- Constant feeling of pressure in the head.
- Excess sweating, tremor.
- Constantly feeling that something dreadful is about to happen.

◆ Indigestion

It is uncertain how this affects the heart.

Probably it results from a reflex action in those nerves which serve both the digestive system and the heart, though there may be direct irritation of the heart by a distended stomach.

The features of indigestion are familiar:

- Bloating, belching.
- Acid, burning sensation after meals.
- Discomfort felt behind breast bone.

Rare

◆ Complications of heart attack

Extra beats are common in the days after a heart attack, often producing few symptoms. They have a different origin from benign extra beats, arising instead from spontaneous beating of the ventricles, the main pumping chambers of the heart. It is usual continuously to monitor the heart's electrical activity in the days after a heart attack looking for just such ventricular extra beats. They can be a warning of the sudden, uncontrolled activity of the ventricles which causes collapse and possibly sudden death.

◆ Excess digoxin

Digoxin is a drug used to treat heart failure and some irregular pulses. In excess it causes:

- Nausea and vomiting.
- Very slow pulse, with extra beats.
- Fatigue.
- Red or green hallucinations.
- Abdominal pains.

Mild cases can be corrected by temporarily dropping digoxin.

Severe cases need intensive treatment in hospital.

◆ Rheumatic carditis

- Fortunately this once-common disease in children is now a rarity in the developed world, but is still prevalent elsewhere.
- Begins two to three weeks after a bad sore throat.
- Joint pains; stiffness flitting from limb to limb.
- Fever.
- Rashes rapidly coming and going.
- Rapid pulse, extra beats.
- Sudden, fidgety movements.

There is danger of permanent damage to the heart valves leading later to heart disease.

The Heart

Heart beats irregularly

People's sensitivity to their heart-beat varies. Some will feel that a very rapid but regular heart rhythm is an irregularity while others are able to focus precisely on the rhythm. A doctor will listen to the heartbeat through a stethoscope while feeling the pulse at the wrist: this often allows a simple rhythm to be diagnosed. Where there is doubt, an ECG recording of the heart is needed.

Probable

◆ Sinus arrhythmia

Careful observation of your own pulse will reveal a change in rhythm as you breathe. The autonomic pathways mentioned elsewhere slow the heart as you breathe out and let it run faster as you breathe in. In some people this is particularly noticeable and may cause alarm.

It is not a disease but an exaggeration of a normal reflex. The reflex is especially noticeable in children.

- Otherwise well.
- Clear relationship to breathing.
- Rhythm changes by about ten beats per minute faster or slower.

◆ Sick sinus syndrome

The sino-atrial node is the trigger in the heart that fires the electrical signal which causes the heart to beat (see *The heart: introduction*, page 181).

So vital is this area of the heart that it has its own blood supply but with age that blood supply can become diseased, resulting in erratic functioning of the trigger.

- Pulse may vary between very fast or very slow.
- Symptoms vary from none at all to fainting to loss of consciousness.
- Treatment is usually a pacemaker.

Possible

◆ Extra beats

Extra beats happening frequently will give the impression of an irregular heart beat. It is difficult to diagnose this situation without an ECG.

Treatment aims to cure the underlying cause. See *Heart makes extra beats*, page 182.

Rare

◆ Pulmonary embolus

A blood clot blocking the circulation to part of the lung and usually arising from a clot in a vein in the calf.

- Sudden feeling of pressure in the chest.
- Breathlessness.
- Possibly sharp chest pain and coughing blood.
- Heart rhythms varying from fast but regular to irregular.

The Heart

Palpitations (including rapid regular heart rate)

Strictly speaking, 'palpitations' simply means an awareness of the beating of the heart but most people use it to mean not just awareness of the heart, but an awareness of some abnormality in the beat. So this symptom is subdivided into: 1 an awareness of a rapid but regular heartbeat; 2 irregular heartbeats; 3 rapid and irregular heartbeat. Extra heart beats (see page182) may also cause palpitations.

There is much overlap between causes, so it is best to check in all relevant sections.

Rapid but regular heart rate

Probable

◆ Fever

Heart rate rises by ten beats per minute per 0.5 degree centigrade rise in temperature so that very high fevers will be accompanied by correspondingly high pulse rates. There is no specific treatment. Relief comes with the disappearance of fever.

◆ Exercise

Any but the gentlest exercise will cause a modest rise in heart rate as the heart responds to the increased demand from the muscles and the lungs for larger quantities of oxygen-rich blood. Pulse rates above 120-130 per minute should be viewed with suspicion as a sign of over-exertion, under-fitness or some combination of the two.

Chest pain appearing on exertion should always be checked.

◆ Emotion

Heart rate increases with excitement or acute emotional turmoil through the mechanism of the autonomic nervous system.

Accompanying features include:

- Dry mouth.
- Rapid breathing.
- Tremor.

Such a response is normal in many circumstances such as fear, sexual arousal, sudden emotional shock. It is part of a co-ordinated system that prepares the body for exertion and to cope with stress. The response becomes abnormal if the individual begins to suffer from chronic anxiety, keeping his or her body in a constant state of increased arousal.

◆ Paroxysmal tachycardia

A term used to cover all those otherwise unexplained episodes of rapid heart beat. There may be underlying causes such as an excess of stimulants such as coffee, alcohol, cigarettes (see *Heart makes extra beats*, page 182); or from heart disease (page 398) or conduction disorders (page 186).

Investigation involves wearing a recording device to capture the rapid rhythm so that its nature can be analysed. Treatment can then be directed appropriately.

- Abrupt onset of rapid heart rate.
- Entirely regular rhythm.
- If rate is fast enough, faintness, lightheadedness.
- Stops as abruptly as it began.

Occasionally the rhythm is so fast or so prolonged that the heart becomes exhausted, causing breathlessness. This requires medical intervention to correct the rhythm.

Possible

◆ Pregnancy

There is a slight but sustained rise in heart rate during pregnancy, by about

The Heart

ten beats per minute. So if your usual rate is 70 per minute it can be expected to rise to 80 per minute. In this way the heart copes with the demands of the growing womb, placenta and baby.

◆ Anaemia

In the anaemic state there is less capacity to transport oxygen around the body. The heart compensates by increasing its speed of pumping. This will only be a noticeable feature in cases of severe anaemia.

Other symptoms are:

- Pallor.
- Slight breathlessness.
- Fatigue.

Anaemia alone is not a complete diagnosis. Further investigation is needed to find the cause.

◆ Heart failure

The early symptoms can be quite undramatic.

- Tiredness.
- Breathlessness on modest exertion.
- Increased heart rate.
- Swelling of ankles.
- Breathlessness lying flat.

Further tests are needed to determine the reason for the heart failure.

See also page 196.

◆ Hyperthyroidism

The over-active gland can cause extra beats or a sustained rapid pulse.
See page 188.

◆ Drugs

There are several over-the-counter drugs which can cause rapid heart rates in a few individuals, including cold remedies containing pseudoephedrine or phenylpropanolamine. Certain anti-asthmatic drugs such as salbutamol may have a similar effect.

Rare

◆ Electrical conduction disorders

These can be thought of as short circuits in the heart which disrupt the usually smooth control of heartbeat (see *The heart: introduction*, page 181). Though relatively rare, there is much interest in these conditions for the light they shed on the electrical circuitry of the heart. There are surgical treatments available to cut the abnormal electrical circuits responsible for the disorder; otherwise they are controlled by medication. One of the least rare of the rare is the Wolff-Parkinson-White syndrome, which strikes most commonly at young adults:

- Recurrent bursts of rapid heart rate.
- Characteristic changes on the electrocardiograph.

◆ Beri-beri

A deficiency of Vitamin B1, common in Third World countries where polished rice is a staple diet. In the developed world it occurs not infrequently in alcoholics with diets deficient in vitamins.

- Tender muscles.
- Rapid, bounding pulse.

The Heart

- Often, swollen ankles.
- Dementia, unsteady gait.
- Rapid recovery is possible if it is recognized and treated early enough.

◆ Bleeding

Serious external bleeding is obvious, but internal bleeding can continue for several hours with few symptoms apart from:

- Increases in pulse rate.
- Thirst.
- Faintness on standing. Eventually there will be:
- Pallor.
- Cold extremities.
- Confusion, collapse.

◆ Myocarditis

Inflammation of the heart muscle, due to a variety of causes, most of which are infections. Some possibilities are viral illnesses, influenza, trypanosomiasis, diptheria.

- Sudden onset of a feverish illness.
- Breathlessness, swelling of ankles.
- Breathlessness when lying flat.
- Rapid pulse.

The diagnosis requires blood tests, ECG recordings and, in difficult cases, biopsy of heart muscle.

◆ Cardiomyopathy

Another wide group of disorders where there is a non inflammatory disturbance of the heart muscle. Many cases are congenital or else related to alcoholism, or due to coronary artery disease.

- Heart failure, tiredness, breathlessness.
- In young people, fainting episodes during exercise.
- Rapid heart rates which may be both regular and irregular.

Diagnosis is by ECG and heart biopsy. These disorders need drug treatment to reduce the risk of sudden serious heart rhythm disturbance. Can run in families.

Rapid irregular heartbeats

Most such rhythms are either atrial fibrillations or atrial flutters. Atrial fibrillation is extremely common in old people. It may be the result of diseased coronary arteries, but frequently there are no other symptoms and life expectancy is little changed. The condition occasionally occurs in bursts in young people, when it is known as paroxysmal atrial fibrillation.

The basic defect is uncontrolled contraction of the atria, the small antechambers where blood first arrives in the heart. In fibrillation, the atria beat at rates upwards of 400 per minute, every one of those contractions sending off to the ventricles, the main pumping chambers, a signal to beat. Fortunately, only a fraction of these signals get through, but still enough to

The Heart

give a heart rate of between 100 to 150 beats per minute. The resulting heart rhythm is totally irregular, as felt at the pulse or as heard over the heart.

Not surprisingly, atrial fibrillation reduces the pumping efficiency of the heart and therefore causes breathlessness and swollen ankles. It also carries a small risk of sending off a blood clot which may cause a stroke or block arteries in the limbs. It is usual to treat fibrillation with drugs, which both slow the rhythm and strengthen the heart. Consideration would be given to reducing clotting of the blood by giving the anti-coagulant warfarin.

Atrial flutter is a less common condition in which the atria beat at a regular rate of between 240-360 beats per minute. This is still too fast to trigger regular contractions of the ventricles, which beat at half or a quarter of the atrial rate (90-180 per minute).

Though strictly speaking this is a regular rapid heart rhythm, frequently the rate keeps changing abruptly, going from 180 to 120 to 90 and back again, giving an impression of irregularity. Atrial flutter is a symptom of serious heart disease and needs hospital treatment.

Episodes lasting longer than a few minutes can exhaust the heart, sending the individual into rapid heart failure, of which increasing breathlessness is a symptom.

The causes below relate mainly to atrial fibrillation.

Probable

◆ Ischaemic heart disease

Blockage or 'furring up' of the blood supply to the heart. This may produce no symptoms other than fibrillation but frequently there will also be angina; see page 216.

◆ Hyperthyroidism

Atrial fibrillation may be the only sign of an over-active thyroid gland, especially in the elderly. Thus it is routine to check for this condition, whose other symptoms include:

- Sweating.
- Tremor.
- Increased appetite.
- Protruding eyes.
- Weight loss

Possible

◆ Mitral stenosis

The mitral valve separates the left ventricle from the left atrium. Stenosis means that the valve has become narrowed and stiff. The most common reason for this was rheumatic fever, which is now rare in developed countries; the process of ageing is the usual reason nowadays. The condition gradually strains the heart, eventually causing heart failure.

- History of rheumatic fever years before.
- Mildest symptoms are just fibrillation.

- As the condition worsens, breathlessness, cough with bloodstained phlegm.
- Eventually swelling of ankles.
- There may be a permanent purple flush over the cheek bones.

Drugs are used to treat mild cases, with surgery to the valve being reserved for more severe cases.

◆ Alcohol abuse

Long-term alcohol abuse weakens the muscle of the heart, allowing various rhythm disorders to result.

◆ Complications of heart attack

In the hours and days after a heart attack the injured heart can produce a variety of disordered rhythms. The most worrying are ventricular tachychardias, where the ventricles go off into bursts of rapid beating which have the potential to turn into totally irregular, life-threatening beating.

Monitoring and dealing with these ventricular rhythms is one major reason for observation in a coronary care unit after a heart attack.

- Rapid thumping in the chest.
- Faintness.
- As the condition worsens, loss of consciousness.

Rare

◆ Pneumonia

This severe chest infection can occasionally set off atrial fibrillation, which disappears after recovery. See page 201.

◆ Endocarditis

An infection of the valves of the heart which usually attacks valves that are already abnormal, for example, after rheumatic fever. Fibrillation is just one of a variety of symptoms.

- Night sweats.
- Malaise.
- Clubbed fingernails.
- Splinter-like lines under the nails.
- Anaemia.

Aggressive long-term antibiotic treatment is needed to eradicate the infection.

◆ Pericarditis

Constriction of the heart by fluid or by fibrous material can give rise to fibrillation.

See *Pericardial effusion*, page 205.

◆ Atrial septal defect

There is a hole between the right and left sides of the baby's heart while it is in the womb. This hole should close at birth, but occasionally remains open. Symptoms can take years to develop, or a murmur may be detected on examination.

- Increased susceptibility to chest infections.
- Breathlessness.
- Palpitations including fibrillation are common.

The Heart

Heart beats slowly

By convention, this is taken as a rate of less than 60 beats per minute. Frequently it is an incidental finding in someone without symptoms, but very slow rates below 40 per minute are likely to cause dizziness, fainting and, in the elderly, confusion.

There are two main causes of very slow rates. The pacemaker of the heart may be sending out a slow rhythm, or there is a block to the pacemaker rhythm so that the ventricles beat at a much slower rate than the signals sent from the pacemaker.

An ECG is needed to diagnose these conditions properly.

Probable

◆ Fitness

A slow pulse is common in athletes and others who take regular physical exercise.

◆ Drug-induced

Digoxin is one drug which causes a very slow pulse if given to excess. Another widely-used class of drugs called beta blockers slows the pulse to around 60 beats per minute but this is an intentional effect and is a sign of correct dosage. Beta blockers are used to treat high blood pressure and angina.

◆ Heart block

Heart block comes from disease of the conducting pathways that transmit the pacemaker signal to the rest of the heart. The ventricles have their own pacemaker which triggers them at 30 to 40 beats per minute, so there may be no dramatic symptoms, even with complete heart block.

The usual reason for this problem is ageing or poor blood supply to the heart. It can also happen after a heart attack.

Symptoms, in increasing order of severity, include:

* None at all, but noticed on an ECG tracing.
* Awareness of a slow thudding heart beat.
* Tiredness.
* Dizzy spells.
* Recurrent abrupt loss of consciousness.

Treatment is with an artificial pacemaker to maintain regular contraction.

Beta blockers

Beta blockers are important in the treatment of heart disease. Sometimes they are also used to quell the symptoms of anxiety: they can stop palpitations and sweats, and are frequently taken by musicians and actors before performances.

The Heart

Possible

◆ Hypothyroidism

An under-active thyroid gland, whose other symptoms include:

- Coarse dry skin.
- Sensitivity to the cold.
- Slow thought, tiredness.
- Gruff voice.

Treatment with thyroid hormone has to be life-long.

◆ Sick sinus syndrome

See also page 184.

Caused by the effects of ageing on the pacemaking area of the heart.

This can cause rhythms from slow to fast and any combination in between.

- Palpitations.
- Dizzy spells.
- Tiredness.

◆ Congenital

Some people are born with a slow pulse, but doctors would judge it prudent to search for other signs of heart disease such as heart murmurs or abnormal ECG traces.

Rare

◆ Cardiomyopathy

A general term for diseases of the heart muscle.

The effect is to cause the rapid appearance of heart failure with either slow or rapid heart rates.
See also page 187.

The Heart

Breathing: introduction

We breathe in order to provide the body's cells with the oxygen essential to their function and to get rid of carbon dioxide, which is produced as a waste product of metabolism. It is no surprise that breathing is affected by all sorts of bodily disorders, often from the lung or heart.

Breathing also helps to regulate the body's acid-alkaline balance. Because the brain controls breathing, disease and also drugs can affect those parts of the brain which, day in and day out, keep us breathing.

This section begins with causes of sudden breathlessness, then continues with breathlessness appearing over relatively long periods.

Causes tend to overlap, so you will see the same diagnoses coming up repeatedly. We make no apology for this: breathlessness is an alarming symptom, and some repetition is helpful.

Heimlich's manoeuvre

There are references to this first-aid technique at several points in this section. It is named after the American physician who has promoted this simple, life-saving procedure, to be used on someone who is choking as a result of inhaling food or other solid objects and is unable to clear the object by themselves.

• Stand behind the person choking.

• Extend your arms in a hug around their upper abdomen.

• With clenched fists make a hard, fast squeeze just under the breast bone.

The manoeuvre forces a blast of air out of the lungs, sufficient to dislodge something stuck in the upper airway. For full details see any modern manual of first aid.

See illustration on page 219.

Rasping, snoring breathing

Also described as stertorous breathing. It is only occasionally a symptom of disease, usually just a nuisance.

Snoring is the result of vibration of the soft palate, which is at the back of the roof of the mouth. The cure is simply a matter of trying out different sleeping postures, or changing the number or firmness of your pillows.

Drinking less alcohol, or if you are overweight, losing weight, may help.

Probable

◆ **Snoring**

See above.

Possible

◆ **Adenoids**

These are pads of tissue at the back of the nose, similar to tonsils. They are probably intended to counter infection which might enter through the mouth and nose. In childhood, adenoids can grow so large that they obstruct nasal breathing.

The child exhibits:

- Nasal speech.
- Snoring.
- Mouth breathing.
- Recurrent ear infections.

Treatment is occasionally surgical removal of the adenoids, if there is no sign of a natural decrease in their size and breathing is significantly affected.

◆ Sleep apnoea

The breathing is obstructed, often at the back of the throat and surrounding structures. It typically occurs in adults, particularly men, who are overweight or have a size 17 collar, or larger.

- Snoring.
- Periods when breathing seems to stop, then restarts with a loud chortling noise.
- Waking unrefreshed in the morning and tired during the day.
- Tendency to fall asleep during the day or even while driving a car.

Treatment is weight loss if required, and if severe, wearing a special mask while asleep. This keeps the airways open. Occasionally, surgery can help.

◆ Stroke

A blood clot or bleeding in the brain causing:

- One-sided paralysis.
- Coma.
- Stertorous breathing, typically if the individual goes into a deep coma.

◆ Alcoholic stupor

Drinking to the point of collapse frequently gives this symptom.

Hoarse, 'wheezy' intake of breath

This is probably a stridor: see *Foreign body*, page 208.

Chest abnormally shaped

Probable

◆ Congenital

Twists of the spine can gradually produce a mis-shapen chest. These can sometimes be treated if spotted early enough.

- Seen from behind, the spine is curved.
- Curve becomes more prominent on bending forward.

Another congenital abnormality gives a funnel-shaped chest with a depressed breastbone. This too can be corrected by surgery which is recommended if there is a risk of the depression pressing on the heart but usually no treatment is needed.

Possible

◆ Chronic obstructive airways disease

A general term covering chronic bronchitis and emphysema.

The continual effort of breathing in these conditions can eventually, in adult life, cause a barrel-shaped chest.

See page 200.

Rare

◆ Asthma

Chronic, severe asthma which is inadequately treated can result in a young adult who has:

- A broad, over-inflated chest.
- Prominent rib margins.
- Prominent breastbone, which gives a pointed appearance to the front of the chest.

The reason is thought to be years of extra effort by the muscles between the ribs, which have to work harder in asthma. They gradually pull the lower ribs into a prominent shape.

This is seen less and less as asthma treatment improves.

◆ Rickets

This disease, due to lack of Vitamin D, can give rise to unsightly prominent joints where the ribs join the breast bone. Now a rarity in developed countries.

Breathlessness, rapid onset

Considered here are attacks of breathlessness which happen rapidly, yet fall short of abrupt suffocation or asphyxia. There should be little difficulty in recognizing the seriousness of the situation, except perhaps with babies and children: with them you should be alert to drowsiness and breathlessness which interferes with feeding.

Probable

◆ Asthma

This common illness is more of a nuisance than a disability for most asthmatics, most of the time. However, asthma can turn suddenly and unpredictably into a life-threatening condition.

Muscle surrounds the airways right down into the lungs. Asthma results from excessive constriction of these muscles, which narrows the airways and increases the effort required to shift air into the lungs. As a cause of chronic breathlessness, asthma is covered in detail under *Breathlessness and wheeze*, page 199, where the common features of asthma are described.

Severe, acute asthma is a potential killer. There is danger for the known asthmatic who underestimates the severity of an attack. There is also danger for someone whose first attack of asthma is severe, unrecognized and who has no standard treatment at hand.

The following signs suggest that asthma is getting out of control and needs prompt medical attention:

- Poor response to usual asthma medication.
- Too breathless to talk in full sentences.
- The chest continually feels 'tighter'.
- Sweating, breathlessness, rapid pulse.
- Neck muscles strain in an attempt to increase breathing.
- As attack worsens, cyanosis (lips going blue), tiredness, pallor, drowsiness, confusion, coma.

Call 999 if this happens. Take (or give) 10 puffs of the reliever medication – typically the blue inhaler.

Deterioration can take several hours or just a few minutes.

◆ Bronchiolitis

This is an infantile equivalent of asthma. It is a winter disease, caused by a particular virus. It occurs in epidemics.

- Initially the baby is snuffly, with a slight cough indistinguishable from a common cold.
- Wheezing begins and worsens over a few hours.
- Breathing produces a crackling sound, also felt through the chest.
- Breathlessness interferes with feeding.
- Breathing becomes rapid, often with grunting.
- At worst, pallor, cyanosis of lips.

First aid: put the child in a steamy atmosphere, which sometimes can improve the situation.

Seek advice from a doctor.

Occasionally, the child needs treatment in hospital with oxygen. Babies with this condition have an increased chance of being asthmatic later in life.

> Children whose parents smoke are three times more likely to enter hospital in their first year with a chest condition than infants of non-smokers.

◆ Croup

This is a viral infection affecting children between six months and three years of age. The child typically has symptoms of a temperature and a 'cold', plus:

- Hoarse voice.
- Intermittent barking cough often worse at night.
- Wheeze which occurs when the child breathes in (stridor).
- Breathing difficulties.

First aid: keep child as calm as possible and seek advice from a doctor.

◆ Chest infection

A severe chest infection or pneumonia can rapidly progress to difficulty in breathing.

- Wet cough, with coloured phlegm.
- High temperature.
- Flaring nostrils.
- Rapid breathing.
- Pain over the affected part of the chest particularly when breathing in.
- Cyanosis (blue colour) of lips and tongue.
- Sometimes bloodstained phlegm.
- Confusion.

The Chest

This is more likely in the elderly or in those who are debilitated for other reasons.

Possible

◆ Heart failure

Predominantly a disease occurring later in life. There is often a history of heart trouble, perhaps heart attack, high blood pressure.

- Early symptoms are tiredness, breathlessness on exertion.
- Swelling of ankles.
- Breathlessness worse on attempting to lie flat.
- You need to stack up pillows in order to sleep.
- In more advanced cases you may wake from sleep with a feeling of suffocation.
- Copious, frothy, pinkish phlegm.
- Relief gained from sitting upright for a few minutes.

This situation may need urgent medical help if it occurs severely.

◆ Pulmonary embolus

A blood clot lodges in the lung. It often arises from a clot which has already formed in a leg (deep vein thrombosis – DVT).

Increased risk factors: long plane journeys; the oral contraceptive pill; immobility – typically in bed in hospital or at home for a pronlonged period.

- Breathlessness.
- Pain on breathing in.
- Coughing up some blood.

Seek a doctor's advice promptly.

◆ Acute on chronic bronchitis

A chest infection can be the minor, extra stress that pushes the individual with chronic bronchitis into severe breathing problems. The already limited effort that someone can put into breathing becomes too little to expel waste carbon dioxide, or to take in fresh oxygen. The result is the equivalent of suffocation over a short period.

- Severe headache.
- Warm, blue hands; rapid pulse; twitching of muscles.
- Agitation, confusion worsening to coma.

This situation needs urgent help.

Rare

◆ Allergic alveolitis

The alveoli are the sacs in the lung where carbon dioxide is exchanged for oxygen. An allergic reaction causes inflammation in these sacs. The consequent swelling interferes with efficient gas transfer.

The commonest cause is an allergy to mouldy hay, known as farmer's lung, and is widespread in areas of non-mechanized farming.

- Breathlessness, wheezing within a few hours of exposure.
- Fever, cough and malaise, joint pains.
- Symptoms take a few days to disappear.

The chronic condition shows:

- Recurrent difficulty in breathing.
- Clubbed (highly curved) fingernails (see illustration page 276).Treatment is to avoid exposure to the cause of the allergy.

Breathlessness over days, weeks or months

This type of breathlessness does not have particularly prominent secondary symptoms, at least not at first. And there are no hard and fast distinctions between all the conditions which share these symptoms, so read this section right through before drawing any conclusions.

Breathlessness that sets in over only a few days or weeks clearly needs investigation.

Breathlessness that appears more gradually can be more puzzling. It should be judged in relation to your usual level of exercise. If your principal form of physical activity is opening the garage door, do not be too surprised at your breathlessness if you have to change a tyre. Remember also that your ability to cope with sudden effort can decline completely unnoticed as long as you are still able to perform your regular activities. For example: shopping trips and gentle strolls may present no problem, but you may be alarmed at how breathless you become climbing stairs. This does not in itself suggest disease, just being out of training.

But there is a pitfall in this: while it is natural to limit exertion to the level you know you can tolerate, that level may actually be abnormally low. The best guide is to compare yourself with others of your age and general fitness. If you are the one who has to rest half-way round a golf course you may have a problem.

Bear this in mind before you jump to conclusions. Ask yourself a few questions. How long since you last did any exercise that made you sweat? Have you gained weight recently? Do you smoke heavily? Honest answers to these questions may be illuminating.

To improve your fitness, aim to achieve shortness of breath and sweating, over a period of 20 minutes, at least three times a week. If you have a heart problem, seek advice from your doctor first.

There are other, everyday circumstances in which breathlessness is normal. Excitement, fear and anger all generate a high breathing rate and may make you feel breathless.

Only after you have excluded all these possibilities is it reasonable to wonder whether your breathlessness is a symptom of illness:

Probable

◆ Coronary artery disease

The arteries to the heart become furred up, reducing blood flow to the heart, and so reducing the ability of the heart to deliver blood efficiently.

- Breathlessness may be the only symptom.

- Angina (chest pain) on exertion.

- When more advanced, the symptoms of heart failure (see page 186).

The diagnosis is made by a combination of exercise ECG and angiography of the heart, where a dye is injected to show up the arteries. Usually treated with an operation to open up the artery with an implanted tube called a stent, or with a graft – coronary artery bypass grafting.

◆ Heart failure

Mainly a problem for older people. The symptoms of heart failure can mistakenly be put down to ageing unless a dramatic or sudden deterioration occurs.

There will often be a history of high blood pressure, angina or heart attack.

Early symptoms are:

- Tiredness, decreased tolerance of exercise.
- Swelling of ankles.
- Loss of appetite.
- Later, breathlessness while lying flat in bed.
- You sleep stacked up on pillows.
- Breathlessness wakes you at night, with a frothy cough; symptoms pass off after you have sat upright for a while.

In the elderly, tiredness alone can be the only symptom of heart failure. Modern treatment has greatly improved the outlook for people with heart failure.

◆ Psychological

A possibility in a younger person: friends or colleagues may notice over-breathing – often the individual leads a stressful life.

- Describes an inability to breathe in deeply enough.
- Otherwise sound health. Reassurance, and thorough investigations, revealing nothing, generally help these cases.

Possible

◆ Chronic obstructive pulmonary disease

Previously known as chronic bronchitis or emphysema (see pages 201 and 74).

- Breathlessness, often with wheeze.
- Usually in smokers.
- Breathing improved by anti asthmatic aerosols.
- The diagnosis needs to be confirmed by respiratory function tests.

See page 397.

◆ Pregnancy

A common feature of middle to late pregnancy, when the womb is enlarged and presses against the diaphragm.

◆ Anaemia

Blood carries oxygen around the body, so that if the volume of blood in one's body drops significantly, breathlessness ensues, together with:

- Tiredness, easy fatigue.
- Pallor on the under-surfaces of eyelids, nail beds.

Symptoms of the disorder which causes the anaemia may also be apparent, for example blood loss, poor diet. Simple investigations should quickly confirm the diagnosis.

◆ Lung effusion

The lungs react to irritation in the same way that the skin reacts to a minor burn. Tissue fluid seeps out, collecting in a pool at the base of the lungs. If this pool grows large enough, it compresses the lung above, reducing its ability to function and causing breathlessness. There are no specific symptoms to indicate an effusion: it has to be detected by medical examination or chest X-ray. There is nearly always some predisposing condition. The commonest are severe heart failure, pneumonia, pulmonary embolus and lung cancer. These cause symptoms considered under *Heart failure*, page 186.

◆ Lung cancer

A tumour may block off a major airway, thereby putting out of action all or part of a lung, and causing breathlessness.

Rare

◆ Skeletal abnormalities

Gross distortions of the chest wall cause the ribs to squash the lungs and heart so that their expansion is restricted.

These deformities, called *Kyphosis* or *Kypho scoliosis*, are discussed on page 270.

◆ Occupational lung disease

A group of occupational lung diseases caused by years of exposure to dust. Common ones are silicosis (miners, pottery workers), Pneumoconiosis (coal miners) and asbestosis.

The symptoms are:

- Progressive breathlessness on exertion.
- Cough.
- Dust control and masks reduce the risks for workers in hazardous industries.

◆ Mountain sickness

The direct effect of the lack of oxygen at altitudes of about 8000 feet or higher. The young and fit are at risk just as much as the unfit or elderly; in fact, possibly more at risk because the young will be climbing faster.

This is a dangerous condition.
Early symptoms are:

- Breathlessness.
- Headache, tiredness.

If ignored these will progress to:

- Profuse bloodstained cough.
- Nausea, confusion.
- Coma.

All cases need descent to lower altitudes; serious cases may also require resuscitation.

◆ Fibrosing alveolitis

The final stage of *Allergic alveolitis* (see page 196), or sometimes of unknown origin.

- Chronic breathlessness.
- Clubbed fingernails (see page 276).
- Cough, cyanosis.

Breathlessness and wheeze

Excluding acute chest infection, considered page 195, this extremely common combination points to narrowing of airways, producing obstructed air flow. Often there is an allergic factor: many asthmatics, sensitive to dust and fumes, exhibit these symptoms for hours, even days on end.

Probable

◆ Asthma

Some 10 per cent of the population suffer from asthma, and the number is believed to be rising. The classic features are:

- Recurrent breathlessness.
- Wheeze and cough.

- In children, persistent night-time cough.
- Common colds that regularly go to the chest.

Doctors are often disinclined to label a child as asthmatic until there is no doubt: it can be a disservice to the child. Helpful treatment is available. See also page 194.

◆ Chronic bronchitis (chronic obstructive airways disease)

Believed to result from years of exposure to fumes, chemicals and smoke, of which cigarette smoke is the main avoidable culprit. The prime features are the gradual manifestation of:

- Increasingly persistent cough.
- Wheeze.
- Breathlessness.
- Large amounts of phlegm ('smoker's cough').

Chronic bronchitis (chronic obstructive pulmonary disease) does not have the same reputation as lung cancer, yet quality of life can be considerably reduced. Perpetual breathlessness, in severe cases, is every bit as miserable as the final stages of cancer. Stopping smoking is vital to slow the damage to the lungs.

Possible

◆ Occupational asthma

This includes many conditions associated with specific industries, in particular those producing flax, sisal, hemp or cotton, animal substances, certain metals, chemicals and organic dusts.

- 'Monday morning breathlessness' on re-exposure to the agent causing the allergy.
- Wheeze, breathlessness.
- Improvement over weekend and holidays when not exposed.

Rare

◆ Drug reaction

The drugs in widest use that can produce this reaction are beta-blockers, used to control high blood pressure or angina; aspirin and similar anti-rheumatic drugs, and a few anti-cancer drugs such as methotrexate, may also be responsible.

◆ Aspergillosis

An infection caused by a fungus called aspergillus, commonly found in rotting and decaying vegetation. For most people, aspergillus is harmless. If the lungs are damaged by previous infection (such as tuberculosis) or asthma, the fungus may cause the following symptoms:

- Recurrent wheeze, cough.
- Feverish episodes.

The diagnosis is determined by blood tests and allergy testing.

Breathlessness and cough

Probable

◆ Chest infection

Recognized by the combination of:

- Cough with yellow or green phlegm.
- Fever, modest degree of malaise.
- Breathlessness plus wheeze.

- All these appear in only a couple of days, often preceded by a sore throat and a common cold.

Antibiotic treatment is usual for these common and not very serious infections.

Possible

◆ Chronic bronchitis

The strict medical definition is: A cough productive of phlegm for at least three months of the year for at least two consecutive years.

It is well known that smokers and workers in dusty environments risk developing the condition. The excessive production of phlegm amounts to an exaggeration of the lungs' defence mechanism against infection and dust: the gooey mucus 'traps' the foreign matter, which the lungs then try to expel by coughing. In permanent overdrive, the lungs begin losing their efficiency. Individuals are at risk of frequent chest infections and, in the long run, progressive shortness of breath.

Though the disease cannot be reversed, further deterioration can be delayed by giving up smoking and by avoiding dust and fumes.

◆ Pneumonia

A serious chest infection, usually of rapid onset with:

- High fever, chills.
- Rapid breathing and cough.
- Phlegm may be rust-coloured or obviously contain blood.
- Aching, or severe sharp pain, in the chest.

Occasionally, especially in the elderly, pneumonia exhibits less clear-cut symptoms, and is suggested by abrupt weakness and fever. Aggressive antibiotic therapy means that pneumonia is no longer the feared killer it once was, though it is still a worry in the elderly or those with pre-existing problems such as heart disease, chronic bronchitis and diabetes.

See also page 201.

Rare

◆ Bronchiectasis

In this disease, once far more common than it is today, the lung structure breaks down, making the lungs susceptible to pockets of chronic infection.

- Initially, frequent chest infections.
- Constant production of large amounts of coloured phlegm.
- Phlegm often bloodstained.
- As it worsens, breathlessness, clubbed (highly curved) fingernails.
- Poor growth in children; fatigue.

◆ Lung cancer

This diagnosis must be considered not only for a cough with breathlessness but for any persistent breathing problem. Adult smokers are particularly vulnerable. See page 209.

◆ Tuberculosis

Now uncommon in developed countries, except in the poor, those with HIV/AIDS, immigrants from the Third World, and those who neglect themselves, such as alcoholics.

The usual features are:

- Malaise, weight loss.

- Cough, often bloodstained.
- Breathlessness resulting from complications.

Treatment, though prolonged, cures the disease.

Breathlessness and feeling tired/exhausted

Though lung disease is usually the cause of breathlessness, it can arise from subtle changes in the condition of the heart, blood or metabolism. Fatigue will then be a prominent symptom, before breathlessness is noticeable. Breathlessness in these situations may result from an imbalance between acid and alkaline chemicals in the body. Major disturbances of regular body functions, such as diabetes and kidney failure, generates excess acid which the body tries to reduce by blowing off more carbon dioxide with heavy deep breathing.

Remember that prolonged or severe breathlessness, for any reason, will eventually cause fatigue simply through exhaustion and a chronic lack of oxygen.

Probable

◆ Anaemia

Blood carries oxygen around the body so that if the volume of blood drops significantly breathlessness ensues, together with:

- Tiredness, easy fatigue.
- Pallor, particularly the under-surfaces of eyelids, nail beds.

Symptoms of the disorder which causes the anaemia may be evident, for example blood loss from heavy periods, poor diet. Simple investigations indicate the diagnosis.

See page 198.

◆ Heart failure

Breathlessness is a frequent symptom in the middle-aged; in the elderly an early indication of heart failure can be unusual tiredness. Once this is recognized, look for other symptoms of heart failure:

- Swollen ankles.
- Breathlessness when lying flat.

See page 397.

Possible

◆ Heart disease

Disturbance of heartbeat with rhythms either too fast or too slow, felt as a flutter in the chest, or as palpitations. These are inefficient rhythms producing breathlessness with fatigue. See page 184.

Other heart diseases, for instance valve problems, cause breathlessness by decreasing the efficiency of the heart. Those with a history of rheumatic fever may find this a problem. In general, these disorders can only be detected by medical examination. See also coronary artery disease in *Breathlessness over days, weeks, or months*, page 197.

Rare

◆ Diabetic complications

Diabetes is the condition that produces a high blood sugar level. The early symptoms are:

- Passing large amounts of urine.

- Thirst.
- Weight loss.

In young people, onset tends to be rapid, over a couple of weeks. In older people it may go unnoticed, apart from slightly increased urine output and a vague sense of tiredness.

Diabetes affecting children and young adults is often caused by a lack of insulin, needed by the body's cells to make use of sugar. Thus, there are high levels of sugar in the bloodstream, yet the cells are unable to use it. But life must go on: the cells' metabolism turns to alternative means of generating energy. The trouble with these is their tendency to generate large amounts of acidic waste products. The body tries to compensate by blowing off large amounts of carbon dioxide, hence heavy breathing.

Meanwhile, sugar in the blood-stream spills out through the kidneys, dragging water with it. The final result is the dangerous state called diabetic ketoacidosis, and is a major medical emergency.

- Dehydration, dry mouth, intense thirst.
- Deep, sighing breathing.
- Sweet smell on breath.
- Confusion, nausea.

Rapid treatment is life-saving. Known diabetics may fall into this state during other stressful illnesses.

◆ Kidney failure

Early symptoms are only:

- Increased passage of urine.
- Tiredness.

Blood tests at this stage allow diagnosis and consequent changes in diet which may give years of reasonable health.

If eventually the kidneys fail there is an array of symptoms, including:

- Tiredness, developing into confusion.
- Deep, gasping breathing.
- Dry, furred tongue.
- Nausea, hiccups.
- Itching, anaemia.

The development of kidney transplantation has revolutionized the treatment of this condition.

Breathlessness and chest pain

Symptoms of this kind are often caused by serious disruption of the output from the heart, or by lung malfunction. If breathlessness is the most prominent symptom, see *Asphyxia*, page 210, or *Breathlessness: rapid onset*, page 194, as well as reading this section. If chest pain is most prominent, look at the sections on heart beat. In view of the importance of these symptoms, some of the information found there is repeated here.

Probable

◆ Chest infection

The gradual appearance of fever, cough and phlegm is often accompanied by a slight ache over both lungs. See page 195.

◆ Heart attack

See also page 213. In a middle-aged person, suspect a heart attack if there is:

- Sudden central chest pain.
- Sweating.
- Pain radiating up to the jaws or into the left arm.
- Breathlessness.

These are the classic symptoms, but in quite a few cases the heart attack is 'silent', meaning that chest pain is not the most obvious feature or may be absent. Instead, a heart attack may be suspected on the basis of:

- Sudden onset of breathlessness as a new symptom.
- Sudden worsening of existing breathlessness.
- Symptoms of heart failure: swollen ankles, breathlessness when lying flat, breathlessness during the night, tiredness.

Recently, there have been major advances in treatment so that early recognition of the problem means a much-improved chance of recovery. It is, therefore, essential to establish the diagnosis as soon as possible. Heart attacks are most common in old people, but are possible at any age; so always take dramatic chest pain seriously.

◆ Pleurisy

The pleurae are the thin membranes that surround the lungs. They become inflamed for a variety of reasons, particularly infection, when you can feel a typical pain.

- Knife-like pain over a small area of the chest.
- Pain worse on breathing in.
- Breathlessness as a consequence of

avoiding deep breathing.

Pleurisy commonly accompanies a chest infection. In this case, it sets in gradually over a few hours. A *Pneumothorax* (see below) causes sudden pleuritic pain as can a *Pulmonary embolus* (see below).

Treatment aims both to relieve the pain and to cure the underlying condition.

◆ Pneumothorax

Collapse of part of a lung, sometimes the whole lung. Quite common and needing appropriate treatment. However, pneumothorax is rarely life threatening, though the pain may be disabling.

Possible

◆ Pneumonia

Suggested by a combination of:

- High fever.
- Rapid breathing.
- Painful cough.

See also page 201

◆ Pulmonary embolus

A blood clot which lodges in the blood supply to a lung. Sudden breathlessness follows the reduction in the lung's efficiency. Pain in the chest is not always a symptom, but will certainly be felt if the affected part of the lung begins to die from lack of oxygen. See page 196.

◆ Lung cancer

This diagnosis should always be borne in mind when unusual breathlessness and chest pain are the symptoms in elderly individuals, particularly those who smoke. See page 209.

◆ Irregular heart beat

Very rapid or very slow heart rates can cause chest pain, with breathlessness a result of low output from the heart. See sections on heart beat, page 184.

Rare

◆ Pericardial effusion

The heart is surrounded by a lining which can become inflamed. This is known as pericarditis. The fluid released from inflammation collects around the heart, interfering with its ability to pump blood effectively. Most often, this condition follows a viral infection. It may also follow a heart attack, or be associated with bacterial infections, inflammatory disorders such as rheumatoid arthritis, or occasionally, trauma.

- At first, the sharp central chest pain of pericarditis.
- Pain seems to radiate to shoulders.
- Often relieved by bending forward; worse lying down.
- Breathlessness, worsening as the fluid builds up.

- Fever may be present particularly if pericarditis has been caused by an infection.

This is not an easy diagnosis, but may be the reason for breathlessness after certain diseases. X-rays and irregular readings recorded by ECG machines may suggest the diagnosis, but it is confirmed with an ultrasound examination of the heart.

◆ Heart tamponade

This is the most severe effect of a pericardial effusion. The condition may begin with pericarditis (above), or perhaps an injury to the heart, such as a stab wound. Fluid or blood gathers around the heart until it is squashed and unable to pump. There are no straightforward or obvious symptoms apart from rapidly increasing breathlessness after the illness or injury which caused the pericarditis; occasionally distended veins in the neck may also be observed.

Treatment is to urgently drain off the fluid.

Chest symptoms – cough introduction

Cough is generally a reflex action of irritated lungs or voice box, or lungs trying to expel phlegm or a foreign body. Most coughs are easily recognizable for the minor problem they are, but sometimes need to be taken more seriously because of duration, pain or associated symptoms. In the very young and the elderly, coughs can be a sign of more serious illness and need more attention.

Dry cough without phlegm

Few of us pass a year without suffering this sort of cough. It nearly always reflects minor irritation of the lungs rather than more serious disease. It passes in a week or so of using simple remedies, such as aspirin or plenty of fluid and avoiding dry atmospheres.

If there are other symptoms of illness, such as raised temperature lasting more than 48 hours, or if the cough becomes chronic, it would be sensible to see a doctor.

Probable

◆ Common cold

Cough, commonly accompanied by other common cold symptoms such as:

- Rapid onset of sneezing and aches.
- Usually cures itself.

◆ Irritant atmosphere

Dry dusty conditions.

- Cough is relieved in normal atmosphere.
- Not otherwise ill.

◆ Post nasal drip

Secretions from the nose or from the sinuses run to the back of throat and provoke cough. Treatment is aimed at the underlying condition, the commonest being chronic sinusitus, hay fever and (in children) adenoid trouble.

Possible

◆ Laryngitis

A common winter illness causing many of the symptoms of the common cold but also:

- Raw feeling in the throat.
- Hoarseness or loss of voice.
- Often develops into chest infection.

◆ Thracheitis

Rather similar to laryngitis, but:

- Raw feeling more in lower neck/upper chest.
- Often 'goes to the chest.'
- Rasping feeling behind breastbone.

◆ Asthma

One of the commonest causes of chronic cough at all ages. The diagnosis, often difficult to make because cough can be caused by so many factors, is suggested by:

- Recurrent wheeze and breathlessness, particularly after exertion. However:
- A frequent, dry, night-time cough may be the first symptom, especially in children.
- Close relative(s) are very often asthmatic, too.
- Associated with eczema and hay fever.

◆ Drug side effect

An unpredictable side effect of so-called ACE inhibitor drugs, increasingly used to treat high blood pressure and other heart conditions.

◆ Acid reflux

Severe acid reflux (heartburn) can spill up from the gullet and into the larynx, causing a cough.

◆ Habit

Not otherwise unwell.

- Worsens if attention given, goes when distracted.
- Worse if nervous.

◆ Whooping cough

The severe form causing paroxysms of cough to the point of breathlessness, followed by a whoop as air is breathed

The Chest

in is now extremely rare, thanks to immunisation.

A milder form, causing a prolonged cough in older children or occasionally adults, is now increasingly recognized.

It settles on its own, though may take three to four months to do so.

Rare

◆ Lung cancer

See page 209.

◆ Tumour or infection of larynx

- Persistent hoarseness, pain in neck, enlarged glands in neck. See page 84.

Cough plus phlegm

Most likely to be caused by a minor infection of the lungs, which in most people will settle rapidly. Those with other pre-existing serious conditions, such as heart disease or diabetes may need antibiotics to control the infection.

Probable

◆ Common cold

After first few days, a 'wet' cough with coloured phlegm, but otherwise feeling well.

◆ Acute bronchitis

Cough, phlegm and wheeze.
- Feeling mildly unwell.
- Some breathlessness.

◆ Chest infection

- Copious cough, phlegm, fever.
- Sweats and feeling unwell.
- Onset over a day or two.

May be accompanied by pleurisy – a knife-like pain between the ribs on breathing in.

Possible

◆ Chronic bronchitis

Cough, phlegm and wheeze for weeks on end, possibly for most of the year. A disease especially of smokers, long-term exposure to dusty atmospheres and of people who live in damp, northern climates such as Britain's.

Don't dismiss the morning 'smoker's cough'; this is your lungs telling you that they are being killed by fumes – their reaction is to push out large amounts of phlegm.

- Frequent episodes of bronchitis, summer and winter.
- Chronic cough.
- Breathlessness eventually becomes a constant feature.

It is essential to give up smoking. This helps to some degree, however late you stop.

◆ Pneumonia

A serious infection of part or all of one lung. You feel very ill.

- Rapid onset.
- Breathlessness or fast breathing.
- General aching, tiredness, cough.
- Sweats – sometimes drenching, especially at night.
- Pain over affected part of lung.

The Chest

Rare

◆ Bronchiectasis

A disease in which the structure of the lungs breaks down, reducing their efficiency.

- Gradual appearance of chronic cough, with copious phlegm.
- Bad breath.
- Chest X-ray needed to confirm diagnosis.

◆ Tuberculosis

Chronic fatigue, malaise, weight loss, anorexia (see page 404). Groups especially at risk are those with HIV/AIDS; low incomes; poor/overcrowded housing; immigrants; alcoholics.

◆ Lung abscess

See under *Cough plus bloody phlegm*, below.

◆ Inhaled foreign body

Typically in children. A child can (unnoticed) inhale a peanut or similar small object. A coughing fit probably follows – which the parent overlooks. Chest infection plus typical symptoms (see page 195) then develops, and never really clears. If these symptoms are neglected, the child becomes listless and run-down after several weeks. Inhaling a foreign body sometimes creates stridor; see *Asphyxia*, page 210.

◆ Pneumoconiosis

A group of diseases in which the lungs become stiffer and stiffer, unable to expand properly.

- Associated with dusty industries such as coal.
- Cough, breathlessness, wheeze, progressive over months and years.
- Finger clubbing: see page 276.

◆ Cystic fibrosis

A childhood disease, caused by inherited genetic abnormality.

- Repeated chest infections, failure to grow.
- Diarrhoea, weight loss.

In some parts of the UK, babies are screened for this at birth.

◆ AIDS

Groups especially at risk are intravenous drug users, homosexuals, bisexuals and heterosexuals with multiple partners, especially those from countries where HIV is commonest.

- Weeks of malaise, weight loss, fatigue, fevers.

Diagnosis confirmed by blood tests. Sputum culture will show unusual organisms.

Cough plus bloody phlegm

A symptom that should not be ignored. In older people (50 plus) and especially in smokers it calls for careful investigation. In younger people there is more likely to be a relatively innocent cause. Even so, they should have an immediate check-up.

Remember that many cases of cough plus bloody phlegm are eventually diagnosed as 'cause unknown' – the symptom simply goes away.

Probable

◆ Chest infection

Yellowish or greenish plegm which contains streaks or blobs of blood, possibly red, possibly rust-coloured. Not an uncommon symptom.

• Mildly unwell with raised temperature and aches.

Possible

◆ Pneumonia

See page 207. The infection causes so much inflammation that blood oozes into the lungs where it mixes with phlegm.

◆ Lung cancer

There is now little doubt that smoking causes most cases of this, one of the commonest forms of cancer. Smokers in particular, and especially smokers in the 50-plus age range, should be alert to the early warning signs because the sooner the disease is diagnosed, the better the results of treatment.

None of these symptoms on their own is absolutely diagnostic of lung cancer, indeed they often prove to be false alarms. However, this is a situation when over-caution is to be encouraged, particularly if you are in the risk group. Combinations of two or more symptoms should arouse increased suspicion.

• A persistent cough, whether dry or with phlegm. Smokers get used to smokers' coughs, making it all the more important to be aware if the cough worsens. An early lung tumour causes this symptom by irritating the lining of the air passages.

• Frequent or unusually persistent chest infections. This can mean that a small tumour is acting as a focus for repeated infection.

• Coughing blood. Even small amounts mixed with phlegm should be investigated and all the more so if the cough produces pure blood. A small tumour can have this effect by oozing blood from its surface.

• Breathlessness – because a tumour has caused collapse of part of a lung.

• Persistent pain or ache in the chest, due to inflammation from a tumour.

• Loss of appetite and weight. For reasons not clearly understood, many cancers cause loss of weight and appetite before the cancer has otherwise shown itself.

Ninety five per cent of lung cancer cases are due to smoking. It is increasingly thought that the remaining five per cent may largely be caused by passive smoking.

◆ Bronchiectasis

See page 208.

◆ Cause unknown

Despite thorough investigation, in some cases the cause remains unknown.

Rare

◆ Heart failure

• Gradual onset of breathlessness, swollen ankles, inability to lie flat.

• Frothy pink sputum, rather than pure blood.

◆ Mitral stenosis

• History of rheumatic fever, see page 263.

• Gradual development of breathlessness, fatigue, dilated veins on cheekbones, giving a 'flushed' appearance, breathlessness when lying flat.

Cough, bloody phlegm and chest pain

Pain in the lungs points to inflammation or injury of the pleura, the thin outer 'skin' that covers the lungs. Inflammation of the pleura frequently accompanies chest infections, when it is called pleurisy.

Probable

◆ Chest infection

See page 195.

Possible

◆ Pneumonia

See page 201. The phlegm is typically rust-coloured (that is bloodstained) rather than containing pure blood and is otherwise green or yellow due to the underlying infection.

◆ Pulmonary embolus

This is a blood clot blocking blood flow to part of a lung. Symptoms may range from mild, knife-like chest pain to collapse.

Increased risk after surgery, in the obese, in those recovering from a heart attack, in women on the contraceptive pill and during pregnancy.

- Coughing blood.
- Pain worse on breathing in.
- If the embolus is large, faintness and sweating, collapse.
- A swollen calf suggests a leg thrombosis (see page 22) as the source of the pulmonary embolus.

◆ Chest injury

Caused by an injury severe enough to damage the lungs directly, or to break a rib, which then punctures a lung.

- Knife-like pains.
- Worse on breathing in.

Rare

◆ Lung cancer with secondary spread to bones

In the later stages of lung cancer, a patient might experience this combination of symptoms.

Cancer of the lung can spread to other parts of the body, for example the bones. If a rib is involved, there will be persistent chest pain, especially at night; a specific tender spot on the rib; and other signs of the disease.

See page 209.

Asphyxia (suffocation)

Obstruction to the flow of air through the mouth, down the trachea or into the lungs. Always look for some simple reversible cause, typically something stuck in the throat. The symptoms of asphyxia are:

- Rapid or abrupt onset.
- Sudden cough, choking and spluttering.
- Rapid cyanosis (bluish colouring) of lips, tongue.
- Panic.
- Stridor, a low- to middle-pitched sound from the larynx, mainly on breathing in. It is also caused by viral infection (*Croup* see page 195).

The Chest

Of course, your first move, if you suspect something trapped in the throat, will be to try to dislodge it. (See Heimlich's manoeuvre, page 219) Then call for help. Then, if you know how, give artificial respiration until help arrives. Usually these situations call for emergency attention as quickly as possible.

Probable

◆ Foreign body

A piece of meat or a similar chunk of firm food is the usual culprit in adults. In children, food can be to blame, but consider also small toys, pen tops, beads, peanuts. The prime signs are:

* Choking.
* Acute stridor: noisy, hoarse, 'wheezing' intake of breath.
* Clutching at throat.

If the foreign body gets past the larynx and makes its way down into the lungs, the coughing and stridor will pass off. In the lungs it will act as a focus for chronic infection, or even a lung abscess. Cough and recurrent infection after a choking fit should be viewed with suspicion because of this possibility.

◆ Swelling of larynx

An acute, severe allergic reaction causes widespread swelling of soft tissues, including the larynx. Call for an ambulance immediately.

Commonest after insect stings or injections. Some people are hypersensitive to specific foods: nuts are commonly to blame.

* Swelling of lips, limbs and throat.
* Acute wheezing.

* Collapse.

◆ Laryngo-tracheitis

A simple laryngitis may occasionally develop into severe swelling. Children whose airways are narrow, and will become obstructed on modest swelling of the soft tissues, are most at risk (see *Croup* page 195).

* Hoarseness developing into stridor (see page 193).
* Laboured breathing, cyanosis (bluish tinge to skin, especially lips).

Possible

◆ Pneumothorax

Lungs are like balloons in some ways, and, just like a balloon, sometimes part of a lung bursts and collapses. Small collapses go unnoticed. Large ones will cause noticeable symptoms and if air continues to leak out from the puncture into the chest, rapid breathlessness will become a problem.

* Sudden, knife-like chest pain.
* Worse breathing in.
* Breathlessness worsening over a few minutes.

Treatment of a large pneumothorax will require emergency treatment in hospital: a needle will be inserted through the chest wall to let out the air compressed inside.

Rare

◆ Epiglottitis

The epiglottis lies just out of sight at the very back of the throat. Infection can cause it to swell until it obstructs the back of the throat. This is an illness found in young children, whose airways are still narrow.

The Chest

This is uncommon now in most developed countries where children are vaccinated against the causative bacteria called *H.Influenzae* (HIB).

- Begins as a simple sore throat.
- Child develops a very high temperature.
- Begins to drool saliva because swallowing is painful.
- Laboured breathing, cyanosis.

If you suspect that your child has epiglottitis it is important not to try to peer down the throat as that can cause complete obstruction. An examination should only be performed in hospital where an emergency tracheostomy can be undertaken.

◆ Diphtheria

A terrible illness which routine vaccination has virtually eliminated from developed countries. A membrane forms at the back of the throat which obstructs breathing. In addition, the germ responsible produces toxic substances that affect the heart and nervous system.

- Begins as a simple sore throat.
- A grey membrane forms at the back of the throat.
- Dramatic enlargement of lymph nodes in the neck.
- Breathlessness, cyanosis.

◆ Tracheo-oesophageal fistula

An abnormality of new-born babies. During embryonic life, the airways and the gullet develop in close proximity to each other. If the trachea opens into the gullet rather than the back of the mouth, food will travel straight from the gullet into the lungs.

- Cough, asphyxia each time the baby feeds.
- Chest infection develops rapidly.

Once recognized, the problem is cured by surgery.

◆ Tumours and cysts

Although these diseases of the larynx or thyroid gland grow quite slowly, they can rapidly increase in size if they start to bleed. The swelling causes obstruction. The diagnosis might be considered in an adult who is known to have a growth and who suddenly becomes breathless.

Chest pain

Though chest pain is commonly and understandably taken as a sign of heart disease, there are many other causes to be considered, not all of them involving the heart. So many vital structures pass through the chest that the list of possibilities is long. There are the gullet, the great vessels coming from the heart, the windpipe and the airways going down into the lungs. Pain may stem from the ribs themselves, the muscles between the ribs or from the nerves. The lungs can ache and inflammation from within the abdomen may give rise to pain in the chest. And certainly, some chest pains, particularly perhaps in born worriers, are psychological. Finally there are pains which remain totally unexplained, even after extensive investigation.

That said, sudden severe chest pain must be taken seriously and needs urgent medical assessment to exclude a heart attack. Advances in the treatment of heart attacks require medical attention to be given within a very few hours of the attack. It is therefore all the more important to get help as soon as possible. It is one area of medicine where doctors, given a classic picture, will back their hunches and treat first, diagnose later, even if immediate test results are negative.

This section is divided as follows:

- A heart attack.

- Sudden chest pain.
- Persistent or recurrent chest pain.

Everyone should be aware of the classic symptoms of a heart attack because early treatment is vital.

- Sudden, severe central chest pain.
- Begins at rest.
- Worse on exertion.
- Pain is crushing, vice-like, gripping.
- May radiate up to the jaws or down the arms, usually the left.
- Breathlessness.
- Sweating.
- Cyanosis (blueness) of lips.

Heart attack

A heart attack occurs when the blood supply to part of the heart is blocked off. Pain comes from the heart muscle in much the same way that cramp occurs in other muscles in other circumstances.

For many years, the treatment was to deal with the complications that can arise, such as heart failure or rhythm disorders (see pages 183). Nowadays, treatment aims to limit the amount of damage to the heart that occurs during the attack, but this calls for treatment within hours or less. This makes it all the more important to get an early diagnosis in hospital.

Not all heart attacks will show all of the

features above: pain is not always a prominent feature, especially in the elderly; some-times there is just:

- Sudden onset of tiredness.
- Irregular pulse.
- Heart failure, with breathlessness and swollen ankles.

In these circumstances, much can still be done to help.

Keep this picture in mind when referring to the sections dealing with other causes of chest pain.

Your doctor does.

Sudden chest pain, possibly a heart attack

Sudden chest pain is always worrying, but just how worrying depends on

associated features. The classical symptoms of a heart attack have been

The Chest

given, but subtleties may help sway the diagnosis. Did the pain come on very suddenly, or over a few minutes? Is breathlessness a feature? Do you feel ill? Does movement make a difference? Were there previous symptoms?

Diagnostic possibilities are different at different ages. Heart disease would not be the first diagnosis for a young person, whereas in an older person it is often difficult to rule out heart disease completely, so tests will commonly be ordered although the symptoms are not completely typical. It is generally safest for a layperson to regard severe chest pain in an adult as a disorder of the heart until proven otherwise.

Doctors will make additional judgements based on the individual's overall condition, including skin colour, pulse, blood pressure or signs of heart disease such as fluid on the lungs or abnormal heart rhythms. An electrocardiogram (ECG) recording of the heart can be helpful; so are blood tests, but these take time, so doctors will often make a diagnosis based on history and examination while awaiting the outcome of investigations.

Probable

◆ Heart attack

See page 213.

Should be suspected on the basis of:

- Sudden onset of severe central chest pain.
- Onset at rest.
- Prolonged and crushing in nature.

Possible

◆ Oesophagitis

Inflammation of the gullet can be extremely painful, with many features resembling a heart attack:

- Central chest pain.
- Spreads up to neck, down arms.
- Sweating.
- Can be difficult to distinguish from heart pain. There may be a previous history of:
- Indigestion, belching.
- Burning pain after food.
- Taking drugs which irritate the gullet such as aspirin.
- Relief with antacids.

However, if occurring for the first time in the middle-aged or elderly, heart disease must be carefully considered.

◆ Nerve irritation

Nerves run in bands between the ribs, encircling the chest. It is quite common for one of these nerves to become irritated, causing pain.

- Sharp chest pain.
- Radiates from the back towards the front of the chest.
- Worse on movement.
- No breathlessness or sweating.
- Pain comes and goes from minute to minute.
- Often one small part of the chest wall is tender.

This condition can be dramatic when it

The Chest

appears but is entirely benign, needing no more than painkillers and rest.

◆ Peptic ulcer

Ulceration in the stomach or upper small bowel (duodenum).

The pain from a peptic ulcer tends to be:

- Confined to the upper abdomen ('pit of stomach' or 'solar plexus').
- Burning in nature.
- Worse at night.
- Appears to go through into the back.
- Preceded by weeks or months of indigestion.
- Possibly blood in vomit.
- Upper abdominal pain on pressure.

Treatment is totally different from that for a heart attack, consisting of intensive anti-acid treatment.

One in ten people will have an ulcer at some time in their lives. This condition used to be commonest in men; now it is almost as common in women.

Smoking, family history, infection with a bacteria (*H. pylori*) and taking certain anti-inflammatory painkillers (such as aspirin, ibuprofen) all increase the risk of developing a peptic ulcer.

◆ Pneumothorax

Sudden collapse of part of a lung.

- Sudden, knife-like chest pain.
- Localized usually to the side of the chest, not central.
- Breathlessness is a possibility.

Rare

◆ Pulmonary embolus

A blood clot lodging in the lungs causing:

- Sudden pressure in chest.
- Discomfort rather than pain.
- Pain, if present, is knife-like.
- Breathlessness.
- Sudden cough with bloodstained phlegm.

Pulmonary embolus is associated with thrombosis of leg veins, giving a painful swollen calf. It can occur after surgical operations.

◆ Dissecting aortic aneurysm

The aorta is the great artery which carries blood away from the heart. If diseased, the walls can weaken, bulge and eventually start to leak. In the days or weeks before this stage there may be warning signs such as:

- Vague upper chest pain.
- Pulsation (feeling of strong, throbbing pulse) in the upper chest.
- Breathlessness through obstruction of part of the lung.
- Hoarseness.

If the aneurysm begins to leak there will be:

- Pain similar to heart attack.
- Possibly vomiting blood.
- Collapse through blood loss.

This condition is very difficult to distinguish from a heart attack by examination alone. The diagnosis is usually made on the result of a chest X-ray.

The Chest

Surgery is possible, depending on the site of the leakage. Frequently fatal.

◆ Pericarditis

Inflammation of the lining around the heart giving rise to:

- Sharp central chest pain.
- Worse on movement.
- Worse on breathing.

Pericarditis may be caused by a viral infection. It can usually be treated and a full recovery is usual.

◆ Pancreatitis

The pancreas lies at the back of the upper abdomen. It is the gland that produces insulin and other substances that digest food. If the pancreas becomes inflamed, these substances are released and start to 'digest' the internal organs with which they come into contact.

Inflammation of the pancreas is most common in alcoholics or in those with gallstones. The very severe pain of pancreatitis can appear to spread up into the chest.

- Pain radiates into the back.
- Nausea and vomiting.

There will be upper abdominal tenderness on examination.

This is a serious condition which calls for intensive treatment in hospital.

Recurrent or persistent chest pain

This means symptoms that come and go over days, weeks or months. Again, the possibilities depend on the person's age, previous medical history and any associated features of disease.

Recurrent chest pain is common and is not always explainable. In young people, the reason often remains obscure, even after intensive investigation.

Probable

◆ Angina

Angina is pain arising from the heart. The reason is nearly always coronary artery disease: that is, 'furring up' of the blood vessels that carry blood to the heart itself. This causes a partial blockage of blood flow, and gives no symptoms until you exert yourself. Then, the heart's increased demand for blood cannot be met, resulting in angina:

- Central chest pain.
- Often radiates to neck or down left arm.
- Comes on with exertion.
- Goes after only a few minutes of rest.
- Worse in cold weather, after meals, emotional stress.

It is common to investigate angina with X-rays which high-light the blood flow around the heart, a technique known as angiography. The information gathered from this test will help the doctor to decide whether to replace the blood vessels to the heart, done in an operation known as coronary artery bypass grafting.

Angina is an important warning sign of heart disease, but in itself it is not usually dangerous and is not a warning of an imminent heart attack. However, angina should always be investigated. It is often treated effectively by angioplasty (where the blocked heart vessel is stretched with a balloon and often a stent put inside the vessel to keep it open). Or it can be relieved by a heart bypass operation. If your angina is getting much worse, contact your doctor urgently. If it is occurring at rest and not relieved by your spray/tablets placed under the tongue, then after 15 minutes you should call an ambulance.

◆ Hiatus hernia

A common condition in which part of the stomach moves up into the chest. As a result the diaphragm – which normally creates a valve-type mechanism – allows gastric acid to cause pain in the upper part of the stomach and the gullet.

Symptoms may be noticed for the first time during pregnancy, or be made worse by it; this is also so if you are obese.

- Pain worse on lying flat or bending over.
- Pain which is burning or searing in nature.
- May appear to radiate up to the neck.
- Burping or belching.
- Relieved by antacids.

Treatment varies from simply avoiding tight clothing and raising the head of the bed, to a range of drugs or, occasionally an operation to tighten up the muscles.

Modern medication, especially drugs known as proton pump inhibitors, are extremely effective for relieving the symptoms of a hiatus hernia.

Possible

◆ Costochondritis

Where the ribs meet the breast-bone there are joints made up of cartilage which can become inflamed. This may occur after injury, out of the blue or some-times in epidemics of a viral infection called Bornholm disease (named after the Baltic island where an epidemic was documented).

- Onset over a few hours.
- Aching on either side of the breastbone.
- Individual joints may be swollen and tender.
- Worse on breathing, or with changes of posture.
- Sometimes a mild fever.

This condition is not dangerous, but may be extremely painful and alarming at the start and can last for several weeks.

◆ Da Costa's syndrome

A kind of cardiac neurosis: a psychological problem of anxiety showing itself as:

- Recurrent pains over the heart.
- Breathlessness out of proportion to effort.

The Chest

- Nervousness.
- Palpitations.

There is no doubt that individuals are genuinely distressed by their symptoms, which are treated by psychological support once heart disease has been ruled out.

◆ Heart rhythm disorders

Very rapid or very slow heart rates can bring on angina, even in individuals with no other heart disease.

- Palpitations.
- Breathlessness.
- Abrupt onset, abrupt finish.

  For details, see pages 184.

◆ Lung disease

Many disorders can give rise to chest pain which may be mistaken for heart disease, including severe infections and cancer. See pages 195.

◆ Gall bladder disease

Lying high up in the right side of the abdomen, a diseased gall bladder can give rise to pain which appears to be in the chest. It is commonest in middle-aged women. There is usually little difficulty in distinguishing this as a cause.

- Pain builds up over a few minutes.
- Lasts for several hours.
- Pain and tenderness mainly under the ribs on the right side.
- May appear to radiate into the chest or to the tip of the shoulder.
- Nausea, vomiting is common.
- Restlessness.

A first attack may be puzzling, but usually a pattern emerges: pain provoked by certain foods, especially fatty ones, with episodes of niggling pain in between major attacks. The usual reason is gallstones, for which there is a variety of treatments, mainly surgical.

Rare

◆ Aortic valve disease

This valve controls blood flow between the heart and the aorta, the major artery from the heart. The valve can become stiff and inefficient; this is known as aortic stenosis, usually a result of ageing, though rheumatic heart disease was once a common cause.

Occasionally, children are born with an abnormal valve. As the valve is so stiff, it has to beat harder to force blood out and this puts a strain on it. For years there may be no symptoms, but with increasing stiffness there will be some combination of:

- Angina.
- Heart rhythm irregularities.
- Breathlessness.
- Fainting on exertion.

The condition produces a characteristic heart murmur that a doctor can detect. The treatment is by heart valve replacement, though other treatments are used in childhood or in the elderly and infirm.

◆ Severe anaemia

It is unusual for anaemia to become so severe without other symptoms, but it does happen occasionally, especially with pernicious anaemia. This starves the heart of oxygen, and angina is the result.

- Pallor or yellowish tinge in pernicious anaemia.
- Sore tongue.
- Tiredness, breathlessness.

Most forms of anaemia respond rapidly to treatment.

◆ Aortic aneurysm

In the days or weeks before this ruptures, there may be intermittent chest pain.

See page 436.

◆ Pericarditis

May account for several days of chest pain.

See page 216.

Heimlich's manoeuvre

Do not perform it on a child under one year of age.

- Stand behind the person choking.
- Extend your arms in a hug around their upper abdomen.
- With clenched fists make a hard, fast squeeze just under the breast bone.

The manoeuvre forces a blast of air out of the lungs, sufficient to dislodge something stuck in the upper airway. For full details see any modern manual of first aid.

The skin and hair

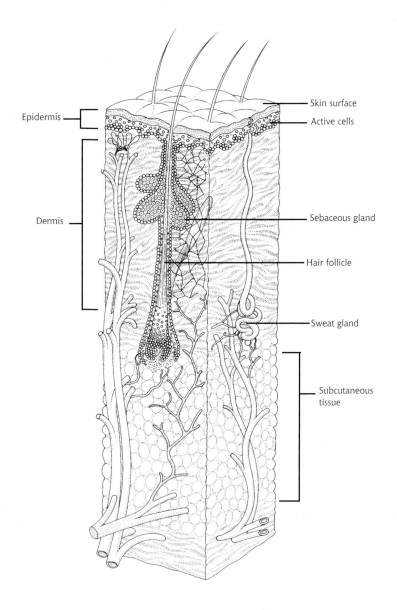

Epidermis

Dermis

Skin surface

Active cells

Sebaceous gland

Hair follicle

Sweat gland

Subcutaneous
tissue

The skin: introduction

The skin is the largest organ in the body, although spread out very thinly. The fact that it can be examined so easily is, as you would expect, especially useful in making a diagnosis. And changes in the skin can sometimes help to diagnose underlying diseases.

Many people are understandably reticent when it comes to discussing or showing changes in their skin – particularly in those areas normally hidden by clothes. Doctors never regard such changes as embarrassing: they think of them only as essential clues to diagnosis.

Rashes

Are analysed here into four key different types, with cross-references to pages where they are covered in detail.

Rashes developing blisters

◆ **Chicken pox**
See page 226.

◆ **Eczema**
See page 317.

◆ **Herpes simplex**
See page 224.

◆ **Herpes zoster**
See page 100.

◆ **Impetigo**
See page 224.

◆ **Pustular psoriasis**
See under *Psoriasis*, page 226.

◆ **Dermatitis herpetiformis**
See page 225.

Rashes of red/purple or black/dark spots under the skin

See *Bleeding 'under' the skin*, page 238.

Rashes extending over most of the body

◆ **Chicken pox**
See page 226.

◆ **Dermatitis herpetiformis**
See page 225.

The Skin

The Skin

◆ **Drug reactions**

See page 230, under *Blue – general.*

◆ **Eczema**

See page 317.

◆ **German measles**

Rubella. See page 130.

◆ **Measles**

See pages 415.

◆ **Porphyria cutanea tarda**

See page 225.

◆ **Psoriasis**

See page 226.

◆ **Scalded skin syndrome**

See page 225.

◆ **Tinea versicolor**

See page 233.

◆ **Urticaria**

See page 242.

◆ **Vitamin A deficiency**

See *Hard skin*, page 242.

◆ **Vitiligo**

See page 233.

◆ **Viral infections**

See page 232, and *Papilloma* or *Wart*, page 236.

(Smallpox is now considered to be eradicated worldwide.)

Rashes in a localised area

See section covering that part of body.

Whiteheads

See *Blackheads and whiteheads/acne*, below.

Pimples

Are covered under *Blackheads and whiteheads/acne*, below.

Blackheads and whiteheads/Acne

Most people have a number of blackheads at any one time and they are not necessarily a sign of any skin abnormality.

They will develop whenever the skin's pores become blocked. If long-standing, or infected, they may become whiteheads, or even become Acne vulgaris, commonly known as acne, or teenage pimples, or 'zits'. The cause of acne is unclear, but changes in hormone levels after puberty and a sensitivity of the grease glands to these hormone levels, resulting in excess grease production, are involved. A bacteria, known as *Proprionbacter acnes*, has a fundamental role and is unique to mankind. Diet plays less of a role than was once thought.

The changes acne makes to the skin are the visible effects of infection and inflammation.

Acne vulgaris

- Starts at puberty.
- Blackheads – pinpricks of black matter and grease – can be seen blocking the entrance to sebaceous glands. The are also known as open comedones. The black matter consists of normal surface skin cells trapped in the grease, and is not dirt.
- Most commonly affects face, upper chest and back.
- Skin may appear greasy.
- Skin bacteria infect the matter in the blocked duct and gland causing local redness, pain and swelling (papules).
- Pus develops, forming pustules (whiteheads).
- This process can continue for years.

If untreated, acne can scar the skin. Modern treatments should improve matters considerably. The cornerstone of treatment is agents that unblock the grease pores around hair follicles. If acne is widespread, treatment by mouth is appropriate and, if severe for example with scarring, refferal to a specialist should be considered.

Blisters

Collections of fluid trapped between different layers of skin. They come in different shapes and sizes. Larger than2/10in/5mm, they are described here as bullae; smaller, as vesicles.

Probable

◆ Injury

Extremes of heat or cold; friction; caustic chemicals; certain plants; some animals; jelly fish; insect bites: all can cause blisters.

- Localized to the site of injury.
- Surrounding skin may be reddened.

◆ Eczema

Often most marked in the skin 'flexures', for example the creases at the elbows, or behind the knees.

- Itching.
- Redness.
- Raised red areas.
- Vesicles.
- Weeping.
- Scaling.
- Crusting.

Eczema vesicles are often not seen, as they have thin walls and are beneath the surface. As in all blistering conditions, the skin is very itchy; and scratching tears the vesicles open. Eczema on the soles of the feet or palms of the hand will produce tense blisters, which persist because the overlying skin in these sites is very thick.

◆ Herpes simplex

This can cause blisters anywhere on the body. They are known as 'cold sores', and occur mostly around the mouth. An infection with the *Herpes simplex* virus is usually minor, but can occasionally be nasty, causing bleeding sores, particularly in and around the mouth. After the first infection, recurrences may occur at times of debility or after exposure to hot sun or cold.

- Skin is locally irritable – a 'tingling sensation'.
- Then reddening and painful.
- Small lumps appear and go on to form vesicles.
- The vesicles burst and crust over.
- The whole cycle takes 10 to 14 days to subside.

  See also *Lips – cracked*, page 77.

◆ Impetigo

A skin infection which is passed on easily by contact.

- Red spots that blister.
- A honey-coloured infected discharge that forms crusts.
- Common around mouth, face and ears.

  See also page 95.

Possible

◆ Chicken pox

See page 226.

◆ Shingles

Herpes zoster. Arises when the chicken pox virus is reactivated after lying dormant for years in the nerves of the area affected.

- Initially, an itchy, localized area of skin on one half of the body.
- Pain develops.
- Reddening occurs; small lumps appear.
- Vesicles form.
- Crusting, followed by healing, sometimes taking up to a month.
- Pain (post-herpetic neuralgia) may be persistent and difficult to treat.

◆ Erythema multiforme

See page 80.

Vesicles and bullae may occur with this disease, which arises from an infection or a reaction to a drug or medicine.

Rare

◆ Pemphigoid

In the elderly.

- Sudden onset of bullae on limbs and trunk. They may arise from reddened or swollen skin.
- Bullae may be filled with blood-stained fluid.

  Requires aggressive treatment, often with steroids.

◆ Psoriasis (pustular)

See page 226.

◆ Dermatitis herpetiformis

A very rare auto-immune disease.

- Itchy rash on the extensor (outer) aspect of elbows, knees and buttocks.
- Multiple intensely itchy, small blisters appear in these areas.

Almost always associated with coeliac disease (see page 137). Treatment of the coeliac disease with a gluten-free diet usually controls the skin condition, but sometimes drug therapy (with dapsone, for example) is necessary.

See under *Methaemoglobinaemia*, page 230.

◆ Pemphigus vulgaris

A very rare but serious condition affecting people usually over the age of 50.

- Crops of widespread blisters known as bullae on the skin and mucous membranes, often starting in the mouth.
- The blisters have very thin walls, so tear easily leaving weeping, reddened and painful skin, which may become infected.

Cannot be cured, but treatment with steroids and antibiotics considerably improves matters. It usually eventually 'burn itself out'.

◆ Porphyria cutanea tarda

Associated with liver damage – often alcohol-induced.

- Exposed skin becomes blistered, scarred and pigmented, after exposure to ultraviolet light.

Treatment includes giving up alcohol.

◆ Epidermolysis bullosa

Several exceedingly rare different types of this inherited disease exist. Bullae develop after minimal injury – typically minor friction – and become infected.

◆ Scalded skin syndrome

Caused by infection in children, and drug sensitivities in adults.

- Sudden onset of malaise.
- Raised temperature.
- Widespread redness.
- Multiple vesicles and bullae.
- Vesicles and bullae join, causing large areas of skin to lift off, like a severe scald.
- May be fatal.

Scarred or pitted skin

In theory, any repeated inflammation or disease process will leave the skin scarred and pitted. In practice, the commonest culprit is acne, the universal plague of adolescence; see page 222. The worst cases leave permanent marks on the face and shoulders.

Scaly skin

True scaling is limited to just a few conditions and diseases.

Excluding the commonest of them, dandruff (see page 265), this leaves:

The Skin

Probable

◆ **Fungal infections**

◆ **Eczema**

See pages 238 and 317, respectively.

Possible

◆ **Psoriasis**

See below.

Rare

◆ **Pellagra**

Vitamin B3 (niacin) deficiency.

• Dementia.

• Severe diarrhoea.

• Scaly changes (dermatitis) of exposed skin.

◆ **Ichthyosis**

See page 246.

Scabs

If the skin surface is damaged and fluid (serum, pus, blood) leaks out (either directly or into blisters which subsequently burst) then golden brown or black crusts – scabs – form on the surface or at the edges of the damaged skin. See also *Blisters*, pages 223.

Probable

◆ **Impetigo**

See pages 224.

◆ **Eczema**

See pages 317.

◆ **Injury**

◆ **Herpes simplex**

See pages 224.

Possible

◆ **Chicken pox**

An infectious disease caused by the same virus that causes shingles (see *Herpes zoster*).

• Crops of spots at different stages.

• Spots are red, raised, form vesicles then pustules (vesicles filled with pus).

• Pustules burst and crust over.

• Fever.

• Malaise.

◆ **Herpes zoster**

See page 100.

Rare

◆ **Pemphigus**

See page 119.

◆ **Psoriasis**

A skin disorder of unknown cause.

• Multiple red lesions of varying size.

• The red areas are covered with thick silver scales.

• If the scales are scraped off, the underlying skin shows multiple tiny bleeding points.

• May occur on any part of the body, but frequently on the back of the knees, elbows and scalp.

- The nails are involved in about half the cases, though the changes can be quite subtle.
- Some individuals develop arthritis (see page 90) in association with the psoriasis.

Pustular psoriasis is an uncommon form of the condition in which pus-filled vesicles (pustules) arise from the affected skin.

When these break down some crusting may occur.

◆ Dermatitis artefacta

Some people suffering from psychological disorders deliberately harm themselves, for example by burning, scratching or even applying caustic fluids. The resulting injuries may well include extensive scabs and crusts, for which there is no clear explanation.

Sometimes child abusers cause similar injuries to children.

Peeling or flaking skin

Occurs in association with many skin diseases, but typically blisters and rashes, whose other symptoms are just as, if not more, noticeable, and which are listed under those headings. And, of course, peeling skin is the eventual and unfortunate outcome of sunburn.

Some skin diseases benefit from sunlight: psoriasis and acne are obvious examples. However, it is now established beyond much doubt that sunbathing predisposes to skin cancer. No sunbathing can be considered entirely safe. You increase your risk considerably if:

- You have fair skin and sunbathe (redheads with freckles should avoid the sun);
- You expose yourself to the sun around the middle of the day;

If you develop any redness of the skin. This means you are burnt. Burnt skin means a higher risk of skin cancer.

It is wise to keep to the following rules when you are on holiday, or during sunny spells:

- Increase your exposure to the sun very gradually.
- Wear T-shirts and hats.
- Use a high-factor sun protection cream. Ensure you use both a UV-A and UV-B filter.
- Cover children well.
- Reapply sun blocks after bathing.
- Avoid the midday sun.
- Protective creams are effective and should be used.

Skin appears pale

See page 392.

The Skin

Skin appears bluish

See page 74.

Skin appears blackened

See *Discolouration of the skin*, below.

Yellow skin

See *Yellowish skin – Jaundice*, page 233.

Localized yellow areas in the skin

◆ Xanthomata
Localized, well-defined deposits of fatty material just below the skin surface. May occasionally be a sign of excess lipids (fats) in the blood, which in turn may predispose to arterial disease. Most commonly seen around the eyes, when the deposits are called xanthelasma.

◆ Gouty tophi
See *Gout*, page 261.

Yellowish skin – Jaundice

See page 233.

Discolouration of the skin

Meaning any abnormal change in the colour of your skin. This can happen because of a local problem, or because of a general ('systemic') disease of one or more of the body's organs or systems.

There are several conditions where changed skin colour is a major feature.

Well-known types of skin discolouration are listed here by the type of colour change and by whether the change is local or general. Obviously, colour changes will usually be more obvious in people with light skins than in those with dark skins.

Not listed here are spots and rashes, which are covered on pages 242-3.

The Skin

Black – local

◆ Mole

Common in adults. They measure from a millimetre or two in diameter, to a centimeter in diameter. Typically brown/black in colour. Some have hairs growing from them. They are harmless, but see immediately below.

◆ Malignant melanoma

A form of skin cancer, usually dark or black, and commonest in fair-skinned individuals who have had lengthy, frequent exposure to the sun. They are increasingly common, very probably because more people take holidays in the sun. The role of ozone-depletion in the atmosphere is less certain, but may be an important factor. Some malignant melanomas are extremely aggressive.

Malignant melanomas start as small black areas and are often difficult to tell from moles. Even a vague suspicion that you may have one is reason enough to show it to a doctor without delay. Early diagnosis improves the chances of successful treatment. Once treated, you may need to be followed up for several years.

The warning signs are:

• New appearance of a pigmented lesion.

• Bleeding within an existing mole (unless there is a clear history of trauma).

• Itching.

• Colour change.

• Change in size or shape.

• Appearance of smaller lesions nearby.

• Ulceration.

• Any one of these warning signs should prompt you to visit your doctor urgently.

◆ Acanthosis nigricans

Black pigmentation in the armpit, the groin, on the face and neck, usually in the elderly. Can be associated with cancer. A similar change commonly occurs in obese patients. Rare, and untreatable.

◆ Dry gangrene

See also *Itching or numbness of the fingers or toes*, page 300. Gradual loss of blood supply to a toe or a foot, or any extremity, may cause this condition. The affected part becomes withered and black and may drop off – typically a frost-bitten toe.

Blue – local

◆ Cyanosis

See *Bluish skin*, page 74.

◆ Mongolian blue spot

A blue/black area typically seen on the buttocks and sacral region in West Indian and Asian children. May often be mistaken for a bruise; can be several centimetres across.

◆ Blue naevus

Occurs anywhere on the body. May be only a few millimetres in size. This is an innocent mole which happens to look blue.

◆ **Livido reticularis**

An exaggeration of the body's normal response to heat and cold: white areas of skin surrounded by a 'chicken wire' pattern of bluish blood vessels.

Blue – general

◆ **Cyanosis**

See page 397.

◆ **Amiodarone**

This drug, for treating heart irregularities, may rarely cause a bluish-grey, slaty discolouration of the skin.

◆ **Minocycline**

Similarly, prolonged courses of this antibiotic, which was a common treatment for acne, can make the skin go permanently slate-grey.

◆ **Methaemoglobinaemia**

Can occur through exposure to certain drugs, for example dapsone, for treating leprosy or dermatitis herpetiformis, or certain chemicals. Some people inherit the condition, which affects the oxygen-carrying capacity of the haemoglobin in red blood cells.

◆ **Ochronosis**

Affects cartilage and other connective tissue, for example the whites of the eyes. The cartilage underlying the skin looks bluish or blue-black, whereas normally the overlying skin colour would predominate.

Caused by an abnormality of amino-acid metabolism called alkaptonuria.

Brown – local

◆ **Pregnancy**

As pregnancy progresses, the nipples, the genitalia and a line down the centre of the abdomen become progressively darker -turning from pinkish to brownish. See also *Chloasma*, below.

◆ **Chloasma**

A brownish, patchy pigmentation of the face that occurs in some pregnant women. Can occur when taking the combined contraceptive pill.

◆ **Venous ulceration**

Long-standing varicose veins in the legs (see page 289) cause brownish pigmentation of the lower legs and feet. Sometimes there is ulceration, too, particularly on the inner side of the ankle.

◆ **Erythema ab igne**

A reddish-brown irregular discolouration which appears after long exposure of skin to heat. May well be noticed on the shins of an elderly person who spends hours in an armchair close to an open fire.

◆ **Seborrhoeic wart**

A flattish, brownish wart, slightly raised above the surrounding skin. Sometimes they occur in considerable numbers. Also known as senile warts because they appear during middle-age and later. Harmless.

◆ Cafe-au-lait spots
Like large freckles; may be multiple. Occasionally associated with 'neurofibromatosis.'

◆ Addison's disease
Caused by long-standing under-activity of the adrenal glands.

Brownish/dark pigmentation of skin, especially skin creases, nipples, genitalia, old scars and gums (in the last, may appear grey).

* Weakness, fatigue.
* Weight loss, anorexia.
* Craving for salt.
* Nausea, vomiting, diarrhoea.
* Low blood pressure.
* Hair loss – occasionally.
* Vitiligo – occasionally. See page 233.

Brown – general

◆ Freckles
May occur naturally or may appear in increased numbers after exposure to the sun. May grow darker than usual and may coalesce, if exposed to sun. Mostly on face, shoulders and arms, but may cover the entire body. Commonest on redheads.

Avoid the sun if you have freckles; see *Peeling or flaking skin*, page 227.

◆ Haemochromatosis
Also called bronze diabetes. An abnormality of metabolism of iron from birth causes:

* Diabetes mellitus, see page 341.
* Bronze skin.
* Cirrhosis.
* Joint inflammation.
* Heart abnormalities.
* Shrunken testes, reduced libido.

Orange – general

◆ Carotenaemia
Eating too much food containing carotene, typically carrots and tomato juice, causes

an orange discoloration of skin. Carotene is the active ingredient of some 'sun-tan' tablets.

Pink – local

◆ Salmon patch naevus
A salmon-pink birthmark.

Can occur anywhere, but often on the neck. Some persist, but most disappear after a few years.

Purple – local

◆ Port-wine stain

A permanent birth mark caused by an abnormality of the capillary blood vessels producing an often extensive discoloured area on the face and neck. Permanent, but can be disguised with make-up.

◆ Kaposi's sarcoma

Bluish-red areas appear on the skin. This is a malignant tumour that used to be seen mainly in Africa, but is now encountered all over the world as one of the complications of AIDS.

Purple – general

Likely to be cyanosis; see page 397.
See also *Blue – general*, page 230.

Redness – local

Described as erythema.

◆ Flushing

As a response to heat, or embarrassment; and in association with the menopause, page 318.

◆ Erythema ab igne

See *Brown*, page 231.

◆ Palmar erythema

Redness of the palms of the hands.
   Seen in alcoholics and in others suffering from liver disease.

◆ Erythrasma

Reddish-brown discolouration of the skin, particularly near skin folds (breasts, armpits, groin). The skin is dry and the areas are irregular and slightly scaly. Caused by bacterial infection.

◆ Paget's disease of the nipple

Localized redness with scaling and inflammation, mimicking eczema. If you notice such changes on the nipple or areola (the pink area around the nipple), see your doctor urgently – the possibility of an underlying breast cancer must be excluded. See also page 326.

Redness – general

◆ Viral infection

Many viruses will cause nonspecific reddening of the skin. Typically, the rash fades soon after the illness settles.

◆ Drug reaction

A diffuse reddening of the skin associated with medication.
   The reddening may be patchy or

blotchy, or widespread. Itching (medical term, pruritus) often accompanies these reactions.

Penicillin and aspirin commonly cause this reaction.

Yellowness – general

This is never a local condition.

◆ **Jaundice**

Yellowish whites of the eyes, and yellow skin gradually progressing to a deeper, browner colour. There may also be itching (with resulting scratch marks),

pale stools and dark urine.

◆ **Uraemia**

See pages 245.

◆ **Mepacrine**

This anti-malarial drug can cause yellowing of the skin.

Whiteness or paleness – local

◆ **Vitiligo**

Destruction of pigment-producing cells (melanocytes) in the skin, giving white patches. In the dark-skinned, these can be quite disfiguring. See also *Addison's disease*, page 231.

◆ **Halo naevus**

Some moles (see *Black*, above) become pale and the area round them loses pigment. Mole and surrounding area are known as halo naevi. Vitiligo (above) may also develop.

◆ **Tinea versicolor**

A fungal infection of the skin.

• Initially, areas of irregular brown colouration.

• Predominantly upper body, arms and neck.

• Later, these patches lose their pigment, giving pale areas.

• Treatable with anti-fungal creams.

◆ **Post-inflammatory**

Any inflamed or damaged skin – say from a graze, a burn, a herpes sore – may lose its usual colour after healing. Normal pigmentation may return after a few months.

◆ **Leprosy**

See page 299.

◆ **Arterial blockage**

See *Peripheral vascular disease*, page 298.

◆ **Phlegmasia alba dolens**

This means blockage of the principal veins draining blood from the leg. Typically after being bed-ridden.

• Initially, malaise.

• Pain in groin and thigh.

• Leg-swelling follows.

• Leg is pale and feels cold.

◆ **Raynaud's phenomenon and disease**

See page 278.

Whiteness or paleness – general

◆ **Anaemia**

See page 366.

◆ **Leukaemia**

See pages 450.

◆ **Albinism**

An inherited abnormality of metabolism that results in absence of pigment in body tissues.

• Fair skin.

• White hair.

• Pink irises of the eyes.

• Problems with sight.

◆ **Phenylketonuria**

Caused by an error of metabolism resulting in an accumulation of chemicals which affect the brain. Children are screened at birth. Treatment involves avoiding foods containing phenylalanine.

• Blond hair.

• Blue eyes.

• Mental deficiency and aggression if untreated.

◆ **Hypopituitarism**

See page 249.

◆ **Shock**

See page 381.

Parasites

Scabies and lice are the principal visible parasites of the human skin and body.
See pages 405.

Linear marks on the skin

These are the causes worth considering of clear, isolated, linear marks on the skin. There are others, but they are extremely rare.

◆ **Lymphangitis**

Infection in a limb can track up the lymphatic pathways to the lymph glands. May be seen on the arm and forearm after a simple injury, even a cat scratch to the hand, for example.

• Site of wound may be apparent.

• A red line extends directly from the region of the wound, continuing up towards the armpit.

• Tender lymph nodes may be felt in the armpit.

Antibiotic treatment is advised, to stop the infection.

◆ **Scabies**

Fine grey lines a few millimetres long.
See page 243.

◆ **Acanthosis nigricans**

See page 229.

White patches

Probable

◆ **Vitiligo**

See page 233.

Possible

◆ **Halo naevus**

See page 233.

◆ **Tinea versicolor**

See page 233.

◆ **Post-inflammatory**

See page 233.

Rare

◆ **Lichen sclerosis et atrophicus**

See page 243.

◆ **Leprosy**

See page 299.

◆ **Morphoea**

See page 242.

◆ **Raynaud's phenomenon and disease**

See page 278.

Miniature red spots

There are two causes worth considering:

◆ **Campbell de morgan spots**

- Tiny and bright red, often raised above the surrounding skin surface.
- Present on the chest and abdomen.
- Commonest in elderly people. Of little significance.

◆ **Spider naevi**

These are essentially red spots with several tiny vessels emanating from the centre. They can appear in children and in adults. Multiple naevi may be a feature of pregnancy and of liver disease; also of hereditary haemorrhagic telangiectasia.

Sores or ulcers

Are described elsewhere in the book in relation to the part of the body on which they occur.

Vesicles

Are small blisters. See page 223.

Wheals

A term describing raised marks on the skin. See *Urticaria*, page 242.

The Skin

Warts

See *Lumps in the skin*, below.

Lumps in the skin

It is best to play safe and report any lump in the skin to a doctor: most are innocent, but some need expert evaluation to rule out the possibility of malignant disease.

The earlier the diagnosis and treatment, the better the outlook. If a lump is pigmented, bleeding, irregular, ulcerated or growing rapidly, all the more reason to see a doctor without delay.

Covered here are lumps that may appear in skin anywhere on the body. Lumps specific to certain parts of the body are covered in the appropriate sections.

Probable

◆ Sebaceous cyst

Sometimes called a wen. A harmless lump caused by build-up of sebaceous material – solidified, waxy, body fluid – in a sweat gland near the surface of the skin. May well start as an unsqueezed zit: which, if it does not become infected, can develop, over many years, into a sebaceous cyst. No relation to cancer.

- Smooth; not tender.

- Frequently multiple on scalp, neck or scrotum.

- Size ranges from a few millimetres to several centimetres.

- A small black mark in the centre, the punctum, marks the entrance to the gland.

◆ Dermoid cysts

These are congenital cysts which develop on the head and neck, and are commonest at the outside end of the eyebrow.

They may also occur as benign tumours elsewhere on the body.

◆ Papilloma

See page 325.

◆ Wart

Caused by a viral infection of the skin. Small, often multiple, pain-free thickening of skin with rough skin on the surface, growing proud of the normal skin.

◆ Verruca

A wart on the base of the foot.

Because the foot is weight-bearing, the wart is pushed into the sole of the foot and can be painful.

Possible

◆ Lipoma

A benign, fatty tumour that may appear as a smooth, often soft, lump in or beneath the skin.

◆ Pyogenic granuloma

Possibly caused by minor injury. A soft, red, fleshy benign tumour which bleeds easily when knocked. Often sited near a finger or toenail.

◆ Ganglion

A local degeneration of fibrous tissue. Appears as a small, firm lump, near tendons or joints. Commonly seen on the back of the wrist. Used to be treated by a blow from the family bible – to disperse the lump. Now, a ganglion is either left alone, drained with a large needle or removed surgically.

◆ Molluscum contagiosum

Caused by a virus.

- Crops of small pink lumps.
- Often on trunk or face.
- Each lump has a depression in the middle.
- They clear up of their own accord.

◆ Vascular malformations

There are many different types: spider naevus, salmon patch (also known as strawberry naevus), port wine stain, Campbell de Morgan spots, and hereditary haemorrhagic telangiectasiae are examples. These are rarely seen as lumps, but a cavernous haemangioma may develop as a lump. It may be extensive, covering part of the face.

Rarely present at birth, but appears during the first few months of life. Normally clears by about six years.

◆ Basal cell carcinoma

Commonly called a rodent ulcer.
See page 96.

Rare

◆ Squamous cell carcinoma

A malignant tumour, commonest in the elderly or those whose immunity is suppressed.

- Often on the head or neck.
- May be an irregular lump.
- May bleed.
- May ulcerate.
- Local lymph nodes may be enlarged.

◆ Malignant melanoma

See page 229.

◆ Secondary tumour

Technical term, metastasis. This is cancer that has spread from a primary site to create tumours elsewhere in the body. Irregular, hard, fleshy nodule(s) or plaque(s) seen or felt in the skin of someone known to have a primary cancer raise the suspicion of metastases.

It is rare for skin metastases to be the first symptom you notice of internal primary cancer, but it is possible.

◆ Lymphoma

One particular type of lymphoma starts in the skin. It is noted as an irregular thickening.

Diagnosis can only be made by taking a sample and examining it under the microscope. See also page 449.

Skin tends to crack

This is a feature of inflammation or infection of the skin. The most common causes are fungal infection and eczema.

◆ Fungal infection

Different fungal infections may affect all parts of the body, but commonly hands, feet (see also *Athlete's foot*, page 300) and groin.

• Discrete, dry, reddened, itchy, painful areas of skin.
• Skin macerates and rubs off.
• Sometimes, associated blisters.
• Some fissuring cracking and thickening of the skin.

Easily treated with anti-fungal creams and ointments.

◆ Eczema

The term is often used interchangeably with dermatitis. May be confused with fungal infections, and vice-versa.

• Diffuse patchy redness.
• Red lumps.
• Weeping, crusting.
• Fissuring, scaling.
See page 248.

Moles

See page 229.

Bubbles from a skin wound

Bubbles and fluid oozing from a wound, or surrounding skin that feels 'crackly' when pressure is applied, suggests a very severe infection known as 'gas gangrene'. Pain, malaise and discolouration will almost always be present. Get medical help immediately.

Bleeding 'under' the skin

Medical term, purpura. In fact, the skin has several layers and the term properly describes blood leaking into surrounding surface tissue. The cause is either an injury which did not pierce the skin surface; or an abnormality of blood vessels, or of blood.

When blood leaks into surrounding tissue, it is broken down and undergoes several changes of colour, from red /purple/black to brown, green and yellow. The significance of purpura ranges from the minimal to an indication of life-threatening disorders.

Probable

◆ Bruise

Bruises can be divided (in order of size) into petechiae, or ecchymosis. If there is also a visible or palpable swelling, the term haematoma is used. Bruising may be caused by direct injury – say a blow with a hammer, or indirect pressure – for example, strangulation.

◆ Senile purpura

- Blotchy, well demarcated purple patches.
- Often seen on legs or arms.
- Part of the ageing process.

Possible

◆ Drug related

May be associated with taking steroids.

- Well-demarcated red and purple blotches.

See your doctor if purpura develops.

◆ Henoch Schönlein purpura

Cause unknown. In adults and children.

- Purpura.
- Urticarial rash.
- Painful joints.
- Abdominal pain.
- Bloody diarrhoea.
- Blood in the urine.

Normally resolves of its own accord, although steroids may be advised. Complications may affect the kidney.

◆ Meningococcal septicaemia

See also *Meningitis*, page 388. A life-threatening condition occurring with or without meningitis. Affects pre-school children and young adults most severely.

- Sudden onset of purpuric rash, which may be extensive or minimal.
- Malaise.
- Fever.
- Rapid deterioration and collapse.
- Death may occur within hours.

If suspected, and certainly if the child has had contact with another case of meningitis, see a doctor urgently.

Rare

◆ Blood disorders

Blood disorders such as leukaemia or aplastic anaemia often show themselves with sudden onset of widespread bruising. See also page 389.

◆ Scurvy

See page 399.

◆ Ehlers-Danlos syndrome

An inherited disease in which the body cannot make normal supporting tissue.

- Markedly 'double-jointed' joints.
- Skin scars easily.
- Bruising is common.
- Skin is soft and velvety in texture.

◆ Disseminated intravascular coagulation

A potentially fatal condition caused by failure of the blood clotting mechanism. Often associated with severe infection. Rarely seen outside hospitals.

The Skin

Boils and carbuncles

◆ A Boil

Is an abscess in a hair follicle. Also known as a furuncle. Prime sites are the neck, armpit and buttocks.

• Local redness.

• Swelling.

• Pain.

• Develops a point and discharges yellow/green pus.

◆ Carbuncle

Is a collection of boils that may interconnect under the skin.

Recurrent boils or carbuncles suggest the possibility of underlying disease, particularly diabetes mellitus, see page 168. Urine can be tested for sugar as a quick screening method.

Another cause of recurrent boils may be poor personal hygiene. Occasionally, the diagnosis of acne vulgaris (see page 223) may have been missed.

Boils and carbuncles will normally come to a head, discharge their fluid naturally and disappear. However, this may take so long or be so painful that it is tempting to lance the boil at an early stage. **Don't**.

It is important that this is done when the boil is 'ripe'. See your doctor or practice nurse to have a boil lanced – if it is done inexpertly, the result may be severe scarring.

Nowadays, antibiotics can often clear boils either before they become too painful or before they discharge.

Bullae

Medical term for a large blister. See page 223.

Corns and calluses

Both words describe harmless thickening of the skin, which develops as a protective measure.

◆ A corn

Typically appears on the upper surface of the little toe, where the toe rubs against shoes.

◆ A callus

Plural, callosities, is a thickening of the skin of the hands or feet. People who go habitually barefoot develop callosities on the pressure-bearing areas of the sole.

Likewise, manual workers develop callosities on the palms of the hands, typically at the base of the fingers.

Flab

Apart from obvious folds of fatty tissue that go with obesity, flab is sometimes used to describe skin which has lost elasticity: you can pick it up in folds, and it fails to return immediately to its original contours.

There are three main causes:

◆ Ageing

With age, skin loses its elasticity. Wrinkles, skin creases and sagging jaw lines are part of the process – and provide limitless work for cosmetic surgeons.

◆ Dehydration

The body needs a certain amount of water in order to function properly. Severe loss of fluid can arise because of reduced intake (for example when someone is in a coma) or increased output (for example with diarrhoea or vomiting).

The result is flabby, turgid skin, which will not unwrinkle when pinched. Naturally, this effect of fluid loss does not happen overnight.

◆ Massive weight loss

If you are obese, and manage, with a commendable spurt of willpower, to lose a large proportion of your weight very rapidly, you may be unjustly repaid with a new problem. The skin needs time to compensate for the loss of fat; meanwhile, huge lax folds of skin develop, particularly on the abdomen, buttocks, thighs and upper arms. Cosmetic surgery may be helpful in some cases.

Hard skin, local or general

The obvious diagnosis is a corn or callus, covered separately on the opposite page. Here are the less self-evident causes.

Probable

◆ Keloid

Describes excessive scarring after cuts or injury and is seen most commonly in black people. The site of the injury hardens, with an overgrowth of hard scar tissue above the level of the surrounding skin. Why some people develop keloid scarring and others don't is a mystery. It is harmless, but severe cases sometimes require treatment for the scar tissue, either by injection or by further surgery.

There is no guarantee that this will lead to a more satisfactory appearance.

Possible

◆ Lymphoedema

◆ Post-phlebitic limb

See *Swollen ankle*, page 289.

◆ Myxoedema

Puffy swelling of the skin, particularly on hands, feet and ankles and around eyes.

May be seen with hypothyroidism, see page 320.

Rare

◆ Vitamin A deficiency

Night blindness.

- Abnormality of the cornea leading to inflammation, scarring and blindness.
- Rough, dry skin.

◆ Morphoea

A localized variant of scleroderma, see below.

- Well-defined, pale areas.
- The skin in these areas is smooth and hard.
- Loss of hair at these sites may occur.
- Ulceration may occur.

◆ Scleroderma

An auto-immune disease.

- Hard, rigid skin develops.
- Tiny red spots (telangiectasia) are evident.

- Skin becomes shiny and smooth.
- Hands become stiff.
- Joints may become stiff.
- Skin of face is affected, making the mouth appear small.
- Face lacks expression.
- Raynaud's phenomenon (see page 278) develops.
- Swallowing is impaired and weight loss follows.

See also *Problems with swallowing plus weight loss*, page 115.

◆ Cancer

Secondary or metastatic cancer deposits (having spread from a primary site elsewhere) can arise in the skin, giving small areas which are hard to the touch. They may be single or multiple.

A somewhat specialized example is a secondary deposit in the navel, called Sister Joseph's nodule, after the nun who first observed it at the Mayo Clinic.

An itchy rash

Probable

◆ Eczema

See page 317.

◆ Urticaria

Commonly called hives. A type of allergic reaction, triggered by various different agents.

Typically, urticaria appears suddenly and dramatically. The wheal may come

and go quite quickly, clearing in one area, only to reappear in another.

- Red, blotchy areas with puffy, paler patches in the middle.
- Some swelling.
- Itchy, often intensely so.

There are several types, grouped according to cause or appearance. One form, dermatographia, is particularly severe: just stroking the skin firmly raises a wheal – you can even draw a picture on the skin. The most common form is allergic urticaria.

Common causes include: plants, chemicals, food, medicine colourants.

◆ Scabies

◆ Lichen planus

Very itchy, flat-topped, purplish bumps on the skin, especially on the wrists and often associated with white patches in the mouth. The cause is usually unknown.

◆ Lice

◆ Insect bites

Can occur as an itchy rash, or with no obvious rash. Details, page 94.

◆ Fungal infection

See page 238.

◆ Pityriasis rosea

Commonest in young people, and may be associated with a viral infection.

- A single, itchy red lesion may appear anywhere on the trunk – the herald patch.
- After a few days, scattered patches of pinkish elevated areas develop. They characteristically lie along the line of the ribs.
- The rash persists for about six weeks.

Usually no treatment is required. Calamine lotion or, in severe cases, antihistamine drugs, may help.

◆ Lichen simplex

You scratch an itchy place. The itchiness goes for a while, but as soon it comes back, you scratch again. A vicious cycle of scratching and itching develops, causing local inflammation. The inflammation causes thickening of the skin, with furrows or lines developing in the chronic case.

◆ Pruritis ani

◆ Vulval itch

These conditions are often characterized by itching plus rash. See pages 316.

◆ Drug reaction

If you are allergic to a drug, the classic reaction is:

- Widespread rash, but predominating on the trunk.
- Patchy reddening.
- Some local swelling.
- Intense itching.

Reactions to drugs can occur even after long-term use.

Rare

◆ Nodular prurigo

- Multiple warty areas.
- Intensely itchy.
- Cause unknown, but possibly initiated by scratching.

◆ Lichen sclerosis et atrophicus

Involves skin around the vulva, anus or penis.

- White, pale skin.
- Clearly delineated.
- Reddened areas within the affected skin.
- Itchy.

When seen on children this may wrongly be attributed to abuse.

Itching – without a rash

Covered here is persistent, severe itching that has become a nuisance. The medical term is pruritus.

Close inspection with a magnifying glass may reveal either of the common causes – scabies and lice. Scratch marks are the obvious evidence of severe itching, and of course they also reveal to the doctor where the symptom is at its worst.

Excluded here are an itching scalp caused by a bad bout of dandruff, covered separately on page 265; and itching in the anal area, covered separately on page 150.

Probable

◆ Scabies

Infestation with the scabies mite, which burrows under the skin.

- Severe itching is noted.
- Mite burrows may be seen as grey lines a couple of millimeters long.
- Burrows are often between fingers or front of wrists.
- Eventually, raised, reddened areas may appear all over the body.
- Scabs may develop because of scratching.

◆ Lice

Commonly known as nits. There are three main types: head lice, body lice and pubic lice.

- Persistent itching.
- Local lymph nodes may enlarge.
- Eggs may be seen on the bases of hairs; or you may see lice themselves: they are quite elusive.
- Spread by direct contact with other infected hairs or skin.
- The pubic louse may cause itching in the anal or vulval regions.

◆ Insect bites including fleas

- Itching at the site of the bite.
- Reddened, hard nodules at the site of the bite appear later.
- Fleas are commonly the culprits; commonest in homes with cats.

◆ Fibreglass

Glass fibres can become invisibly embedded in skin, causing itching. Protective clothing should be worn.

◆ Senile pruritis

The elderly sometimes complain of itching for which no cause can be found: it may be the result of the ageing process.

◆ Threadworm

See *Worms*, page 144.

- Itching and irritation around the anus.

Most children have this common complaint at some time. Treatment is simple, and available either directly from the chemist or from a doctor.

◆ Strep infection

Commonest in young children. A bacterial infection of the anal skin causing a chronic, itchy anal condition.

Possible

◆ Pregnancy

Many women complain of itching in the last months of pregnancy. Local causes such as thrush need to be excluded.

◆ Liver disease

◆ Jaundice

Any condition which causes jaundice, typically, liver disease, may also cause intense itching. The itching may arise before the yellow skin colour is noticed.

◆ Drugs

Some drugs, for instance, penicillin and aspirin, can cause severe allergic reactions, with itching. And some of the narcotic drugs, including cocaine and heroin, may cause itching, sometimes related to impurities.

◆ Psychological

Itching without any cause found after full examination and investigation may be a sign of underlying psychological problems.

Rare

◆ Dermatitis herpetiformis

See page 225.

◆ Uraemia

High levels of urea in the blood are one of the end results of untreated renal (kidney) failure. A number of symptoms may be present:

- Dry, coated tongue.
- Breath smelling of urine.
- Hiccups.
- Nausea and vomiting.
- Dry, yellow-brown skin with a whitish 'frost'.
- Marked itching.
- Anaemia.

◆ Blood disorders

A number of blood and related diseases may cause severe itching. They include: Polycythemia rubra vera; lymphoma; Hodgkin's disease; leukaemias.

Pruritis

The medical term for itching.
See pages 27-8, 68-9, 150-1, 242-3, 244-5, 300-1, and 316-7.

Skin feels clammy

If associated with coldness, look at Itching or numbness, page 300.

Dry skin

The two simple explanations are inflammation, or failure of the sweat glands to work normally.

Probable

◆ **Eczema**

See page 317. When not in a phase of acute inflammation, patches of skin affected by eczema may feel dry and rough to the touch.

◆ **Fungal infections**

See page 238.

Possible

◆ **Heat (sun) stroke**

Prolonged physical work in hot conditions or staying too long in the sun puts anyone, even the fit athlete, at risk of heat stroke.

- Commonest in the very young and the elderly. Symptoms may develop rapidly.
- Dry skin, hot to the touch.
- High temperature.
- Weakness.
- Thirst.
- Headache.
- Confusion.

- If untreated, can be fatal. It is important to protect yourself against the sun:

- Wear hat, shirt; apply sun block; maintain a high fluid intake (no alcohol).

- Keep cool by taking frequent showers or swimming; avoid exposure to the midday sun.

If you suspect this condition, seek medical help urgently.

◆ **Hypothyroidism**

See page 320.

Rare

◆ **Uraemia**

See page 245.

◆ **Vitamin A deficiency**

See page 242.

◆ **Ichthyosis**

A group of inherited disorders of the skin, in which the skin is thickened, dry and flaky. Often the inner aspect of skin overlying joints (typically armpits and elbow creases) is spared.

- Very occasionally, these changes, appearing in later life, may be associated with underlying malignant disease.

Body odour

This is possibly the vaguest and most subjective symptom of all. Doctors and dentists see many people who believe that they smell, or that some part of them smells, even though no one else has commented.

Some people seem to be abnormally sensitive to smells.

And some people, notably small children, have a virtually non-existent sense of smell.

Serious underlying disease is very rarely the reason for offensive body odour. If you put aside obvious cases of body odour caused by stale sweat, and if you also exclude psychological cases, where the smell is a belief rather than a physical fact, body odour usually comes down to three relatively common possibilities:

◆ Athlete's foot

A fungal infection of the feet with reddened, itchy, painful areas between the toes, fissuring and cracking. The feet and shoes give off a characteristic cheesy odour, which is sometimes strong enough for others to smell, even if the shoes are on.

◆ Bad breath

See *Halitosis*, page 82.

◆ Offensive discharges

for example vaginal discharge.

...and one rare possibility:

◆ Fish odour syndrome

One of several rare metabolic diseases. The first three are easily remedied by self-help and commonsense use of over-the-counter medications. The last needs specialist treatment and advice on odour-concealment.

The Hair

Lifeless hair

Loss of 'body' or 'life' in the hair is to some extent inevitable with advancing years. It is also seen in association with medical conditions that cause baldness. Severe stress, such as that caused by major, prolonged illness, can also affect the quality and thickness of hair. Vitamin deficiency and severe undernourishment will also affect hair quality

Loss of hair or baldness

Also known as alopecia.

Hair loss, known as 'male pattern alopecia' – in other words balding – is part of the normal male ageing process and is characterized by:

- Recession of the hairline at the forehead and temples.
- Thinning of the hair on the crown. It becomes frizzy and loses 'body'.

- A gradual meeting of the hairless areas so that hair remains only on the sides and back of the head.

Though women are not prone to baldness, thinning and hair loss happen in most women as they get older.

Abnormal hair loss can of course be a sign (in women as well is in men) of scalp disease, or more generalized disease.

The Hair

Stages of male baldness

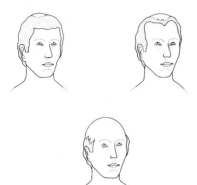

Most such cases, as this section shows, are fairly easy to distinguish from normal baldness.

Probable

◆ Eczema or dermatitis

Any inflammatory skin condition may cause loss of hair in the affected areas.

- Complete patches of hair loss.
- Skin is itchy, inflamed, weeping and may have some crusting.

There is often some dermatitis or eczema elsewhere on the body, though this could be a localized contact sensitivity on the scalp (for example, from a hair dye).

◆ Alopecia areata

The commonest cause of patchy baldness.

- Local areas of total baldness, often only a few centimeters across.
- Normal 'baby smooth' skin.

- Several patches may occur together.

Regrowth normally occurs spontaneously after a few months, but if there has been damage to the pigment cells deep in the skin, new hair can be white when it reappears. This is often seen at a time of stress, such as bereavement.

◆ Childbirth

Many women notice changes in hair substance and texture before and after childbirth: Scalp hairs normally live for about three to seven years. Hairs are continually reaching the end of their life, entering the 'falling out phase', which lasts a few weeks.

During pregnancy, however, no hairs switch into this falling-out phase and so hair density gradually increases, resulting in a lovely thick head of hair by the end of the pregnancy. After childbirth, all those hairs that would have naturally fallen out over the previous nine months do so at once, resulting in a somewhat dramatic shedding of hair, which can be quite alarming.

In rare cases, the original texture of the hair is never restored.

Possible

◆ Injury

Burns, skin loss or even deep cuts can damage hair-bearing skin, so that hair may never re-grow.

Generally speaking, hair does not grow on scar tissue. The only solution is to hide such areas by expert combing and styling.

The Hair

◆ Trichotillomania

Nervous playing with the hair leaves it twisted, broken or with bald patches.

◆ Psoriasis

- Hair loss in areas of psoriasis on the scalp.
- Silvery, scaly red patches seen in scalp.
- Other signs of psoriasis seen elsewhere on body; see page 226.

◆ Iron deficiency

- Generalized hair loss or thinning.
- May improve after taking iron supplements.
- See also *Iron deficiency anaemia*, page 394.

◆ Hypothyroidism

- See page 320.
- Hair is sparse.
- Hair may be dry and thin.

◆ Post-menopausal change

Hair texture may change in and around the menopause due to alterations in hormone balance. The role of hormone replacement therapy in protecting against or reversing the effects of the menopause is a subject of continuing research.

◆ Ringworm

Medical term tinea capitis. A fungal infection of the skin of the scalp.

- Circular bald patches.
- Scaling of the skin.
- Brittle hair stumps remain.

  Treatment can be creams or tablets.

Rare

◆ AIDS

Hair loss may be noted in the later stages of AIDS.

◆ Hypopituitarism

Under-activity of the pituitary gland may show itself in many ways, including:

- Absence of sexual function (absence of libido).
- Absence of periods in females.
- Pale skin.
- Hair loss.
- Visual defects.
- Weight gain and fatigue.

  See also page 390.

◆ Anagen alopecia

Some drugs affect hair during their growth phase, notably anticancer 'cell poisons' given as courses of chemotherapy. Vitamin A toxicity (for example with the powerful acne drug, roaccutane) may rarely cause diffuse hair loss. After stopping the drug, hair usually grows again. Anticoagulant therapy is another, not uncommon cause.

Site of pituitary gland

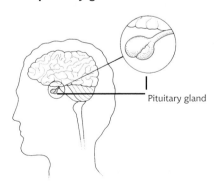

Pituitary gland

Dandruff

The cause of this very common condition is sensitivity to a yeast known as Malassezia furfur. It lives on the scalp of about one person in four. About 10 per cent of people become sensitive to it and the result is dandruff. The only way to remain clear is to use an anti-yeast shampoo, even if only once a fortnight.

The worst cases are accompanied by itching of the scalp. Sometimes a steroid-based scalp application may be necessary. Rarely other conditions, such as psoriasis are diagnosed.

Unwanted body hair

It is one of nature's many ironies that while baldness is almost universally an unwanted male symptom, unwanted body hair is almost exclusively a female symptom.

Covered here is hirsutism in its specific sense of a male pattern of hair distribution on a woman.

Probable

◆ Normal pattern

Patterns of hair growth on face, limbs and body vary according to country or region of origin.

Individuals should compare themselves with others from a similar ethnic background before deciding that they have abnormally hairy bodies. For example, Japanese and Chinese women have very little body hair, whereas Mediterranean people may have much more.

Possible

◆ Polycystic ovaries

Otherwise known as the Stein-Leventhal syndrome.

- Hairiness.
- Obesity.
- Acne.
- Absent or very infrequent periods.
- Ovaries have multiple cysts.

◆ Menopause

Women going through the menopause may note increased amounts of hair, typically fine hair that appears on the face.

Rare

◆ Drugs

A number of drugs may increase either fine hair on the face or body hair elsewhere. They include:

- Some steroid preparations.
- Hormone treatments, including the pill.
- Minoxidil, used to treat raised blood pressure, but now also used as a hair restorer.
- Some anti-epileptic drugs.

◆ Anorexia

Severe wasting conditions can cause an excess of hair growth.

The most common situation is anorexia nervosa, where an excess growth of fine downy hair, known as lanugo hair, occurs, typically on the face.

◆ Acromegaly

In addition to its other features (see page 426), women with acromegaly may have increased body hair.

◆ Cushing's syndrome

May be caused by a disorder of the adrenal gland, or by taking steroids.

- Round, 'moon' face.
- Fat deposited on back (buffalo-hump).
- Fat deposited on body (not legs).
- Muscle fatigue.
- Easily bruised skin.
- Stretch marks.
- Bone pain.

Women also note:

- Increased body hair.
- Periods stop.
- Enlarged clitoris.

Men may suffer from:

- Impotence.
- Acne.

◆ Turner's syndrome

A genetic disorder where an apparently female person has only one female chromosome, instead of the two needed for normal female development.
   Changes include:

- Very short stature.

- No secondary sexual characteristics (with total absence of periods).
- Short web-necked appearance.
- Broad chest with widely separated nipples.
- Deafness.
- Hirsutism.

◆ Congenital adrenal hyperplasia

Excessive growth of the adrenal glands from birth

- Mild hirsutism.
- Enlarged clitoris.
- Fused labia.

May appear at a later age with:

- Acne.
- Early false puberty.
- Enlarged clitoris.
- Absent or scanty periods.

Site of adrenal gland

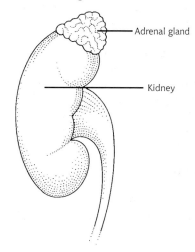

Adrenal gland

Kidney

The skeletal and muscular symptoms

The bones, joints and muscles: introduction

This section covers the body's 'chassis': the frame on which the tissues hang. Connected to the bones are the muscles whose expansion and contraction, lengthening and shortening, provides movement. They have many common problems.

In this section the usual order of symptoms has been varied in order to begin with some key general symptoms of muscles and bones occurring elsewhere in the body. We then move to specific bone, joint and muscle symptoms as experienced in different parts of the body, working from the shoulders downwards. Finally, under the heading *Fingers and toes*, are grouped symptoms affecting the outer reaches, or extremities, of the body, which are vulnerable in certain special ways.

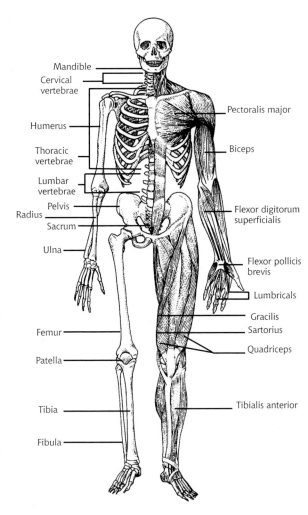

Mandible
Cervical vertebrae
Humerus
Thoracic vertebrae
Lumbar vertebrae
Pelvis
Radius
Sacrum
Ulna
Femur
Patella
Tibia
Fibula

Pectoralis major
Biceps
Flexor digitorum superficialis
Flexor pollicis brevis
Lumbricals
Gracilis
Sartorius
Quadriceps
Tibialis anterior

Wasting and loss of power in the muscles

Muscular wasting, or atrophy, results from either damage to the nerve or blood supply to a muscle; lack of use because of illness or injury; or primary muscle disease.

Probable

◆ Injury

The body's normal protective response to immobilization of the affected part. One of the best examples of this is a damaged knee. The knee is held slightly flexed, and you try to prevent movement for a few days. By the end of a week, you may well see some wasting of the quadriceps muscle at the front of the thigh. The weaker the muscle, the less safe the joint feels, and a vicious circle of disuse and further wasting then continues. This is why careful medical assessment and controlled exercises to maintain muscle bulk are important for all such injuries.

◆ General body wasting

Bed-bound patients can develop generalized disuse atrophy (wasting) of these muscles. This can be aggravated by the underlying condition.

Possible

◆ Carpal tunnel syndrome

See page 274.

◆ Injury of a nerve or nerves

See page 299.

◆ Diabetes

See *Diabetic neuropathy*, page 297.

◆ Alcoholic neuropathy

See page 298.

◆ Rheumatoid arthritis

See page 261.

Rare

◆ Motor neurone disease

A disease of the nervous system. There are several forms, but the main features are:

- Progressive onset of muscular weakness, accompanied by muscle wasting.

- Small muscles of the hand are affected first.

- 'Flickering' contractions of parts of muscles.

The disease progresses relentlessly, ultimately affecting speech, swallowing and breathing muscles.

◆ Duchenne's dystrophy

This is a primary muscle disease affecting boys, which starts during the first few years of life.

- Wasting and weakness of back and pelvic muscles; affects both sides of the body.

- Failure of function affecting both sides of the body leads to a 'waddling' gait while still mobile.

- Gradual degeneration leading to inability to walk and general immobility.

- Immobility leads to the muscles shortening, and deformity becomes inevitable.

- The outlook is poor.

◆ Subacute combined degeneration of the spinal cord

See page 300.

Skeleton and Muscles

Cramps, aches and pains in the muscles

Most are of little significance. If they die away within a few days they should not be taken seriously, unless they are recurrent.

Probable

◆ Simple cramp

- Sudden onset of muscle spasm, often while asleep.
- Muscle, often the calf, feels hard due to contraction.
- Relieved by massage.
- Often residual discomfort for a few hours.

◆ Viral or bacterial infection

Fleeting muscular pains are a common accompaniment of any infection. Most settle within a day or two. No specific treatment is required, apart from that for the underlying infection.

◆ Injury

A direct blow to a muscle can cause painful local swelling and bruising. Indirect injury, for instance straining to lift a heavy object, can make muscle fibres stretch and tear. Repetition of the movement reproduces the pain. Treatment for both is painkillers and resting the affected muscle.

Possible

◆ Intermittent claudication

See *Peripheral vascular disease*, page 298.

◆ Spinal stenosis

The spinal cord runs through a bony tunnel within each of the vertebrae of the back. In later life this tunnel often becomes narrowed, squeezing the spinal cord.

- Pain felt in the muscles of the buttock, thigh or leg, worse when walking.
- Pain often improves when bending forwards.
- Usually affects adults over the age of 50.
- Associated with back pain and is due to wear and tear, degenerative change in the back, or associated with long-standing disc prolapse problems.

◆ Biomechanical imbalance

Loss of salt, typically after strenuous exercise, can precipitate painful cramps.

◆ Polymyalgia rheumatica

- A disease of the elderly.
- Painful, upper limb muscles.
- Extreme muscle stiffness, particularly in the morning, where you have to roll out of bed
- Malaise.
- Fever.

Rare

◆ Drugs

A number of drugs are known to cause muscle pains. The most widely used drugs associated with this are statins.

Skeleton and Muscles

Others include lithium, alcohol, amphetamines and suxamethonium (used for general anaesthesia).

◆ Dermatomyositis

A disease associated with disordered immunity. May very rarely be associated with cancer.

- Inflammation and pains in multiple muscle groups.
- Muscular weakness.
- Rash often around eyes and on the backs of hands.

◆ Polymyositis

Can be associated with many diseases, including collagen disorders and lung cancer. May remit and relapse.

- Progressive, painful inflammation of muscles – worse when used.
- Affects muscles in a variable manner, but those affected are weak.
- Fever.
- Malaise.
- Rapid heart rate

◆ Cushing's syndrome

Caused by an excess of corticosteroids, and often the result of doctors giving steroids to treat other diseases such as rheumatoid arthritis.

- Weight gain, except for limbs.
- Moon face.
- Buffalo hump.
- Muscle weakness.
- Purple lines (striae) on abdomen, back and upper thighs.

- Osteoporosis.
- Diabetes.
- High blood pressure.
- Hair grows on body.
- Occasional psychiatric disorders.

◆ Primary aldosteronism

A very rare disease, also known as Conn's syndrome, caused by excess secretion of the chemical aldosterone by the adrenal gland.

- Muscle weakness.
- Excessive thirst.
- Excessive urine output.
- High blood pressure.

◆ Tetanus

Caused by the organism *Clostridia tetani* and acquired by contamination of open wounds. The damage is done by a very powerful toxin that attacks the nervous system. Symptoms may take two weeks or more to develop.

- Local muscular weakness near site of infection.
- Facial muscles go into spasm: the individual appears to be forcing a grin.
- Muscles of the body go into spasm at the slightest stimulus.
- Fever.

Tetanus still claims victims, even when cared for in specialized units. Immunization is the essential precaution, and needs to be repeated every ten years until you have had at least 5 tetanus vaccinations.

Skeleton and Muscles

Poor or absent muscle control

See *The brain and nervous system*, pages
348-382, especially *Convulsions*, page 358,
and *Paralysis*, pages 377.

Involuntary twitching or trembling muscles

See page 409.

Painful bones

Pain in bones can be either localized – to
part of one or more bones – or generalized.

Types of fracture

Probable

◆ **Injury**

Is it broken?

Signs of a break (fracture) are:

• Pain at the site of injury.

• Possibly deformity – the limb looks bent.

• Loss of function – typically inability
to bear weight.

Simple

Depending on the site and force of
the injury, skin, nerves and blood
vessels may be involved.

Obviously, urgent medical attention
is needed.

Persistent pain following an injury,
particularly when accompanied by
swelling, should raise the suspicion of
a fracture. Seek medical help.

Compound

Lesser injury may not cause a break,
but can still cause pain and loss of
function. See also *Subperiosteal
haematoma*, next page.

Incomplete

Bones swollen or misshapen

Probable

◆ Callus

New bone formed after a fracture.

- Previous, definite bone fracture.
- Forms within a few weeks.
- The larger the bone, the greater the amount of callus.
- Pain-free when bone is fully healed.

◆ Subperiosteal haematoma

- A direct injury to bone, typically the shin, but no fracture.
- Clear history of local injury.
- Swelling (bruising) noted almost immediately.
- Painful for several weeks after the injury.
- A hard lump still apparent weeks or months afterwards.

  Common in those who play 'rough and tumble', or contact, sports.

◆ Osteoarthritis

See page 281.

◆ Osteoporosis

See page 259.

Possible

◆ Secondary cancer

There is the possibility of localized bone pain being caused by a secondary (metastatic) deposit in someone with cancer. So if an individual has a known cancer elsewhere in the body, this possibility needs considering. In an otherwise fit person, it becomes a rare rather than possible diagnosis.

◆ Inflammatory arthropathies

A term for joint inflammation, e.g. rheumatoid arthritis or ankylosing spondylitis, See pages 268.

◆ Acute osteomyelitis

A bone infection which, if suspected, requires immediate treatment. A primary site of infection elsewhere in the body may be apparent, the bone being affected by bacteria carried in the bloodstream.

- High, persistent fever.
- Sudden onset of pain in bone with swelling, which may not be obvious.
- Overlying redness and swelling of the soft tissues, not the bone.
- Extreme pain on movement.
- Rigors.
- Malaise.

◆ Chronic osteomyelitis

May occur after untreated or inadequately treated acute osteomyelitis; or after a compound fracture (where there is a fracture and a cut down to the bone).

- Thickening of bone.
- Wound (sinus) discharging pus.
- Local pain.
- Inflammation around wound.

◆ Malunion of fracture

Failure of adequate reduction – meaning a poorly joined break.

Sometimes this occurs despite careful realignment or setting of the broken bone.

It may give the appearance of deformity or swelling.

◆ Paget's disease of the bone

See page 407.

Rare

◆ Rickets and osteomalacia

See page 269.

◆ Acromegaly

General enlargement of the skeleton caused by excessive growth hormone from the pituitary gland. Jaws and hands appear especially large.

◆ Benign tumour of bone and cartilage

Both bone and cartilage in any part of the body may give rise to benign tumours which present as:

* Pain-free hard lumps.

* Smooth surfaces.
* Slow-growing.

◆ Cancer of the bone or cartilage

Individuals with known cancer of other organs of the body (for example breast or lung) may develop secondary tumours (deposits) in the bones.

* Chronically and progressively painful.
* Pain may be very localized.
* A lump may not be present.

Other symptoms of advanced cancer may be present, but sometimes bone secondaries are the first indication of an as-yet undiagnosed cancer. This is why localized pain in a bone without a history of injury should be followed up with your doctor.

Primary malignant bone tumours are rarer than secondary tumours. They may form at any age, and there are several different types.

◆ Tuberculosis

See page 427.

Bones breaking easily

Meaning fractures occurring without an obvious history of injury. They divide into two types: those which are the result of disease (pathological) and those in apparently normal bones (spontaneous or stress fractures).

Spontaneous or stress fractures may occur because of repeated bending, as when athletes train; or after repeated compression, for instance jumping and running, that acts on the spine.

* Local pain.
* Local swelling.
* Relieved by rest over a few days.
* Pain recurs when activity is repeated.
* May not be seen initially on an X-ray.

Typical sites include the small bones of the foot (metatarsals); upper arm bone (humerus); upper thigh bone (neck of femur); knee cap (patella); and spine.

Skeleton and Muscles

Humerus

Spine

Thigh bone
or femur

Knee cap

Metatarsals

In pathological fractures, the bone is abnormally weak because of either local abnormality (for example, malignant tumours, tuberculosis, osteomyelitis) or general abnormality (for example, osteoporosis, osteomalacia).

These abnormalities can be congenital (for example, brittle bone disease) or acquired (rheumatoid arthritis). Also, if a bone is unused, it becomes thinner and is prone to break.

Probable

◆ Osteoporosis

The inclusion of osteoporotic fractures under pathological fractures is a little controversial, but the simple fact remains that osteoporotic bone is not normal bone. Gradual thinning of the bone, particularly in elderly females, may result in broken bones without significant injury. A fracture of the neck of the femur is very common. The symptoms are:

- Pain in the groin/hip (after or causing a fall).

- Apparent shortening of the leg.

- Inability to bear weight on the affected side.

- The foot on the affected side may be turned outwards.

Most commonly treated with an operation to realign and fix the broken bone.

Other common sites of osteoporotic fractures include the wrist (breaks easily after a mild fall) and the upper backbone (thoracic spine) which often breaks on its own, causing pain and the stoop often present, particularly in elderly ladies.

Skeleton and Muscles

Skeleton and Muscles

Possible

◆ Osteomalacia

See *Rickets and osteomalacia*, page 269.

◆ Disused bone

Bone requires regular use to maintain its normal structure. If unused because of paralysis (for instance by a stroke, multiple sclerosis or spina bifida), the bones become weak and may even break when the individual is being carried, or turned in bed.

So, bone pain in any bedridden or partially paralysed individual may be caused by a fracture.

◆ Bone cancer

Whilst uncommon in someone not known to have cancer, severe bone pain following a minor injury should be taken seriously in someone known to have cancer, and bone cancer in particular.

See page 258.

Rare

◆ Paget's disease of the bone

See page 407.

◆ Osteomyelitis

◆ Benign bone tumours

◆ Brittle bone disease (osteogengesis imperfecta)

There are several types. In the severest form, fractures develop in the womb and at birth. In the milder form, fractures occur later in life. This is a hereditary disorder of connective tissue, often found in many members of a family. It prevents bones and other tissue forming properly.

The symptoms may include:

• Bones fracture with minimal injury.

• Whites of the eyes appear blue.

• Teeth may be deformed.

• General deformity because of repeated fractures.

Other possible symptoms include hearing loss, teeth problems and easy bruising.

◆ Marble bones

Also known as osteopetrosis. A very rare, inherited condition, in which bones become even more solid and hard than usual.

As well as an increased likelihood of fractures, growth may be affected.

Inflamed or aching joints

Virtually any generalized disease, such as influenza, gives symptoms of aching in joints and muscles. These are often fleeting, moving from one joint or muscle to another. Many diseases have major or primary involvement with joints, the most significant of which are:

Probable

◆ Viral infection

Any viral infection, such as the common cold or influenza, will give vague joint pains.

• General malaise.

• Fever.

- Cough, runny nose.
- Muscle pain.
- Joint pain.
- Normally cures itself in a few days.

Some viruses can lead to joint swelling for a longer period of time e.g. german measles (rubella), slapped cheek disease (parvovirus) and glandular fever.

◆ Osteoarthritis

See page 281.

Possible

◆ Gout

Caused by excess uric acid in the blood. May be caused by heavy drinking; medication (for example, bendroflumethiazide used to treat high blood pressure); a kidney problem; certain diets high in 'purine foods' (for example, marmite, game meat) and other rarer causes.

- One joint is affected at a time ('monarticular'); most commonly it affects the big toe joint first.
- Sudden onset.
- The joint is hot, shiny, red and excruciatingly painful.
- There may be malaise and fever. Attacks recur and involve other joints. Each attack may last around one week.
- Gouty tophi, lumpy collections of uric acid crystals, form in the skin, particularly on the ears and adjacent to joints.

The high levels of uric acid, if untreated, can cause kidney stones and kidney failure. Blood tests or taking a sample of fluid from the swollen joint help to confirm the diagnosis.

Lifestyle changes and medication can control the symptoms.

◆ Rheumatoid arthritis

The commonest type of chronic, generalized inflammatory joint disease. It is actually a connective tissue disease and it may be hereditary. Symptoms are caused by persistent inflammation of the synovial membrane, which lines the joint capsules. Commonest in young women. Treatment consists of pain relief and reduction of inflammation. Recent advances in medication have revolutionized treatment.

In the later stages, severe cases may need surgery to improve function impaired by deformity.

An immunoglobulin called rheumatoid factor is commonly present in the blood of affected individuals. Features include:

- Painful swelling of joints (often symmetrical).
- Early morning stiffness.
- Progressive joint deformity. (See also sections on specific joints.)
- Progressive loss of function.
- Lumps may appear in the skin and around joints.
- Osteoporosis may develop.
- Anaemia.
- Muscle wasting.
- Higher risk of heart disease later in life.

Skeleton and Muscles

◆ Ankylosing spondylitis

See page 268.

◆ Sickle cell disease

An inherited disease found in those of African origin. The red blood cells become sickle-shaped when low amounts of oxygen are available. These sickle cells are less pliable than normal cells and so block up capillaries (small blood vessels) causing damage to organs because of lack of oxygen and poor blood supply. Some individuals are less affected – they are described as having sickle cell trait.

Those with full-blown disease have recurrent attacks of severe pains, in limbs and abdomen – sickle crises.

Features of the disease include:

• Anaemia.

• Increased predisposition to infection.

• Joint pains.

• Fever.

• Jaundice.

• Abdominal pains.

Treatment is mainly aimed at relieving the symptoms. Blood transfusions, administering oxygen and strong painkillers are mainstays.

Rare

◆ Septic arthritis

This is a very serious condition and should be seen by a doctor the first day it is noticed. A joint becomes infected with a bacteria. Most commonly this occurs after joint surgery (such as a joint replacement) or in a joint damaged by arthritis.

Distal interphalangeal joint

Distal interphalangeal joint

Symptoms include:

• Painful, swollen, hot and possibly red joint. Usually only one joint is affected.

• Fever.

• Frequently feeling unwell.

Treatment is a course of antibiotics lasting many weeks, often starting in hospital on a drip.

◆ Juvenile idiopathic arthritis

This is the childhood form of rheumatoid arthritis and similar conditions.

◆ Reiter's syndrome

Occurs in adults, mainly in men. It occurs a few weeks after a bowel infection (such as. salmonella), or a sexual infection (such as chlamydia).

There will be the following three symptoms:

• Urethritis – burning on passing water, often with a discharge.

• Conjunctivitis .

- Arthritis – pain and swelling of two or three joints, for example a hip, knee or ankle.

◆ Psoriatic arthritis

Occasionally, arthritis can be a complication of psoriasis, a skin disease.

- Various joints, in different parts of the body, are affected.
- The distal interphalangeal joints may be the only ones involved.
- Possibly nail pitting.

◆ Gonococcal arthritis

One of many complications of the sexually transmitted disease gonorrhoea.
In males the main symptom is:

- Urethral discharge.

In females up to 75 per cent may have no symptoms. Those that do may have:

- Pain on passing urine.
- Vaginal discharge.
- May develop in one joint with symptoms of infective arthritis (see opposite).

◆ Systemic lupus erythematosis (SLE)

See page 417.

◆ Rheumatic fever

◆ Haemophilia

See page 399.

◆ Syphilis

See page 344.

Skeleton and Muscles

Swollen joints with nodules

Probable

◆ Bursa

Many joints have sacs, like empty balloons, overlying their surfaces. If damaged, these fill with fluid and enlarge. They feel like smooth, fluid-filled swellings and may be uncomfortable and irritating. In particular, the bursa in front of the knee may become swollen after kneeling: commonly known as housemaid's knee.

◆ Osteoarthritis

See page 281.

Possible

◆ Rheumatoid arthritiis

See page 261.

◆ Gout

See page 261.

Rare

◆ Charcot's joints

Joints that have lost the sense of pain and position. If the joint is damaged, it can become progressively more deformed, as degeneration occurs rapidly. The joint looks as if it should be very painful, possibly with extreme swelling and deformity. Fluid, bony protuberances and loose pieces of bone may easily be felt in and around the joint. Dislocation is not uncommon. The commoner causes include syphilis, spina bifida, indeed anything that can damage the peripheral nerve system, including diabetes and alcohol.

Skeleton and Muscles

Painful joints

See *Inflamed or aching joints*, page 260.

Stiff joints

See *Inflamed or aching joints* page 260.

Painful shoulder

Probable

◆ Frozen shoulder

Commonest in later middle age.

- Slight injury to shoulder joint may or may not have occurred.
- Subsequently progressive pain and stiffness.
- Pain starts at shoulder tip and runs down outer arm towards the elbow.

Can be very disabling, with reduced movement of the shoulder and pain when moving it, or lying on it at night.

Tends to cure itself over a year or so, but may be treated with physiotherapy or a cortisone injection to encourage movement of the shoulder.

Called 'frozen shoulder' because someone with this condition tends to hold their shoulder very still, due to the pain.

Possible

◆ Painful arc syndrome

Most common in a middle-aged or later middle-aged person.

- Pain at shoulder tip.
- Variable in intensity; worse at night.

Dislocation of the shoulder

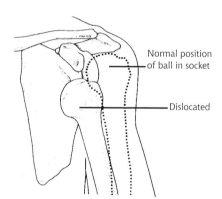

Normal position of ball in socket

Dislocated

- Limited shoulder movement.
- Local area of tenderness – can be identified with one fingertip.
- Pain worse over part of the 'arc' made by raising the arm from the side.

◆ Rotator cuff tear

Tendons lying at the upper part of the shoulder can tear or rupture without warning. Tends to occur with pre-existing wear and tear changes, and so typical of the elderly.

- May be associated with a fall or lifting.
- Sudden onset of pain.
- Arm cannot be moved outwards.

◆ Dislocation of the shoulder

A common injury in 'contact' sports. The shoulder is a ball and socket joint. Forceful injury makes the ball, which is found at the top of the humerus (upper arm bone), slip out of its socket.

- Pain on movement.
- Loss of shoulder contour.
- 'Ball' (humeral head) may be felt below the outer end of the collar bone.
- Arm is held out from the body at elbow.

◆ Rheumatoid arthritis

The shoulder joint can be affected in patients with rheumatoid arthritis. See page 261.

◆ Fractured collarbone (clavicle)

The shoulder bone is known medically as the clavicle and may break as a result of direct or indirect injury.

- Pain at the point of the break.
- Pain on arm movement: often the individual holds the affected arm with the opposite hand to prevent movement.
- Deformity at fracture site.

◆ Fractured humerus

The upper end of the humerus can break in a number of ways, but the damage is almost always the result of a direct blow or a fall.

- Pain when attempting to move shoulder or arm.
- Often, substantial tracks of bruising down arm.
- Variable amount of deformity – dependent on the degree of displacement.

◆ Polymyalgia rheumatica

◆ Osteoarthritis

See page 281.

Rare

◆ Ruptured biceps tendon

In the elderly. The top end of the biceps muscle runs over the top of the humeral head. Changes due to wear and tear can make it rupture.

- Sudden onset of pain at shoulder tip.
- Flexing arm against resistance allows upper end of biceps (now unattached) to bunch up and become visible in the upper arm.

◆ Tuberculosis

See page 427.

◆ Internal bleeding

Anyone who develops pain at a shoulder tip after abdominal injury, when lying flat, must be urgently investigated for internal abdominal bleeding.

It is thought that blood from the bleeding point tracks up to the diaphragm, from where pain is referred to the shoulder, which shares the same nerve supply.

Skeleton and Muscles

Cannot straighten back

See *Painful back*, below.

Round or hunched shoulders

See *Kyphosis* and *Scoliosis*, covered under *A lump on the back*, page 270

Painful back

The back is taken here as the area from the neck down to the tailbone (the coccyx). All of us will have at least one episode of back pain during our lives caused by either injury or disease.

Back pain lasting more than two to three weeks and which does not respond to simple painkillers must be reported to a doctor.

Pain may prevent you from straightening up, but may also be felt when in a 'normal' upright posture.

Probable

◆ Muscular

Tearing or bruising of muscles or ligaments.

- Distinct history of injury – typically a blow, pulling or pushing.
- Dull ache initially, but the pain increases.
- Pain is local.
- Worse on movement, typically coughing or deep breathing.
- Resolves after a few days.
  May need strong pain killers.

◆ Acute back strain

May develop after a sudden twisting or bending movement, or lifting even a very small object.

- Often in the lower back.
- Often very painful at start, then less so.
- Worse on movement – may be impossible to move initially.
- Difficult to say exactly where the pain is.
- Lifting the leg straight while lying flat may aggravate the pain.

Normally responds to gentle mobilisation and pain killers, though improvement can take many weeks.

A physiotherapist, osteopath or chiropractor may be able to help.

◆ Chronic back strain

Low back pain that recurs. The individual has had similar episodes over a number of years and will be aware of the types of activity that cause it and relieve it. Symptoms can be made worse by obesity.

- Similar symptoms to acute back strain, but may be less intense.

Prolapsed intervertebral disk

Spinal cord

Prolapsed disk

Gelatinous centre pressing on nerve

Disk

Vertebra

Nerves

Skeleton and Muscles

◆ Osteoarthritis

The wear and tear disease. Particularly vulnerable are weight-bearing joints such as hips and low lumbar spine, but any joint can be affected.

- Intermittent, non-specific low back pain.
- Worse after standing and at the end of the day.
- Relieved by rest.

However, it is possible that discomfort remains even whilst lying in bed.

Gradually, as the joint becomes stiffer, pain decreases, and some mobility is lost.

◆ Sciatica

Really a symptom itself, rather than a diagnosis, and a common one for many who suffer from bad backs. Caused by pressure on the sciatic nerve, which has its origins in the lower back. Can, rarely, be caused by actual damage to lumbo-sacral nerves, lumbar spine and the sciatic nerves.

Persistent sciatica needs investigation as it can indicate serious underlying disease.

- Pain originates in low back or buttock.
- Pain radiates down the back or side of the thigh, calf and sometimes into the foot.
- Tingling or numbness may also be noted in the leg.
- Symptoms can be made worse by raising and straightening the leg.

◆ Cervical spondylosis

See page 126.

Possible

◆ Kidney infection

Pain usually on one side of the loin, the area on either side of the backbone, between the ribs and hip. Often, the pain is severe and associated with fever and urinary problems, such as pain on passing urine and passing small, frequent amounts. Requires antibiotics urgently.

◆ Prolapsed intervertebral disk

Often known as a 'slipped disc' (as are acute and chronic back strains and sciatica). The fibrous disc that acts as a buffer between the vertebrae has a gelatinous centre. Age or injury can cause this centre to bulge out, applying pressure on the nerves which emerge between the vertebrae and supply sensation to the body.

- Minor episodes of backache are an early warning.
- Sudden onset of severe back pain when bending or stooping: you may be unable to stand.
- Sciatica (page 267) may be present.
- Coughing and straining make the pain worse.
- Numbness or tingling may develop in a leg or foot.
- Very occasionally, a slipped disc may cause urinary retention. This is a medical emergency.

The symptoms may subside in a few days or weeks; although a few may persist.

Numbness or tingling

If you have numbness or tingling in the feet or legs or in the genital region, and/or your ability to pass water seems to be affected, seek medical help urgently.

◆ Shingles

Initially, skin irritation.

- Red spots develop, in a band a few inches wide on one side of the body.
- The spots develop into fluid-filled vesicles which burst and form crusts.
- Can become very painful.

If suspected, can be treated with one of several anti-viral drugs, best given before the spots develop.

Tends to cure itself.

Shingles is caused by the chicken pox virus. Those who have not had chicken pox can catch it from someone with shingles.

◆ Coccydynia

Pain associated with the coccyx or tail bone.

- Persistent pain after a fall.
- Pain aggravated by local pressure.
- Pain aggravated by sitting.

◆ Scoliosis

See page 270.

◆ Kyphosis

See page 270.

◆ Osteoporosis

Thinning of the bones often caused by ageing. In women, this is especially a post-menopausal problem.

- Occurs in otherwise fit individuals.
- Increasing deformity as age increases.
- Shortening of the vertebral column; height loss.

◆ Ankylosing spondylitis

Essentially an inflammatory disorder, affecting the spine and sacroiliac joints – commonest in males during the late teenage years.

It tends to occur in families.

- Intermittent backache or buttock pain at the early stage.
- Intermittent stiffness.
- Symptoms worst in the early morning, improving with movement and exercise.
- As the disease progresses, swelling and stiffness of other joints may develop.

Skeleton and Muscles

* Occasionally, eyes, heart, and lungs may be affected.

Rare

◆ Cancer of the spine (primary or secondary)

The spine is a well-recognized site of secondary cancer – meaning cancerous growth which has spread from another (primary) site. Anyone developing the following should see a doctor without delay (although most of these symptoms are **not** due to cancer):

* Severe continuous pain in the back that wakes you at night.
* Pain radiating from the back to the limbs.
* The development of pain, weakness or altered sensation in the limbs.

Other symptoms of cancer, including weight loss, malaise and loss of appetite may also be evident.

◆ Benign tumour of the back

Although benign tumours rarely give rise to pain, large ones, or ones adjacent to pressure areas, for example, at the level of a trouser waist band, may do so.

Even if you think it is benign, report it to a doctor.

◆ Discitis

An infection develops in the intevertebral disc (see illustration, page 267). The pain often gets gradually worse over weeks. Can be difficult to diagnose. Sometimes it is associated with fever symptoms, weight loss or feeling generally unwell.

Treatment is antibiotics for many weeks, usually starting in hospital.

◆ Rickets and osteomalacia

Both represent similar disease processes in children (rickets) and in adults (osteomalacia), and are caused by lack of Vitamin D.

The symptoms of rickets are:

* Skull deformity.
* Knee, ankle and wrist thickening.
* Enlargement of the bony cartilages of the chest ('rickety rosary').
* Lower limb deformities.
* Rarely, spinal curvature and pain.

The symptoms of osteomalacia are:

* General bone pain.
* Backache.
* Muscle pain.
* Loss of height due to vertebral collapse.
* Stress fractures.

◆ Gastro-intestinal or abdominal disease

A number of unusual conditions may cause back symptoms, although very rarely in isolation.

Inflammation of the pancreas and peptic ulcer may cause pain (often centrally in the small of the back). Inflammatory bowel disease such as Crohn's disease or ulcerative colitis can cause back pain, either by referred pain from the diseased bowel or because of the joint inflammation that, rarely, may be associated with them. An aneurysm (swelling) of the large aorta artery can cause back pain together with pulsation in the abdomen.

◆ Tuberculosis

See page 427.

Skeleton and Muscles

A lump on the back

Probable

◆ Benign tumour of skin structures

Meaning a harmless lump, such as a lipoma or sebaceous cyst, which may occur in the skin anywhere in the body. Common features are:

- Pain-free.
- Slow increase in size.
- Otherwise sound health.

◆ Infection

- Often sited on the upper back.
- Painful.
- Red.
- Localized swelling.
- Pus may ooze out.

Any infection may eventually become an abscess – a collection of pus. Often, it may discharge itself, but occasionally surgical drainage may be needed. Sometimes a cellulitis (see page 290) develops, which requires antibiotics. If recurrent infections occur, then a doctor should ensure that diabetes is not to blame.

◆ Normal bony prominences

Occasionally, a previously unnoticed lump may become apparent. This often occurs after a loss of weight. The spine itself is a rather knobbly structure.

Possible

◆ Kyphosis and scoliosis

Deformities of the spine causing humps. Kyphosis:

- Spine is unusually curved.
- Curve of the upper spine is exaggerated when viewed from side.
- Hump-back appearance.
- Some pain.

There are various causes including: bad posture, osteoporosis, osteoarthritis, ankylosing spondylitis, or rare congenital disease. Scoliosis is a sideways deformity of the spine:

- Sometimes a family history.
- Spine appears to curve more to one side when looked at from behind, particularly when person bends forwards.
- Some pain.
- May be associated with any disease that affects the spine.

Rare

◆ Spina bifida

A congenital abnormality recognized at or soon after birth.

◆ Cancer

People with known malignant disease may develop secondary growths in either the skin or skeletal structures of the back. Pain, irregular contour and rapid growth are ominous signs.

Usually the cancer will have already made itself known.

◆ Tuberculosis

Unrecognized tuberculous infection of the spine or other bone(s) can cause

Skeleton and Muscles

sudden collapse of the affected part so that a bony lump can be felt. This may be known as a kyphus (and is a specific type of kyphosis – see page 270).

- Develops rapidly.

- Often associated with general malaise and occasional fever.
- Pain is often slight in the early stages, but can then become severe and constant.

Back pain, women only

Probable

◆ Period pain

Also called dysmenorrhoea.

- Low abdominal and back pain associated with periods.
- Occurs at each period and settles.
- Otherwise fit.

◆ Mittelschmerz

Low back and abdominal pain developing in the middle of the menstrual cycle.
    Believed to be associated with ovulation.

Possible

◆ Pelvic inflammatory disease

Infection of the female genital tract. If suspected, requires treatment to minimize the risk of infertility later.

- Fever.
- Low back and low abdominal pain, ranging from severe to very slight, or even non-existent.

- Vaginal discharge – yellow/green/brown.
- Discharge is often smelly.
- Possibly malaise and fever.

Rare

◆ Cancer of the cervix, ovaries and womb

- There may be chronic, unremitting back or lower abdominal pain.
- Possibly offensive, bloody vaginal discharge (in cases of the uterus and cervix).
- Abdominal swelling: fluid collects in the abdominal cavity.

Other symptoms associated with malignant disease may be present:

- Weight loss.
- Anorexia.
- Anaemia.
- Malaise.

Painful elbow

A number of structures around the elbow can give pain. The elbow joint is made up of three bones: the humerus, the radius and the ulna. A number of muscles and tendons attach near the joint, and nerves pass close by.

A direct blow can, of course, break or bruise the bone: the olecranon is the most prominent part and is often damaged. The lower end of the humerus may be broken. The upper end of the radius may be broken indirectly if you fall on an outstretched hand: force is transmitted up the arm to its top end.

The symptoms of a fracture are:

- Local pain.

- Local swelling.

- Loss of function- flexing/ extending and twisting the forearm.

- Deformity may not be particularly noticeable.

Bruising can give similar symptoms, but the pain disappears relatively quickly and function returns.

One other elbow problem lies outside our conventional analysis of probable, possible and rare: knocking the 'funny bone'.

The funny bone is not in fact a bone, but a nerve called the ulnar nerve, which runs round the back of the medial epicondyle. If you knock it:

- Exquisite pain on the medial epicondyle (and not knowing whether to laugh or cry).

- Pain and altered feeling (tingling) sensed down the forearm to the hand (mainly on the little and ring fingers), lasting a few seconds.

Probable

◆ **Tennis elbow**

◆ **Golfer's elbow**

These are 'repetitive strain injuries',

The elbow bones

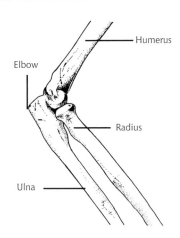

Humerus

Elbow

Radius

Ulna

typical of tennis players and golfers, but more commonly seen in anyone who uses their arms repetitively.

- Local pain: in tennis elbow, the outer side of the elbow is involved; in golfer's elbow, the inner side.

- Pain worse on certain movements, for instance turning a door handle, shaking hands, lifting, serving at tennis;

Patients are often middle-aged. May be treated with rest, physiotherapy or more rarely now with a local injection of anaesthetic and steroid; occasionally surgery may help. Acupuncture may also be of benefit.

Rare

◆ **Loose bodies**

Pieces of bone may chip off and lie free in the joint as a result of injury, degeneration (perhaps from osteoarthritis), inflammation (perhaps from rheumatoid arthritis) or some unknown cause.

- Intermittent pain in joint.
- Joint locks.
- Cannot always fully extend or flex the elbow.
- Associated symptoms of other disease.

If symptoms persist or progress, surgical removal of the loose body may be necessary.

◆ Infected bursa

The bursa is a sac, like an empty balloon, that lies under the skin over the olecranon. Injury – a blow or friction – to the olecranon makes the bursa fill with fluid, which can then be seen as a lump on the point of the elbow. This is often pain-free.

Occasionally, enlargement is associated with other disease such as gout or rheumatoid arthritis. If the overlying skin is damaged (cut or grazed), then the fluid may become infected.

Painful wrist

Probable

◆ Sprain

Usually the result of a twisting or bending injury.

- Uncomfortable on movement, but no real limitation.
- No specific local tenderness.
- Will settle within a few days.

◆ Colles' fracture

Common in post-menopausal females who fall on to an out stretched hand. The ends of the radius and ulna are broken.

- A 'dinner fork deformity'.
- Pain in wrist.
- Deformity: lump on back of wrist.
- Pain on movement.
- Swelling can be extensive.

Requires realigning and immobilization in a plaster.

Colles' fracture

◆ **Scaphoid fracture**

After falling on to an outstretched hand.

• Pain in wrist.

• Swelling.

• Pain on movement.

• Local pain at base of the back of the thumb.

If this fracture is untreated, the scaphoid, a small bone in the wrist, will degenerate, causing early osteoarthritis. Suspected scaphoid fractures must be immobilized initially, and X-rays reviewed after a week or so.

Possible

◆ **Osteoarthritis**

See page 281.

◆ **Rheumatoid arthritis**

See page 261.

◆ **Carpal tunnel syndrome**

Although mainly causing symptoms in the hands and fingers, carpal tunnel syndrome may cause pain in the wrist and forearm too. Pressure on nerves passing to the hand through the wrist gives rise to tingling and numbness.

Common in pregnancy and pre-menstrually, or when fluid retention is a symptom.

See also *Swollen hands*, opposite page.

Rare

◆ **Tuberculosis**

See page 427.

Swollen wrist

See *Painful wrist*, page 273.

A swelling at the wrist

Probable

◆ **Ganglion**

A small, usually pea-sized or larger, fluid-filled swelling adjacent to the wrist joint, capsule or tendon sheath.

• Localized smooth lump, normally on the back of the wrist.

• Cystic.

• Can shine a light through it.

• Mild discomfort; worse if knocked.

Usually no treatment is required. Occasionally removed by surgery.

Used to be treated by firm blow from the family bible – not recommended these days.

Possible

◆ **Osteoarthritis**

See page 281.

◆ **Rheumatoid arthritis**

See page 261.

Rare

◆ Pseudogout

Caused by calcium crystals collecting in the joint. In hours, the joint becomes red, hot, painful and swollen. Treated with strong painkillers. Usually settles down in a few days.

◆ Septic arthritis

See page 283.

Unusually large hands

If these have increased in sized in adulthood, this may be a feature of *Acromegaly*, page 258.

Swollen hands

Probable

◆ Normal variation

Intermittent swelling of one hand, or both, is a common, noticeable symptom.

You may find it difficult to remove rings, or a wrist strap may make an indentation on the wrist. May be worse in hot weather or, for women, pre-menstrually.

◆ Pregnancy

Particularly in the later stages, the body's normal response is to retain fluid. This tends to make the hands look puffy. It is important to have your blood pressure and urine checked by your midwife/GP to ensure that your blood pressure has not risen during pregnancy.

◆ Injury

Swelling would be a normal response to direct physical insult, for example, bruising, or a fracture or a tendonitis.

Carpal tunnel syndrome

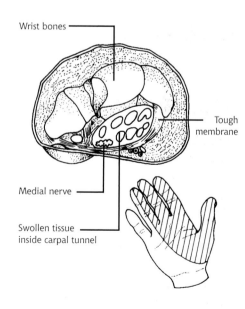

Wrist bones

Tough membrane

Medial nerve

Swollen tissue inside carpal tunnel

Skeleton and Muscles

Possible

◆ Hypothyroidism

Carpal tunnel syndrome (page 274) can be feature of this condition, which is caused by an under-active thyroid gland. (Do not confuse this with hyperthyroidism, an over-active gland.)

Other symptoms are:

- Skin becomes dry and rough.
- You 'feel the cold'.
- Voice becomes gruff, features coarsen.
- Weight gain, constipation, slow speech, slow thought.

The disorder is easily treated. For further details, see *Hypothyroidism*, page 68.

Rare

◆ Axillary vein thrombosis

Blockage of the main vein in the armpit or upper arm. May have no apparent cause, or occurs after vigorous exercise.

- Swelling of entire arm.
- No pain, but there may be a dull ache.
- Superficial veins of arm may appear more prominent because the deep veins are blocked.

◆ Lymphoedema

Primary or secondary.
See page 291.

Trembling hands

See *Trembling or shaking hands*, page 409.

Clubbed or curved fingers or nails

This means that:

- The end part of the finger becomes rounded.
- The nails appear larger and more curved lengthways and side to side.
- The angle between the nail bed and the skin on the back of the finger is lost; see illustration, right.

If the fingers have been clubbed since birth, and there are similar finger-shapes in the family, then the symptom is not significant. But if clubbing develops during life, it may well be associated with other diseases, some of which are listed below. It

Clubbed fingers

is rare for clubbing alone to be the first indicator of these diseases. Medical science has not yet explained this phenomenon.

Diseases of which clubbed fingers is a symptom:

- Lung diseases such as bronchiectasis, lung fibrosis (fibrosing alveolitis), cystic fibrosis, lung cancer.

- Heart disease: congenital heart disease, endocarditis.

- Gastro-intestinal disease: Crohn's disease, cystic fibrosis, liver cirrhosis, ulcerative colitis.

- Malignant disease.

  See relevant sections for further details.

Problems with fingernails

It is said that over 60 diagnoses can be made from examining the nails alone. The appearance of the nail may be a clear sign of certain diseases, and the commonest variations are listed here along with the disease with which they are associated.

- Bitten fingernails: may, of course, be no more than a habit, or may point to an underlying tension, even anxiety or depression, particularly if of recent onset.

- Paronychia (sometimes known as 'a whitlow'): an abscess of the fingertip, which becomes red, tender, tense and throbbing; pus may accumulate. Often needs to be released by a surgical incision. Antibiotics may be required.

- Transverse fissures (lines): quite common after any illness and may be present for many months.

- Transverse ridges: often in association with eczema.

- Sub-ungual haematoma: discolouration after injury. The classic injury to a nail is a hammer blow, or an object dropped on the toes.

Within a few minutes, a blue, then a purplish, then dark brown or black area

Paronychia – a 'whitlow'

may appear. The toe feels painful and throbs, because blood, which causes the discolouration, builds up pressure under the nail.

The symptoms are easily relieved by piercing the nail over the haematoma with a heated sterile needle, allowing the blood to escape. This should be done by a health professional, as it would be unsafe to do this in the presence of a finger fracture.

- Pale nails or leuconychia: in association with pale mucosa and conjunctiva in the eye this symptom suggests anaemia.

- Bluish nails: suggests cyanosis. Often accompanies lung or heart disease. Examine also the lips and the ears – breathlessness may be a feature.
- Koilonychia or spoon-shaped nails: iron deficiency, anaemia.
- Glomus tumour: an exquisitely tender, red or violet coloured area a few millimetres across under the nail.
- Pitting of the nails: often occurs in association with psoriasis.
- Onycholysis: the nails separate from the nail bed – another feature of psoriasis, particularly at the end of the nail.
- Fungal infections of the nails give a markedly thickened, irregular and discoloured nail. The nail loses its usual colour, becoming uniformly cream-coloured and opaque. Other fungal infections may be present elsewhere.
- Onychogryphosis: enormous overgrowth and thickening of (mainly) the big toe nail, most commonly seen in the elderly. Advanced cases end up looking like a ram's horn.
- Brittle nails: may be due to excess manicuring and application of polish and polish remover.
- Splinter haemorrhages: longitudinal areas of redness that look like small splinters at the tips of the fingernails:

may be associated with infection of the heart lining. Heart murmurs, malaise, shortness of breath, fever and anaemia are other signs.

- White lines: short, white lines are frequently seen across nails. The exact cause is unclear. They may be a sign of a blow to the nail, or may appear after an illness. They are of little significance.

Other diseases associated with nail deformities are:

- Lichen planus: a rare, itchy skin disease that also affects the nails.
- The whole skin may be affected. The nails (in about 10 per cent of cases) become flaky, striated (lined), spoon-shaped, or may be destroyed.
- Alopecia areata: hair loss from the scalp, in patches. The nails may be pitted.
- Nail-patella syndrome: a rare hereditary disease. Rudimentary or absent nails and small or absent patella (kneecap).
- Paronychia congenita: nails are thickened, as is the surrounding skin.
- Dystrophic epidermolysis bullosa: irregularity and thickening of the nails which makes the skin blister easily in response to injury.

Extremely cold or frozen fingers

This symptom occurs with *Chilblains and Frostbite*: see under *Itching or numbness of the fingers or toes*, page 300.

◆ Raynaud's phenomenon

The hands go cold and painful. The fingers change colour, first white, then blue, then when they recover, red. The condition can occur on its own (Raynaud's disease) or arise from other causes, such as drugs (beta blockers); connective tissue disorders (SLE, scleroderma, see page 242); use of vibrating tools; or sometimes the presence of an extra rib in the neck.

Swollen or misshapen fingers

Probable

◆ Pulp space infection

Infection, typically after a prick from plant or needle in the soft tissue at the finger tip.

- Swelling.
- Pain.
- Redness.
- Throbbing.

    May require drainage or antibiotics.

◆ Trigger finger

Thickening or inflammation of part of a flexor tendon in a finger or thumb causes:

- The digit to 'stick' when bending or straightening.
- May 'unstick' with a snap, spontaneously, or:
- May need to be forced to straighten.

If a finger or thumb is severed, place it in a clean, sealed plastic bag or wrap it in clean material or clingfilm, surround it with ice, and rush to the nearest hospital. (Do not put the ice directly next to the finger as this can damage it). With new microsurgical techniques, it is sometimes possible to save the digit.

Swollen or misshapen fingers

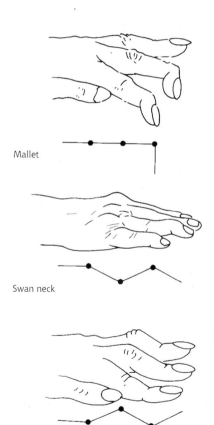

Mallet

Swan neck

Boutonniere

- A small tender nodule may be felt at the base of the digit on the palm.
- This nodule can be felt clicking as the digit is flexed.

Recovery may be spontaneous, but persistent symptoms can often be treated with a cortisone injection or sometimes surgery.

◆ Heberden's nodes

Caused by osteoarthritis.

- Distal interphalangeal joints (see illustration page 262) are painful.
- Bony overgrowth makes the joints appear enlarged and knobbly.

Possible

◆ Mallet finger and thumb

Damage to the tendon (extensor) which attaches to the dorsal surface of the end bone of each digit. The damage may be caused by injury to the end of the digit, or indirectly, after a wrist fracture.

Occasionally, it happens in association with other disease – such as rheumatoid arthritis.

- Terminal phalanx of digit appears bent but cannot be straightened.
- Splinting for six weeks may help cure cases caused by direct trauma.

In other situations, surgery may be needed.

◆ Rheumatoid arthritis

This disease affects the fingers and hands in a number of ways, including:

- Ulnar deviation of the fingers: the fingers appear to drift towards the

side of the little finger, and the knuckle joints appear pronounced.
- Swan neck deformities; see illustration.
- Boutonniere's deformities; see illustration.
- Drop finger: the finger cannot be extended at the knuckle joint.
- Mallet thumb; see above.

◆ Dupuytren's contracture

A fibrous contracture of (commonly) the little and ring fingers, which cannot be completely straightened.

- Sometimes the fingers are so bent that cleaning of the hand is a problem.
- Thickening can be felt on the palm side of affected fingers and on the palm.
- Usually of unknown cause, but has been linked with excessive drinking, and with certain drugs. It may also be hereditary.

◆ Gout

A generalized disease that may affect joints and skin. In the fingers and hands, the following may be seen:

- Tophi: lumps in the skin containing waxy, yellow material.
- Deformed joints of fingers and hand.

Rare

◆ Flexor sheath infection

Infection in the sheath surrounding the tendons that bend the fingers (flexor tendons).

- Entire finger is red and swollen.
- Pain.
- Loss of function.
- Pain worse on movement – finger is held crooked – the most comfortable position.
- Infection (untreated) may spread back into the palm of the hand.

This is an orthopaedic emergency, needing immediate treatment to prevent long-term loss of function and deformity

◆ Ischaemic contracture

Also known as Volkmann's contracture. Direct or indirect injury to the blood supply of the forearm damages muscle, making it atrophy and shrink.

- Pale or bluish-looking skin on hand.
- Thin forearm.
- Hand is clawed – fingers flexed at both finger joints.
- Sensation diminished.
- Fingers can only be straightened when the hand is flexed at the wrist.

- Only able to grip when hand is flexed.

◆ Congenital deformities

- Present at birth.
- Failure of development – part or all of the fingers and hand may be deformed or absent.
- Syndactyly or webbing: fusion of adjacent fingers.
- 'Extra' digits: ranging from small lumps of flesh to entire digits (usually on the outer part of the limb).

◆ Congenital contracture

- Present from birth.
- Fingers may be bent.
- Thickened tissue may be felt on the surface of the palm.
- May only affect one digit.

◆ Malignant tumours

See *Lumps in the skin*, page 236.

◆ Benign tumours

See *Lumps in the skin*, page 236.

Skeleton and Muscles

Painful hip

Likely to have different causes at different ages. Pain is often felt in the groin or the front of the hip, and may radiate down the thigh and to the knee. In children (who may not complain of pain) a limp may be the only evidence of pain.

Accidental dislocation is excluded from this section because the cause – severe injury – is obvious.

Probable

◆ Osteoarthritis

From about 50 years of age. Osteoarthritis is a problem of growing old – of degeneration. All of us are affected to some degree by this form of arthritis, sometimes described as 'wear and tear arthritis'. Some pre-existing conditions predispose to an early appearance of osteoarthritis, including congenital dislocation of the hip, infective arthritis, Perthes' disease (see below), and slipped epiphysis (see below) – the risk is increased if the diagnosis is missed or treatment delayed.

- Pain radiating from groin to knee.
- Initially after exercise, progressing to pain at rest or disturbing sleep.
- Progressive stiffness of leg.
- Difficulty in putting on shoes and socks.
- Progressive limp.
- Apparent shortening of leg.

Treatment is first aimed at relieving the pain (painkillers); then at improving function (exercises and physiotherapy); eventually, severe cases may require joint replacement.

◆ Fractured neck of femur

See information on pathological fractures under *Bones breaking easily*, page 258.

Possible

◆ Irritable hip

Typically in children.

- Pain in groin or front of thigh, often to the knee.
- Limp.
- All movement of hip limited by pain.

This diagnosis tends to be made if investigations for other causes lead to nothing. The hip settles with bed rest and, occasionally, traction. A child who develops a limp when there was none before (and no obvious reason such as

Slipped epiphysis

Normal position of epiphysis

Slipped epiphysis

injury) should be taken to a doctor the same day in order to exclude other more serious problems, for example infection.

Rare

◆ Perthes' disease

The blood supply to the femoral head is compromised, and it dies. The course of the disease is up to four years. Surprisingly, the symptoms can be quite slight.

- Patient aged five to ten years, occasionally older or younger.
- Intermittent ache in hip.
- Intermittent limp.
- Painful movements.

It is important to distinguish between this serious disease and irritable hip.

◆ Slipped epiphysis

- Hip pain and limp.
  Diagnosis is by x-ray.

◆ Congenital dislocation of the hip

See *Dislocated hip*, below.

Dislocated hip

May be congenital (hereditary) or acquired, or caused by infection.

◆ Congenital dislocation (CDH)

CDH tends to run in families and arises because of an abnormally-shaped hip socket, combined with lax joint ligaments. Breech birth (when the baby's feet, rather than the head, come out of the birth canal first) increases the likelihood. Babies with family histories of CDH, or who have been in the breech position during pregnancy are often screened a few weeks after birth by ultrasound scan to ensure that this condition is not present.

Symptoms before walking:

- Asymmetry of hip, seen at skin creases.
- Legs will not part fully.
- The baby may be late to start walking.

Symptoms after walking:

- Asymmetry of legs.
- Limp.

If both hips are dislocated, the waddling gait could pass as normal, in which case the dislocation will go undetected, causing damage. So the problem needs to be recognized at an early stage.

Treatment is with different forms of splint. If untreated, the limp remains, and the hip joint is progressively distorted and damaged. Ultimately, severe osteoarthritis develops and hip replacement may be needed as an adult.

◆ Acquired dislocation

Acquired dislocation of the hip is caused either by injury or infection. Typically, a car or motorcycle accident, in which the individual is sitting with the knee bent, results in the femoral head being pushed backwards out of the acetabulum. Extreme force is needed.

- Extreme pain.
- Deformity in extreme cases.
- Leg is shortened and twisted inwards.
- The knee is slightly bent.
- The leg cannot be moved.

The femoral head can be replaced in the acetabulum, but recovery can be a lengthy process, often because there are other injuries.

Much less commonly, the hip may also dislocate forwards; also centrally, when the femoral head pushes through the acetabulum into the pelvis.

◆ Septic arthritis (infection of hip)

Occurs most commonly after hip surgery, but can arise on its own in adults and children.

Untreated infection in any joint requires urgent orthopaedic attention to remove pus and clear the infection, as the joint surface and surrounding structures can be rapidly destroyed.

- Features include:
- Pain (of variable intensity).
- A limp.

Skeleton and Muscles

- Eventually, loss of function.
- Malaise.
- Fever.

Neglected, or mistreated, episodes of infective dislocation may mean surgery at a later date to correct deformity.

Bow-leggedness

This is in most cases an innocent variation of the normal, occuring in childhood. Most children grow out of it.

- Feet together.

- Knees splayed.

May also, but much more rarely, be seen in rickets (page 269), osteoarthritis (page 281), and Paget's disease (page 407).

Limping

Limping can be a symptom of many disorders and is caused by pain, or deformity or both.

Look for a specific site of pain or deformity, and then refer to that section.

Pain when walking

Look at pages 254-256 first, then consider alternatives in the following pages

covering leg and knee; also the preceding pages covering hip.

Walking with a waddling gait

See *Congenital dislocation of the hip*, page 283 and *Duchenne's dystrophy*, page 253.

Painful leg or thigh

See the general bone and muscles symptoms, page 254, also back symptoms, page 266.

Paralysed leg

See pages 377-378.

Vein or veins standing out in leg

See *Varicose veins*, page 289.

Skeleton and Muscles

Swollen leg

See *Swollen ankle*, page 289.

Weak leg

See *Wasting and loss of power in the muscles*, page 253.

Leg unusually white

This may indicate sudden blockage of an artery – a medical emergency – as a result of *Peripheral vascular disease*, page 298.

Knee pain after injury

The precise cause of the pain will be governed by the force of the injury, and its site – so 'probable', 'possible' and 'rare' are not relevant here.

The knee is made up from: bones – lower femur, upper tibia, patella; ligaments – medial and lateral collateral, anterior and posterior cruciate; the joint capsule; the menisci medial and lateral; and the surrounding soft tissues. All can be damaged.

The most significant injuries are listed below, plus their symptoms and an indication of the type of injury that may cause them. All require immediate treatment.

Delaying treatment, especially if the injury is severe, will increase the risk of complications. All injuries to a joint increase the risk of early onset of osteoarthritis.

◆ Dislocation of the knee

Enormous force is needed to disrupt the knee joint, including its capsules and ligaments.

- Severe pain.
- Marked deformity.
- Marked bruising.
- Nerves and arteries to the leg may be damaged.

◆ Dislocation of the patella

See *Locked or locking knee*, page 286.

◆ Femoral condyle fractures

May be sustained after a fall from a height.

- Severe pain in the knee, which cannot be moved.
- Immediate swelling and deformity.

◆ Ligamentous tear

Can be complete or partial, and is often

missed, the symptoms of swelling, pain and reduced function being put down to 'sprain'. Often the worse the damage, for example, a complete rather than a partial tear, the less the pain. If someone has a severe injury to the knee which still allows some movement, the knee should be assessed for stability by an expert when symptoms have settled and before any sporting activities are started again.

◆ **Fractured patella**

Probably caused by falling on to knee, or by a direct blow.

- Immediate swelling.
- The knee is bent.
- May be unable to straighten leg, either because of pain or disruption of the straightening mechanism.

◆ **Supracondylar fracture of the femur**

Caused by severe, direct injury.

- Severe pain – knee cannot be moved.

- Immediate swelling and deformity.

◆ **Fractured tibial plateau**

Caused by a direct blow or a fall from a height.

- Severe pain – knee cannot be moved.
- Immediate swelling and deformity.

◆ **Upper tibial epiphysis and apophysis**

Injury to the upper lower leg, below the knee cap (the shin just below the knee), can damage the point of attachment of the quadriceps tendon to the tibia.

- Knee swollen, particularly below kneecap.
- Local tenderness at the upper tibia.
- Raising the leg when it is straightened is painful or impossible.

A similar condition in young adults, which develops spontaneously, is known as Osgood Schlatter's disease.

Swollen knee

See *Knee pain afer injury*, page 285, *Knee locked or locking*, below; *Inflamed or aching joints*, page 260.

Locked or locking knee which may collapse

The knee joint gets fixed at a particular angle. If it is completely locked it is not possible to straighten it. Some knees lock intermittently: they may appear to 'catch', and then to straighten. These symptoms invariably suggest a problem within the knee itself, either a damaged cartilage (meniscus) or a loose body, which might be bone or cartilage. If injury to the knee predates the symptoms, it is important to remember exactly how it happened.

Probable

◆ Ligament damage

The most common reason for the knee to lock, collapse or give away is damage to one of the internal ligaments. Symptoms are often similar to those of damage to the cartilage; see *Torn medial meniscus*, below.

◆ Torn medial meniscus

Typically the meniscus is crushed and twisted between femur and tibia. Common in footballers and rugby players.

- Often immediate pain at the inner aspect of knee.
- Knee may lock – cannot be fully straightened.
- Swelling of the joint within a few hours.

After the first incident, symptoms may subside, only to recur with increasing frequency.

Possible

◆ Loose body

- Trapped between femur and tibia.
- Intermittent sudden pain on climbing or descending stairs.
- Inability to straighten leg.
- Swelling, due to fluid, may accompany each attack.

Each attack resolves as the loose body moves from between the joints.

The loose body may be felt in the joint, often above or at the side of the patella.

◆ Osteoarthritis

Degenerative or osteoarthritic changes in the joint can cause formation of loose

Knee injuries:

Fractured patella

Star-shaped fracture   Transverse fracture

Ligamentous tear

Medial ligament   Cruciate ligaments

Supracondylar fracture of femur

Correcting the fracture

Skeleton and Muscles

Skeleton and Muscles

bodies; see page 287. Common in later middle age, and onwards.

Rare

◆ Recurrent dislocation of the patella

Anatomical peculiarities, which are often, in fact, normal variants of the ligaments, muscles, tendons or bones around the knee may allow the kneecap to slide side-ways. Commonest in young females.

- Kneecap may appear very mobile from side to side.
- Knee gets stuck in a bent position (maybe only briefly), causing the individual to fall (collapsing knee).
- Kneecap can be felt to one side, and then moves.
- May occur in both knees.

◆ Torn lateral meniscus

Less common than a torn medial meniscus; see page 287. Symptoms are the same, except pain is on the outer side of the knee.

◆ Discoid lateral meniscus

An abnormally-shaped lateral meniscus slips between the femur and tibia and the knee gives way. A 'clunking' sensation is experienced. Eventually, surgery will be needed.

◆ Chondromalacia patella

Degeneration of the cartilage at the back of the kneecap. Young females are often affected.

- May have had recurrent patella

Knee joint

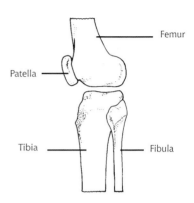

dislocation (see above) or a knee injury.

- Intermittent pain at the front of the knee, with swelling.
- Occasional locking of the knee.
- Knee occasionally gives way.

◆ Osteochondritis dissecans

The lower part of the articular surface of the femur (the condyle) may be damaged after injury. Part of the articular cartilage flakes off, creating a loose body.

The individual is often in his or her late teens.

- Intermittent ache.
- Intermittent swelling.
- Intermittent locking.
- Knee feels unstable, as though it will collapse.

'Knock' knees and bow legs

In the great majority of cases, knock knees are a normal feature of childhood. As the child grows, the knees gradually begin to look normal, usually by the time the child is seven.

- Feet appear splayed.

- Knees press against each other. Doctors often watch the leg shape over a period of six months to see how the appearance changes.

- May also, but rarely, be seen in rickets (page 269); osteomalacia (page 269); Paget's disease (page 407); and Charcot's joints (page 263).

Bow legs

Bow legs are common in infants. If the child is lying flat, with feet together, and there is a gap of more than 2 in/5 cm between the bottom of the femurs at the knee, an X-ray may be a useful precaution to exclude rare causes, such as rickets and problems of bone development.

Bowing on one side only should always be investigated by doctor.

Skeleton and Muscles

Painful knee

See *Inflamed or aching joints*, page 260; *Locked or locking knee*; page 286; *Painful hip*, page 281.

Swollen ankle

Can be one or both sides.

Probable

◆ **Acute or chronic injury**

See *Weak and painful ankle*, page 291.

◆ **Isolated dependent oedema**

The calf muscles play an important role in helping to prevent the ankles from swelling. When they are not used regularly, the feet and lower legs tend to swell with fluid (oedema). This commonly occurs when sitting for long periods on a plane, and is common in the elderly who sit for long periods of the day. It can be improved by keeping mobile and by raising the legs up on a stool. Support stockings can also help. It is important also to consider other causes of ankle swelling such as *Heart failure*, and other causes listed in the possible/rare sections below.

Possible

◆ **Varicose veins**

Enlarged leg veins caused by damage to valves in the veins.

Skeleton and Muscles

Blood fails to return to the heart at the proper rate and stays in the leg. This in turn can cause a swollen ankle and lower leg, often only on one side.

- Varicose veins visible.
- Increases during day or after exercise.
- Discomfort rather than pain.
- Disappears when leg is elevated, and at night.
- May be associated with ulcers, particularly inner-ankle swelling.

Long-standing varicose veins cause brownish discoloration of the lower legs and feet. Sometimes described as varicose eczema.

◆ Deep venous thrombosis

Blockage of the veins by a thrombosis or blood clot deep inside the leg. May occur for no reason; or after an operation or prolonged bed rest. More likely in the elderly, the obese, smokers, and those on the contraceptive pill or with known cancer. If suspected, requires urgent medical attention.

- Sudden onset.
- Initially no pain, then mild/moderate discomfort.
- Calf and sometimes the thigh also swell.
- Pain may be aroused by pressure on the back of the calf.
- Swelling is persistent and does not decrease.

If a piece of the clot moves from the legs to the chest, there will be chest pain and shortness of breath. (See also *Pulmonary embolus*, page 210) If the clot to the lung is large enough, death can follow in rare cases.

◆ Post-phlebitic limb

For months or years after a deep venous thrombosis (above) the limb may remain swollen and tender. Ulcers may develop at the ankle, plus discoloration of the skin.

It is best treated with support bandages.

◆ Cellulitis

A bacterial infection of the soft tissues. It may be localized in part of the foot, ankle or leg, or it may spread. Caused by a simple puncture wound, or by bacteria gaining access through broken skin on the foot or ankle (for example, via an ulcer or Athlete's foot).

- Redness; swelling.
- Can be very painful.
- Skin may be shiny, due to stretching.
- Malaise.
- Fever.

Rest and antibiotics will be needed to treat this condition.

◆ Heart failure

If the heart fails to pump as well as it should, the body retains fluid. At worst this can cause congestion of the lungs, which makes breathing difficult. A mild case may cause ankle swelling.

- Swelling on both sides.
- Legs feel cool.
- May be intermittent.
- May be associated with shortness of breath.

- In bad (and untreated) heart failure, swelling may progress all the way up the leg.

Associated symptoms can include distended neck veins and cyanosis. The symptoms can be treated with diuretic and other heart tablets.

Rare

◆ Anaemia

Ankle swelling may be the first symptom noted by an anaemic individual. This is because anaemia may precipitate mild heart failure (see opposite).

◆ Lymphoedema

Obstruction to drainage of fluid via the lymphatic system. It may be primary (no underlying cause); the result of congenital abnormality; or it can arise from absence of the lymphatic system in that limb.

A congenital form, known as Milroy's disease, also exists.

Secondary lymphoedema can be caused by operation on the lymph glands in the groin (for example to control malignant disease), obstruction to the lymph glands (for example by cancer) or by parasite infection – filariasis.

- Firm swelling.

- Does not vary in size.
- Infection or inflammation may develop; see *Cellulitis*, oppsite.
- Skin becomes thickened.
- In severe cases the skin may acquire the texture of elephant hide – elephantiasis.

◆ Missed fracture

Occasionally a small fracture of an ankle bone may go unrecognized at the time of injury, resulting in long-term swelling, pain and instability.

◆ Nephritis

Damage, acute or chronic, to the kidneys caused by disease, not injury, may also cause swelling of the ankles. Other symptoms may include:

- Puffy face (particularly around the eyes).
- Protein and/or blood in urine.
- Malaise.
- Shortness of breath.
- Nausea and vomiting.

◆ Hypoproteinaemia

Low levels of a protein known as albumin can cause ankle swelling. This can occur in kidney disease, liver disease or in conditions that affect the amount of protein absorbed by the gut.

Skeleton and Muscles

Weak and painful ankle

Almost always the result of injury, such as a twist (often caused by slipping on a step) or jumping from a height. The ankle joint is made up of three main bones: the tibia, fibula and calcaneum. Each may be damaged. The injury also damages the soft tissues (ligaments, tendons and muscles) surrounding the ankle. Pain originates from these structures. The ankle feels 'weak' and likely to 'give away'. The symptoms only relate to the affected ankle.

Ankle injuries should be regarded seriously, since even untreated sprains can cause long-term disability. Pain killers, rest and physiotherapy are often appropriate treatments if there is no fracture.

Probable

◆ Acute trauma (sprain)

- Clear story of injury.
- Painful to stand or bear weight.
- Swelling, local or general.
- Swelling appears after a few hours or the following day
- Ankle feels as though it will 'give away'.

◆ Achilles tendonitis

The Achilles is the tendon that joins the calf muscle to the back of the foot. It often gets inflamed in those who do plenty of walking, particularly in sedentary, older athletes taking up sport again, or after a recent calf injury. *Overpronation* (see page 294) predisposes to Achilles tendonitis. The tendon is often painful, worse on walking/running and can become swollen. Treatment consists of rest, stretches, painkillers, physiotherapy and treatment of the overpronation, if present.

The Achilles tendon can rupture. Usually, this happens whilst walking or exercising, and no cause is found. It is more common in those who have had Achilles tendonitis and in those taking long-term steroid medication. There is a sudden onset of

Bones of the foot and ankle

Fibula

Tibia

Calcaneus

severe pain on the back of calf/heel associated with a snapping noise, as if a shot has been fired. Often, there is immediate difficulty with walking and the area swells.

Possible

◆ Chronic injury

- Injury some time in past – weeks, months or even years.
- Symptoms have persisted for some time.
- Feeling of 'weakness' or 'about to give away' predominates.
- Pain not so intense as with acute trauma.
- Swelling after exercise.

Rare

◆ Fracture

In general, the symptoms are very obvious and confined to the affected bone.

- Pain severe.
- Unable to bear weight.
- Immediate swelling.
- Bruising within a few hours.

A break to the lower end of the tibia will cause symptoms on the inner aspect of the ankle; to the lower fibula on the outer aspect; to the calcaneus (heel bone) on both sides and at the back over the heel.

Unusually large feet

Probable

◆ **Normal variant**

Most individuals worried about their foot size have no physical abnormality or underlying disease. The size of their feet merely reflects the variation in size that would be expected in any population. And many people worry that their feet are too small.

Rare

◆ **Acromegaly**

See page 258.

Skeleton and Muscles

Flat feet

The term really means flattening of the arches. It can be a postural problem, in association with knock knees and a short Achilles' tendon. It may occasionally be congenital, in association with spina bifida, but this is rare. It may also develop as a result of general lack of fitness, say after being bed-ridden. The muscles and tendons that support the arches become wasted and flat feet develop.

- Feet look flat – no arch on instep.
- Shoe soles wear badly.
- Pain is rare, but may develop later in the foot and leg muscles.

Most commonly, no cause for flat feet is found, and unfortunately specialists can offer little in the way of help.

The French believe in encouraging very young children to walk in barefoot on different surfaces (sand on a beach is a favoured one), to help develop the arches. Flat feet often run in families.

Treatment is rarely needed, although instep supports may be of some help.

Painful arches of feet

See *Flat feet*, above.

Overpronation

This condition is increasingly being recognized. It is commonest in those with flat feet. Pronation is the slight inward rolling motion the foot makes during normal walking or running and helps to accommodate movement. Some people, however, roll more than normal. The arch of the foot then flattens, and this causes excessive stress and pressure on the soft tissues of the foot.

Over-pronation can aggravate foot pain; plantar fascitis; Achilles tendonitis; shin splints; knee, hip and and back problems. It can often be treated effectively by wearing special insoles (orthotics).

Painful feet

Probable

◆ Verruca

Also called a plantar wart; caused by a viral infection, hence outbreaks in schools and swimming pools.

- Local tenderness on sole of foot, where the verruca is pushed into the surface.

- The plantar wart is visible and there may be several – normally on the weight-bearing areas.

- May vanish spontaneously.

> Most schools no longer undertake verruca checks. There is no need to prevent a child swimming because he or she has a verruca. As this is a viral infection, the body will eventually overcome it, and the verruca will go.
>
> Only painful or unusually troublesome verrucas need to be treated. An old, hard verruca is not very infectious. Treatments bought over the counter from a chemist work best, but take many weeks to take effect.

Hallux valgus

Normal position of big toe

Morton's metatarsalgia

Neuroma

First metatarsophalangeal joint

Possible

◆ Plantar fasciitis (policeman's heel)

An inflammation of the layers of membrane, called fascia, which lie in the sole of the foot.

- Common after the age of 40.
- Local tenderness underneath the heel.
- Worse on walking/running.
- Often associated with Overpronation (see opposite)

Commonest in occupations requiring individuals to be on their feet for long periods – a penalty of being a policeman or traffic warden. Treatments include a heel raise, foot stretches, physiotherapy, orthotics and occasionally a steroid injection.

◆ Hallux valgus (see diagram)

The big toe becomes deformed, commonest in women beyond middle age.

- Big toe tip points to outer side of foot.
- Base of big toe is prominent.
- The end of the metatarsal bone points to the inner side of the foot.
- A lump of bone is therefore felt under the skin.

The overlying skin becomes thickened and painful (bunion) as does the bone on the sole of the foot.

May eventually need surgery.

◆ Hallux rigidus

Caused by osteoarthritis of the first metatarsophalangeal joint.

- Pain on movement.

- Bony outgrowths may develop, appearing as lumps around the joint.
- Thickened skin may develop on the upper surface of the joint.
- Range of movement of the joint is eventually limited by stiffness and pain.

Rare

◆ Claw toes

See *Pes cavus*, below.

◆ Morton's metatarsalgia

Affects the middle-aged.

- Enlargement of the nerve (neuroma) between the heads of metatarsal bones.
- Local pain between two toes, worse if foot is squeezed from side to side.
- Tingling of the two toes affected
- May require a cortisone injection or surgery.

◆ Pes cavus

The opposite of a flat foot: the arch of the foot is raised. Often associated with curling of the toes (claw toes). Thought to be caused by imbalance of the muscles that support the arches, and most likely to be seen in those with neurological disease of the lower limb, for instance poliomyelitis, spina bifida, cerebral palsy.

- Curled or clawed toes.
- High arch on instep.
- Callosities eventually develop on pressure points.
- Metatarsalgia (pain on the metatarsal heads) may develop.

Skeleton and Muscles

Skeleton and Muscles

Swollen feet

See *Swollen ankle*, page 289.

Ulcerated or infected feet

Probable

◆ Ingrown toenail

The big toe is the one almost always affected. The side of the nail cuts into the toe tissue causing local infection (paronychia).

Caused by ill-fitting shoes and cutting the nail too short. or picking at the nail.

- Outer side of nail most commonly affected.
- Often on both feet.
- Recurrent pain.
- Recurrent infection – with redness, swelling and pus.

May ultimately need surgery to nail bed.

◆ Athlete's foot

See *Itching or numbness of the fingers or toes*, page 300.

◆ Verruca

See page 294.

Possible

See under *Dermatitis*, page 301; *Diabetic neuropathy*, page 299; and under *Peripheral vascular disease* on page 298.

Rare

See under *Alcoholic neuropathy*, page 298; *Multiple sclerosis*, page 298; *Raynaud's disease*, page 278; *Buerger's disease*, below; *Frostbite*, page 301; *Syphilis*, page 344.

Buerger's disease is painful ulceration caused by obliteration of blood vessels in the limbs; particularly in young male smokers of eastern European origin.

Corns on the feet

See page 240.

Fingers and toes

Collected here is a group of symptoms which can particularly affect the fingers and toes (but also the arms and legs): parts of the body at the outer reaches of the blood's circulation. The nose and ears are similarly placed, and certain symptoms such as numbness, itching or discolouration (for example chilblains) can affect them just as they do the fingers and toes.

Numb fingers and toes

The onset of numbness in any part of the body should be taken seriously. It is not a common symptom in isolation and may be an accompaniment to underlying disease. Its main danger is that the 'warning sign' of pain is not present: therefore skin damage, skin breakdown and ulcers may develop because the individual cannot feel the discomfort. This is particularly common over pressure points (heel, medial and lateral malleolus, sole of the foot).

Numbness of fingers and toes accompanied by back pain is a serious symptom, and should be reported to your doctor immediately. It can be a sign of direct pressure applied to a nerve by a disc or from a bone injury.

Pressure points of the feet

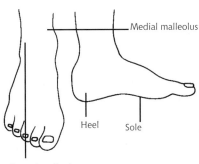

Medial malleolus

Heel   Sole

Lateral malleolus

Possible

◆ Cervical spondylosis

See page 126.

◆ Diabetic neuropathy

A long-standing complication of diabetes. Neuropathy means disease of the nerves. If you have diabetes, you may notice:

- Some tingling and pain (lower limbs).
- Stocking anaesthesia (numbness over a leg to the knee – the area covered by a stocking).
- Some muscle wasting and weakness.
- Painless ulceration over pressure points on feet.

- Cellulitis (see page 290), associated with ulcers.
- Occasionally only one nerve may be affected, causing numbness, muscle wasting and weakness in one limb.

Other neurological symptoms of diabetes may be:

- Radiculitis – localized scalding and painful sensory changes.
- Irregular shape to pupils.
- Impotence.
- Failure of orgasm.
- Nocturnal diarrhoea.
- Feeling of dizziness on standing or changing position (postural hypotension).
- Loss of sweating in lower limbs.

Skeleton and Muscles

◆ **Multiple sclerosis**

Used to be known as disseminated sclerosis. Nervous tissue in the central nervous system is affected.

Features may include:

- Numbness and tingling in hand(s) or feet (allowing ulcers to develop if pressure points are not treated carefully).
- Visual disturbance (poor vision, double vision).
- Weakness in limbs.
- Loss of postural sense.
- Vertigo.
- Bladder disturbance.
- Tremor.
- Speech disturbance.
- Swallowing difficulties.

May take several years to be diagnosed as it remits and relapses. The outlook is mixed: some unfortunate cases suffer, eventually, from paralysis and disability; in many, symptoms remain mild and many can be helped with medication.

◆ **Peripheral vascular disease**

As individuals age, the arteries begin to 'fur up' with fatty and calcified deposits: a normal part of the ageing process, known as atherosclerosis. In certain individuals, particularly smokers and those with a genetic disposition, the arteries fur up more extensively and at a younger age. Progressive atherosclerosis will result particularly in reduction of blood supply to the legs, with:

- Cold limbs (predominantly the legs).
- Legs may appear pale if lifted in the air.
- Cramp-like pain, particularly in the calf muscles, on walking any distance (intermittent claudication).
- Pain settles when walking stops.
- Occasionally sensory changes, including numbness.
- Pulses may not be felt in the usual places.

◆ **Alcoholic neuropathy**

Most chronic alcoholics have damaged nerves, giving:

- Numbness in the lower limbs. Ulcers may develop.
- Tingling in the lower limbs.
- Burning in the lower limbs (especially in the feet).
- Weakness of the lower limbs.
- Wasting of the muscles of the lower limbs.

Walking will be affected. The problems can be reversed by giving up alcohol; proper diet; taking B vitamin supplements.

Rare

◆ **Guillain-Barré syndrome**

Also known as acute inflammatory polyneuropathy.

An illness affecting the peripheral nervous system. It can occur at any age, often one to three weeks after an acute viral or bacterial (for example, food poisoning) infection.

- Initially, tingling in the hands and feet.

- Weakness develops in the arms and legs and ultimately, in severe cases, the muscles controlling the lungs. Sometimes the individual needs artificial ventilation.

- Loss of sensation may be severe or minimal.

- Facial weakness is a possibility.

Gradual improvement takes place over weeks or months: Most people make a full recovery.

◆ Frostbite

See page 301.

◆ Leprosy

Essentially a disease of underdeveloped countries acquired by close contact with an infected individual over a prolonged period.

Under these circumstances, the diagnosis will probably be obvious. One of the early signs is numbness and tingling in the ends of the arms and legs. There are many other symptoms.

Skeleton and Muscles

Altered sensation in the fingers and toes

Any disease or injury of a nerve can cause altered sensation in the area of the skin supplied by that nerve. It can take many forms, from tingling, through pins and needles and burning, to complete absence of sensation if the nerve is destroyed.

Probable

◆ Disease or injury of a nerve or nerves

Perhaps the commonest form is pressure neuropathy – or nerve palsy. This can occur if you fall asleep in an awkward position. Nerves usually affected are the ulnar (at the elbow); the radial (at the upper arm); and the peroneal nerve by the knee. Common to all these palsies are:

- Initial numbness on waking in the area served by the nerve.

- Initial loss of function of the affected part.

- Within a few minutes, sensation returns.

- At first this is a mild tingling, but it progresses to painful pins and needles.

- After several more minutes, or longer, the sensations settle and full function returns.

Occasionally, if the local pressure on the nerve has been unduly prolonged, full function may take weeks to return.

◆ Cervical spondylosis

See page 126.

◆ Carpal tunnel syndrome

See page 274.

Possible

◆ Diabetic neuropathy

See page 297.

◆ **Multiple sclerosis**

See page 298.

◆ **Peripheral vascular disease**

See page 298.

◆ **Alcoholic neuropathy**

See page 298.

Rare

◆ **Subacute combined degeneration of the spinal cord**

SACD for short. This is a result of Vitamin B12 deficiency, caused by a number of factors, the most significant being pernicious anaemia.

Other causes include poor diet, extreme vegetarianism and malabsorption, Damage is done to parts of the white matter in the spinal cord, giving:

- Pins and needles (paraesthesia) in the feet (hands and arms rarely affected).
- Inability to feel vibration and to sense position – affecting legs and body.
- Weakness in the legs; muscle wasting.
- Unsteady gait.

Obviously other symptoms of the disorder causing SACD may also be present.

◆ **Guillain-Barré syndrome**

◆ **Frostbite**

◆ **Leprosy**

See pages 298, 301 and 50, respectively.

Tingling fingers and toes

See *Altered sensation in the fingers and toes*, page 299.

Itching or numbness of the fingers and toes

In an otherwise normal individual.

Probable

◆ **Athlete's foot**

A fungal infection of the feet.

- Irritation between the toes.
- Burning and itching between the toes.
- Some redness, as a result of inflammation.

- Crusting and further infection can take place.
- Smelly feet.
- Cracking of skin, particularly between the toes.

◆ **Chilblains**

Damage to blood vessels in the skin caused by exposure to cold. Treated best by slow rewarming.

- Local pain in fingers or toes.
- Itching and burning at first, followed by:
- Swelling.
- Local discolouration (reddish/ purple) at the site of pain.
- Blister formation.

Possible

◆ Dermatitis

Acute dermatitis – inflammation of the skin – may be caused by an allergy to chemicals (for instance, deodorants or washing powders). So dermatitis can be caused by socks washed in a detergent to which an individual is allergic.

- Irritation.
- Burning.
- Inflammation, including weeping and crusting skin.

Symptoms confined to areas which come in contact with the source of the allergy.

Rare

◆ Frost bite

In prolonged below-freezing temperatures, all extremities are at risk, including ears, nose, toes and fingers. People with poor circulation, typically the elderly, or those who lose heat fastest (for instance children) are most at risk.

- Initial pain and tingling in affected part.
- May become numb (pain-free) – a bad sign.
- Discolouration: may at first be reddish purple, but when the affected part becomes white, then the frostbite is serious.

If untreated, the frostbitten areas will develop gangrene – death of tissue – because blood is no longer supplied. Ulcers develop and rapidly become infected. Urgent medical help is needed to supervise the rewarming of the affected part, and to minimize the final damage.

Skeleton and Muscles

The reproductive and sexual organs

Introduction

This chapter is divided into symptoms in women, symptoms in men and symptoms when the two come together in sexual relations. The sexual organs are shown in the diagram below.

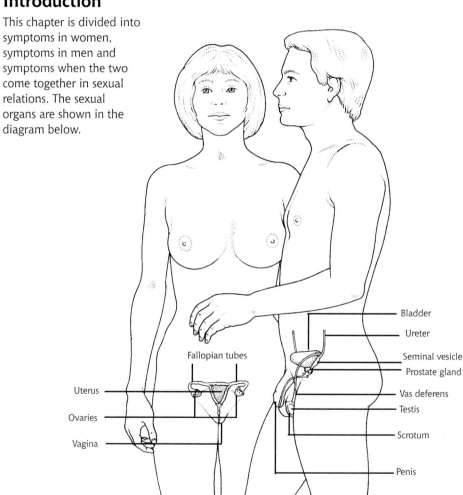

Fallopian tubes

Uterus

Ovaries

Vagina

Bladder

Ureter

Seminal vesicle

Prostate gland

Vas deferens

Testis

Scrotum

Penis

Symptoms in women

Menstruation

During the monthly cycle, the lining of the womb thickens and prepares to accept a fertilized egg. If conception does not take place, the lining breaks down and is shed – this is the menstrual discharge. This complex process involves hormones from the brain, the ovaries and the egg, all directed towards a common goal: a successful pregnancy. It is aptly said that menstruation is the womb crying for want of a pregnancy. Problem-free menstruation depends on a healthy balance between mind and body: it is more likely to be upset by psychological factors than most other bodily functions.

The length, frequency and heaviness of menstruation vary from person to person and from month to month, and this is not necessarily a symptom of abnormality. Sudden changes are a different matter and should be heeded.

Pre-menstrual tension

Feelings of tension and stress are just two from an array of physical and mental changes, which appear up to two weeks before menstruation and which go on after bleeding begins. Among the many possible symptoms, the commonest are:

• Feeling bloated.

• Irritability and tension.

• Tiredness.

• Headache.

• Tender breasts.

• Depression.

No one reason satisfactorily explains the symptom, nor is there any agreed or predictably useful treatment. Possibilities include Vitamin B6, evening primrose oil, herbal treatments, and alternative or complementary therapies. Hormonal preparations are also used, such as the contraceptive pill. Other drugs such as diuretics, SSRI antidepressants or tranquilliser medications have also been tried with varying degrees of benefit. The use of symptom diaries where women record their feelings can identify other gynaecological symptoms or psychiatric symptoms which may in turn lead to specific treatments or cures. Some women find that simply knowing that they have a real condition, albeit one which medicine is relatively ignorant about, enables them and their families to adjust to their symptoms.

Painful periods

Lucky is the woman who has no pain with her periods. For most, levels of pain vary widely, as does the amount which different women tolerate. Pain can certainly be regarded as abnormal when time is regularly lost from work, or when periods are accompanied by debilitating cramps, faintness and vomiting. In older women, these symptoms should be investigated, particularly if previously acceptable periods become intolerable, and are accompanied by pain on intercourse or heavy bleeding.

Probable

◆ Unknown origin

Painful periods are common in young women, for the first few years of menstruation possibly related to release of prostaglandin hormones and muscle contraction in the wall of the womb.

- Typically the pain begins 12-24 hours before bleeding and continues for the first one or two days.
- Pain is usually felt in the lower abdomen, tops of legs and lower back.

Anti-inflammatory drugs which counteract the effects of prostaglandins (ibuprofen, aspirin, mefanamic acid), can help. The contraceptive pill is also useful and usually lightens and shortens the periods.

Possible

◆ Endometriosis

A condition where tissue identical to the lining of the womb is found outside its normal location; commonly in the ovaries, fallopian tubes, and pelvis. It 'bleeds' in synchrony with menstruation.

- Commonest in women in 20s and 30s.
- Pain often lasts throughout the period, but can occur before or after.
- Often pain deep in the pelvis on intercourse.

- Sometimes causes difficulties with fertility.

Treated with hormones such as the contraceptive pill, or others which stop the periods. Surgery is sometimes required to destroy or remove endometriosis tissue.

◆ Pelvic inflammatory disease

Usually sexually acquired, for example, chlamydia infection.

- Can follow IUCD (coil) use, termination of pregnancy, or childbirth.
- Accompanied by pain deep in the pelvis on intercourse.
- Sometimes with vaginal discharge or other STD symptoms.
- Periods may be irregular.
- Risk of infertility and ectopic pregnancy.

Treatment with antibiotics. Essential to treat partner and contacts to prevent re-infection.

◆ Fibroids

A condition where benign growth of the muscle wall of the womb occurs.

- Commonest in ages 35-50, especially non-Caucasians.
- Associated with heavy periods and sometimes fertility problems.
- Sometimes swelling or a lump is felt in the lower abdomen.
- Can become suddenly painful due to twisting or interruption of blood supply.

Many women need no treatment as fibroids regress after the menopause. Alternatively, can be treated with hormones that induce a menopausal state. Occasionally treated by surgery.

Heavy periods

The amount of blood lost during a period is very variable, but as a rule of thumb heavy periods are defined by blood loss which interferes with life. Loss of blood clots or flooding is a common feature, as are periods lasting longer than a week or accompanied by anaemia (felt as tiredness or observed as pallor in the complexion).

Probable

◆ Dysfunctional bleeding

This refers to an abnormal pattern of bleeding in the absence of any structural abnormality in the reproductive organs.

* Is common at the beginning and end of reproductive life, and may be associated with failure to ovulate.
* May respond to hormone treatment or may resolve with time as a teenager or with menopause later.

Possible

◆ Fibroids

See opposite.

◆ Pregnancy and miscarriage

Sudden or severe bleeding in any woman of childbearing age can relate to pregnancy or its complications.

20-40 per cent of all pregnancies miscarry, mostly in the first 12 weeks. Heavy bleeding or a 'late' period may be a miscarriage.

Pregnancy may or may not be accompanied by other symptoms such as nausea, vomiting, missed periods, breast tenderness.

Consider the possibility of contraceptive failure.

A urine test for pregnancy should be done. Pregnancy is also sometimes tested for with an ultrasound scan or, rarely, a blood test. A negative test may become positive if it is repeated after an interval.

◆ Endometriosis

See opposite.

◆ Pelvic inflammatory disease

See opposite.

Rare

◆ Thyroid disease

Under-active glands are associated with heavy periods.

◆ Abnormal blood clotting

Heavy menstrual flow may result from any condition which makes the blood clot less well than it should. Also look for:

* Easy bruising.
* Gums which bleed easily.
* Pallor.
* Enlarged lymph glands.
* Blood in urine, vomit or from bowels.

◆ Tumours of the cervix and womb

Though heavy periods are a possible symptom, these diseases are more likely to cause: irregular bleeding or post coital bleeding, unusual discharge, or post-menopausal bleeding.

Routine investigation of heavy periods will discover these tumours.

Irregular periods

Irregular periods are common at the beginning and end of a woman's reproductive life. Other causes of irregular periods need to be distinguished from bleeding between periods (inter-menstrual bleeding), bleeding after intercourse (post coital bleeding), and bleeding after the menopause (post menopausal bleeding), which are all potentially serious symptoms.

It is best to report irregular bleeding to a doctor in order to establish whether the cause is important. If tests are suggested, these might include an ultrasound scan, hysteroscopy (looking into the womb with an endoscope), colposcopy (examining the cervix with a microscope) or endometrial biopsy (sampling the lining of the womb). Irregular periods may also be infrequent or become absent, so it is advisable to cross check with the section on this topic.

Probable

◆ **Dysfunctional bleeding**

See page 305.

◆ **Breakthrough bleeding on the contraceptive pill**

See page 310.

◆ **Hormone replacement therapy**

May need investigation to exclude other gynaecological causes.

May be used as treatment for irregularity before the menopause.

Possible

◆ **Pelvic inflammatory disease**

See page 304.

◆ **Polyps of the cervix or womb**

See page 310.

◆ **Cervical erosion**

See page 310.

◆ **Atrophic vaginitis**

See page 311.

Rare

◆ **Cancer occurring anywhere in the female sexual organs**

Whilst cancer is rare, it is serious. Early diagnosis improves outlook and can offer a complete cure. Routine investigation of irregular bleeding should discover this.

Absent or infrequent periods

This section concerns women who have had previously normal periods. In the case of periods which have never started, see *Delay in beginning menstruation*. In young women, stress is so often the reason for absent or infrequent periods that further investigation is usually unnecessary, except for reassurance, or to exclude pregnancy. Irregularities in women in their late 30s or early 40s are likely to have a physical or hormonal cause. In particular, women with infrequent periods should be examined to make quite sure that normal but infrequent periods are just that, and are not in fact occasional, abnormal episodes of bleeding from the womb or cervix.

Bleeding out of the blue, without your usual pre-menstrual symptoms, should definitely be investigated. Absent or infrequent periods may first be noticed as irregular periods, so it is advisable to cross check with the section on this topic.

Probable

◆ Pregnancy

It is a useful and proven medical rule of thumb that, if in doubt, any woman of child-bearing age with absent periods should have a pregnancy test if intercourse has taken place.

After any missed period, you should be on the look-out for other symptoms of pregnancy, such as: morning sickness, tender breasts, lethargy, weight gain, passing urine more frequently than usual or appetite changes. Have a pregnancy test if you are uncertain.

◆ Stress

An extremely common reason, especially in young women.

Stress is caused not just by obvious emotional turmoil but major changes in lifestyle, such as changes of job, travel, illness. Even what appears to be 'everyday' stress, such as preparing for

exams, can be sufficient to stop periods.

In conditions of obvious tension, the absence of periods for two or three months should not be a worry, as long as a pregnancy is excluded.

Investigations are rarely needed, unless symptoms persist for more than six months.

◆ Exercise

- Commonly seen in athletes or fitness fanatics.
- Associated with osteoporosis in the long term.

◆ Major weight change

Both excessive weight gain and dieting leading to weight loss will disrupt periods, because they affect some brain centres.

The most extreme form is anorexia nervosa: typically there is a distorted body image, self-induced vomiting, laxative abuse, and excessive exercising all resulting in significant weight loss.

◆ Breast feeding

Periods can stop or are scanty during breast feeding, since breast feeding hormones delay the normal return of the menstrual cycle.

It is, however, possible to become pregnant while breast feeding, for ovulation may still occur.

Possible

◆ Menopause

- Commonest age of menopause is 51.
- Premature menopause due to

ovarian failure can happen from the age of 30 onwards.

- Often preceded by irregular periods.
- Sometime there is a family history of early menopause.

◆ Raised prolactin

Prolactin is a hormone that normally contributes to the production of breast milk.

Absent periods, plus a milky discharge from the breasts, suggest an excess of prolactin. Can be caused by a tumour in the pituitary gland at the base of the brain.

Some drugs can cause it, for example, major tranquillisers used to treat mental illness or anti-emetics.

Blood tests and MRI scanning of the pituitary help with diagnosis.

Can be treated by medication or sometimes surgery.

◆ Polycystic ovarian syndrome

- Infrequent or absent periods.
- Excessive body hair.
- Acne.
- Weight is critical, commoner and more severe in the overweight, but can effect women of normal weight.
- Associated with infertility, diabetes, and increased risk of heart disease.

Diagnosed with blood tests and ultrasound scanning.

Treated with weight reduction, drugs which modify hormone levels and antidiabetic drugs. Rarely surgery.

◆ Post-pill absent periods

Commonest in women whose periods were irregular before they began to take oral contraception.

- Otherwise sound health.
- Periods return after three to six months.

If you have not had a period for more than six months after you stop taking the pill, seek professional advice.

◆ Serious general disease

The strain of another serious physical such as cancer or a major psychiatric illness or drug addiction may well cause absent or infrequent periods. Other symptoms of serious illness might include:

- Weight loss.
- Tiredness.
- Chronic cough.
- Fever, diarrhoea.

Periods should return after recovery.

Rare

◆ Thyroid disease

Over-excitability or lethargy, combined with disturbed periods, may suggest an over - or under-active thyroid gland.

◆ Adrenal disease

A possibility if absent periods are accompanied by:

- Hairiness.
- Weight gain.
- Weakness.

Delay in beginning menstruation

By the age of 16, most Western girls are menstruating, and it is reasonable to be concerned about those who are not.

Probable

◆ Normal but delayed

This is likely if there is:

- Normal development of breasts and pubic hair (including armpits).
- Normal growth.
- Family history of menstruation starting late.

In addition, hormone tests would be normal. In these circumstances, it is a matter of 'wait and see', sometimes using hormones to kick start the system.

Possible

◆ Hormone disorders

Suggested if the girl has the following symptoms:

- Short stature.
- Poor development of breasts.
- Either an absence or an excess of body hair.
- Obesity.
- Very severe acne.

Investigation of the girl's hormones, and treatment with hormones, may be needed.

◆ Anorexia nervosa

See page 396.

Rare

◆ Obstruction to menstrual flow

A membrane across the vagina can block the discharge of normal menstrual blood. There is normal sexual development and recurrent lower abdominal pain at period time.

- A bulge may protrude from the vagina, containing menstrual blood.
- Treatment is simply the removal of the membrane.

◆ Genetic disorders or congenital malformation

There are a wide range of disorders which can lead to malformation of the womb, ovaries and vagina, or even a complete absence of these organs. There are no characteristic symptoms: it is a matter for specialist assessment, after all other causes have been excluded.

Reproductive &
Sexual Organs

Bleeding between periods or after intercourse

The older the woman, the greater is the significance of this symptom. Causes are frequently obvious to the trained eye: you should always obtain your doctor's

advice with this pattern of abnormal bleeding.

Check that the cause is not blood in your partner's semen.

Probable

◆ Breakthrough bleeding on the pill

- Often when commencing the pill or the first few cycles.
- Remainder of the cycle is normal.
- Scanty, painless show of blood for a day or two.
- Often occurs about the same time each month, usually towards the end of the pill packet.

If this appears for more than a few months, a change of pill may be advised. This bleeding does not, however, mean that the pill is not working. Don't stop taking the pill because of the bleeding: finish the packet normally.

◆ Erosion of the cervix

A harmless and treatable alteration of the surface of the cervix, sometimes associated with pregnancy, or the contraceptive pill use.

- Heavy, clear vaginal discharge.
- Bleeding after intercourse.
- Brief, irregular blood-spotting between periods. Blood appears on underclothing and lavatory paper unexpectedly.

Treatment involves cauterizing that part of the cervix, an outpatient procedure.

◆ Hormone imbalance

Caused by changes in natural hormone levels during the cycle.

- A possibility in young women.
- Regular, scanty, inter-menstrual bleeding.

- Periods are otherwise normal.

The diagnosis is made only after the other possibilities have been ruled out.

◆ Ovulation bleeding: mittelschmerz

Occurs at the time of ovulation, midway between periods when an egg is released from the ovary.

- Sometimes accompanied by lower abdominal pain.
- Sometimes followed by a change in the nature of vaginal discharge.
- Doesn't occur when on the combined contraceptive pill.

Possible

◆ Polyp of the cervix

A small fleshy outgrowth from the cervix, which causes no other symptoms, and which may be visible to a doctor during an internal examination. Polyps usually need to be removed, though they are rarely cancerous.

Unusual in young women.

◆ Inflammation of the vagina

May be due to infection.

In post-menopausal women, when vaginal skin becomes thin and raw and is often accompanied by: dryness of the vagina, itch, and sometimes a thin, watery, blood-tinged discharge.

Treatment aims to eradicate the infection, and put female hormones back into the walls of the vagina, with oestrogen cream or hormone replacement therapy (HRT).

◆ Cancer of the cervix

Cervical cancer is one form of cancer that should be largely preventable by having regular cervical cytology (smear) tests. There is also an effective vaccine which can be given to girls before they become sexually active.

It is associated with infection by the *Human papilloma virus* types 16, 18 and 33. Commoner in women with many sexual partners, those who have sex at a young age, those who have many children, or those with HIV or other STDs.

There is a pre-cancerous stage (cervical intraepithelial neoplasia or CIN) which has no symptoms but can be detected by having regular cervical cytology tests – at least every three years. If abnormal, women are advised to have a more detailed examination of the cervix with a microscope (colposcopy). If needed, simple outpatient treatment may be given during colposcopy to destroy the abnormal cells. Sometimes the pre-cancerous stage reverts to normal without treatment.

Cervical cancer in its early stages may have no symptoms, but later may present with:

- Bleeding after intercourse or bleeding between periods.
- Unusual vaginal discharge.
- In advanced cases there may be pain in the pelvis or pain from secondary spread to adjacent structures, or other parts of the body.

Early treatment is simpler and can be curative, whilst more advanced disease carries a worse outlook and requires more extensive intervention.

◆ Cancer of the womb

See page 312.

Rare

◆ Urethral caruncle

See page 312.

Bleeding after the menopause

Bleeding which occurs more than a year after periods have apparently finished is a very important symptom, which should not be ignored, even if it happens only once, or if the blood looks pink rather than the usual full red. Always seek medical advice if this occurs. There can be confusion with bleeding in urine, or from the anus or bowel, so be prepared for your doctor to examine those regions, too.

Probable

◆ Atrophic vaginitis

Thinning of the vaginal lining associated with menopause.

- Associated with dryness of the vagina, soreness and pain with intercourse.
- Pinkish discharge is commoner than outright bleeding.
- Responds to oestrogen creams or HRT.

Reproductive &
Sexual Organs

◆ **Polyp of the cervix**

See page 310.

Possible

◆ **Cancer of the womb**

About 10-20 per cent of women with bleeding after the menopause will have cancer of the lining of the womb (the endometrium).

Pain is a sign of advanced disease. The first symptom is usually painless bleeding.

Diagnosis is confirmed by sampling the endometrium – usually as an outpatient or sometimes under anaesthetic (D and C – dilatation and curettage).

Treatment is usually by hysterectomy and radiotherapy.

If it is caught early, the outlook is positive, but in advanced disease the prognosis is poor, underlining the need to report post-menopausal bleeding as soon as possible.

◆ **Cancer of the cervix**

See page 311.

Rare

◆ **Urethral caruncle**

This occurs when the outlet from the bladder, the urethra lying just in front of the vagina, becomes swollen and inflamed. The treatment is usually surgical.

• The swollen area is painful to touch.

• Pain when passing urine.

• Pain on intercourse.

Bleeding from the vagina

This topic refers to bleeding which is unexpected. Menstrual problems are dealt with under specific headings.

Probable

◆ **Miscarriage**

Pregnancy is a possibility for any woman of childbearing years who experiences unusual vaginal bleeding. There is often great difficulty in deciding between a miscarriage and an ectopic pregnancy (see opposite). Miscarriages up to the twelfth week after conception are common, occurring in up to 20-40 per cent of pregnancies. They are emotionally traumatic. The chances are increased in the presence of:

• A missed period.

• Tender breasts, morning sickness.

• Lower abdominal pain.

◆ **Ectopic pregnancy**

Occurs if a fertilized egg implants not within the womb, but somewhere else, usually inside the fallopian tube. Typical symptoms include:

• Usually one or two missed periods, abdominal pain which may be severe, then vaginal bleeding. Sometimes the bleeding is internal and if heavy may cause may cause faintness, or shoulder tip pain.

• Risk factors include a history of pelvic

inflammatory disease, endometriosis or use of the contraceptive coil or progesterone-only contraceptive pill.

This is a life threatening emergency. Treatment is usually surgical, involving removal of the pregnancy and sometimes the tube. Occasionally an early ectopic is treated with a drug called methotrexate or by observation without the need for an operation. Later fertility can be affected.

Possible

◆ Complications late in pregnancy

In an established pregnancy, bleeding suggests a possible abnormality of the placenta. Painless bleeding happens if the placenta is lying too low in the womb (medical term: placenta praevia). Painful bleeding, especially after 26 weeks, may mean that part of the placenta has detached from the womb (abruption). In either case, a full and urgent obstetric assessment is essential.

◆ Disease of the cervix

A possibility if the symptoms include any of the following, each of which is dealt with under specific headings:

- Heavy vaginal discharge.
- Irregular bleeding.
- Bleeding after intercourse.

◆ Disease of the womb

This is the likeliest cause of vaginal bleeding after menopause, an extremely important symptom.

◆ Atrophic vaginitis

See page 311.

Rare

◆ Abnormal blood clotting

See page 305.

Discharge from the vagina

Normal discharge from the vagina is clear, or slightly yellow. It varies in volume and consistency during the monthly cycle, reaching a peak at the time of ovulation, which is roughly mid-cycle. Vaginal discharge is also increased by sexual activity and ejaculation of semen into the vagina during intercourse. If you have a coil fitted, the amount of discharge may increase. Any change in the amount, consistency or smell of the discharge from what you would normally expect can be considered abnormal.

Probable

◆ Thrush

Caused by a yeast infection – usually *Candida albicans*, which commonly live in small numbers around the genital area. Symptoms occur when the yeasts multiply and inflame the skin. Usually not sexually transmitted and a male partner does not need treatment unless he has the symptoms. Risk factors include diabetes and having recently taken antibiotics.

Typical symptoms include:

- Vaginal itching, white discharge (sometimes 'curd' like), and redness or soreness in the vulva and vagina.

Can be self treated with pessaries, creams or tablets which kill the yeasts.

Consider the possibility other STIs, especially if the symptoms do not settle with treatment.

◆ Bacterial vaginosis

Caused by an imbalance of the normal bacteria in the vagina with an overgrowth of anaerobic types, typically *Gardnerella vaginalis*. Not thought to be sexually transmitted, so partners do not usually need to be treated.

- Produces a smell, sometimes described as fishy or cheesy.

Treated with an oral antibiotic – metronidazole or clindamycin cream in the vagina.

Consider the possibility other STIs, especially if the symptoms do not settle with treatment.

Possible

◆ Atrophic vaginitis

See page 311.

◆ Erosion of the cervix

See page 310.

◆ Polyp of cervix or womb

See page 310.

◆ Vaginal infections and other sexually transmitted infections (STIs)

Chlamydia and rarely trichomonas or gonorrhoea.

Needs specialist assessment, tracing of sexual contacts and treatment.

Always seek medical advice if you suspect an STI.

◆ Pelvic inflammatory disease

See page page 304.

◆ Foreign body

Probably the commonest is a tampon lodged deep inside the vagina. Young girls sometimes push small things inside themselves. Occasionally condoms slip off and are retained in the vagina.

- Yellow or green discharge, increasingly heavy.
- Very smelly.
- Possibly fever.

Tampons and the like are easily removed; children may need a specialist's help.

Rare

◆ Tumour

Growths in and around the vagina may be a rare cause of a persistent discharge, but should be visible on gynaecological inspection. Occasionally, tumours of the womb, cervix and ovaries can present with a discharge.

◆ Sexual abuse

This upsetting possibility needs to be considered for girls who have recurrent or unusual vaginal discharges. Signs of sexual interference might include:

- Tears, bruising around the vagina or back passage.
- Disturbed behaviour.

Reproductive & Sexual Organs

This highly charged topic needs the utmost care, both to avoid false conclusions and yet to uncover hidden misery. If suspected, the case, should be placed in professional hands.

Vaginal protrusion and swelling of the vulva

Probable

◆ **Prolapse of the womb**

Occurs typically in women who have had children, or after the menopause, due to weakening of the muscles in the pelvis and around the vagina.

- The cervix is felt as a firm lump, coming down into the vagina.
- Worse on coughing, straining.
- Lessens on lying flat or relaxing.
- Surgical repair is possible.

Possible

◆ **Prolapse of the bladder or rectum**

Bladder prolapse is felt in the front of the vagina.

- Usually causes leakage of urine on coughing, laughing.
- Rectal prolapse is felt at the back of the vagina.

  Surgical repair is possible.

◆ **Vulval varicosities**

Seen in pregnancy where the veins and tissues in the vulva become engorged with blood. Usually resolves after childbirth.

◆ **Labial cysts, Bartholin's cyst**

- Presents as a swelling on the vaginal lips, usually on one side only.
- Commonly gets infected and may be painful or discharge pus.

  May need antibiotic or surgical treatment.

◆ **Genital warts**

See page 343.

Rare

◆ **Tumour**

The growth could arise from the womb, or the walls of the vagina or adjacent organs; gynaecological examination will pinpoint this.

Reproductive & Sexual Organs

Vaginal odour

Probable

◆ **Normal**

Some vaginal odour is unavoidable, and is probably a sexual cue.

Possible

◆ **Infection**

- Suggested by odours which are very smelly, or fishy.

- Accompanied by itch and discharge.

  For causes, see section above on discharge from the vagina.

◆ Foreign body

See page 314.

◆ Psychological

- An odour, but your partner or doctor smell nothing unusual.
- A worry that the odour is obvious to others or feeling the need to wash or clean the genital area too frequently.

  A sympathetic ear may allow worries to be expressed, typically about the fear of STIs or cancer.

Rare

◆ Cancer

Cancer of the cervix, womb, or even the bowel, may cause a persistent, foul-smelling vaginal discharge, bleeding, and pain.

Things should not reach this stage unless warning symptoms have been neglected, such as unusual vaginal bleeding, discharges and changes of bowel habit.

Vaginal pain

The causes overlap with those symptoms described under *Painful sexual intercourse*, see page 339.

Probable

◆ Infections

See under causes of *Vaginal discharge*.

◆ Atrophic vaginitis

See page 311.

Possible

◆ Vaginismus

Spasm of the muscles around the vagina which contract so tightly that intercourse is difficult or impossible.

Treatment involves psychological techniques to improve relaxation and sexual confidence.

Rare

◆ Cancer

Cancer growing within the vagina can cause pain, but it is highly unlikely to be an early or sole symptom.

Previously there is likely to have been: bleeding after intercourse, between periods or after the menopause. Usually there will be discharge which may be bloodstained.

Vulval itch

Probable

◆ Infection

- Rapid onset of intense itch.
- White or coloured discharge.

  Most commonly due to *Thrush*, see page 313.

Possible

◆ Allergy

The sensitive skin in and around the vagina may itch because of allergy to over-vigorous washing, bubble baths, vaginal deodorants or condoms. Diagnosis is arrived at by cutting out all possible irritants, and then testing each one individually. Special low-allergy condoms are available.

◆ Threadworms/crab lice

Threadworms are extremely common, particularly in childhood. Itching is intense, especially at night and usually felt in and around the anus.

Crab lice are sexually transmitted and may be visible on close inspection in the pubic area; consider the possibility of other STIs if you find them.

Treatment of both is straightforward.

◆ Eczema/psoriasis

Common skin disorders, causing:

- Dry, flaking areas.
- Psoriasis spreads around back passage.
- Usually skin elsewhere is affected.

Rare

◆ Lichen sclerosis (LS) or leukoplakia

LS is typically whitish or shiny, thin-looking skin, sometimes with cracking and soreness.

Leukoplakia is whitish skin with thickening.

Commonest in the elderly, but LS can also occur in children.

Specialist assessment and follow up is essential as complications can include cancer.

◆ Cancer

Skin cancer may present the following symptoms:

- An itchy sore.
- Slowly grows.
- Bleeds.

Treatment is usually curative, but the earlier the diagnosis, the better.

◆ General disease

Several disorders may cause generalised itch. Specific features might include:

- Swollen lymph nodes – suggest infection or lymphoma.
- Jaundice suggests liver disease.
- Changes in volume of urine produced suggests diabetes.
- Widespread skin involvement due to other skin diseases.
- Joint pains suggesting rheumatological diseases.

See also *Itching – without a rash*, page 244.

Pain in the pelvis

Pains in the lower abdomen are common in women, and are frequently difficult to diagnose. Apart from gynaecological causes (problems in the womb, tubes, ovaries and vagina), there are other pelvic organs to consider: the intestines, and the bladder. In addition pain from other abdominal organs, such as the kidneys, can be referred to the pelvis; as can pain from irritation of nerves in the back. Diseases of

Reproductive & Sexual Organs

the major arteries which run through the lower abdomen can also be implicated. The abdomen is also a sensitive index of emotional turmoil, at all ages and in both sexes. Pain associated with the following symptoms suggest a gynaecological cause:

• Painful periods.

• Unusual vaginal discharge.

• Abnormal vaginal bleeding.

• Pain on intercourse.

• Infertility.

See the sections referring to these symptoms for further details. Symptoms pointing to a non-gynaecological cause are:

• Diarrhoea, constipation or bleeding from the bowel.

• Frequent or painful urination or the presence of blood in the urine.

• Pain varies depending on your posture – suggests a muscular or back cause.

• Pulsation in your abdomen, pain in your legs on walking.

• Depression, anxiety or relationship problems.

Your overall condition may point to one of the many non-gynaecological diseases which can cause recurrent abdominal pains.

Your doctor will rely on the pattern of symptoms, and the results of tests, before making a diagnosis.

Hot flushes

Probable

◆ Menopause

Known also as 'the change', or 'the change of life', and linked to the drop in levels of oestrogens present in the blood. It marks the end of fertility. Average age of the menopause is 51 years, though this varies. In addition to hot flushes, symptoms include:

• Periods become irregular with variable flow before stopping.

• The skin of the vagina becomes drier and thinner – see *Atrophic vaginitis*, page 311.

• There is atrophy of other oestrogen dependant tissues in the genital area and breasts, leading to urinary

leakage – stress incontinence, and prolapse, see page 315.

• There is weakening of the bones, leading to osteoporosis and risk of fractures.

Some features are more controversial, perhaps a reflection of personal adjustments to this major event in a woman's life:

• Loss of sexual desire.

• Depression.

• Irritability.

Hot flushes usually continue for about two years; a few unlucky individuals continue to have them for more. This is not a symptom of disease. For some women, it is a relief for periods to end; for others, it is a matter of deep emotion: the beginning of old age. The reaction of the majority of women lies some where between the two, and is intimately connected with support from their partners and families, and their own self-esteem.

Overall about 80 per cent of women manage without any medical intervention. For others, hormone replacement therapy (HRT) is an effective treatment for the symptoms of the menopause, relieving hot flushes, vaginal dryness and slowing the development of osteoporosis. Whether it relieves the psychological symptoms is more controversial. A decision about HRT needs detailed discussion with your doctor about the likely benefit versus the adverse risks, such as increased breast cancer risk in long term users. Women wanting mainly to reduce the risk of osteoporosis have the option of other non-HRT treatments.

Alternative or complementary therapies are widely used to good effect.

Possible

◆ Overactive thyroid gland

Symptoms include:

- Sweating, increased appetite, weight loss.

- Intolerance to heat.
- Hand tremor.
- Consistently rapid pulse, possibly palpitations.
- Protruding eyes (in some cases).

Treatment aims to reduce the output of thyroid hormone from the thyroid gland.

Rare

◆ Persistent fever or sweats

It is worth considering whether any of the many causes of fevers or sweats might be responsible. The subject is covered in detail elsewhere, but your suspicions might be aroused by:

- Hot flushes occurring with in the presence of a measurable fever.
- Hot flushes beginning abruptly while periods are still normal and regular.
- Drenching sweats at night.
- Malaise, weight loss.
- Symptoms starting after foreign travel to areas of endemic disease, such as malaria zones.
- Occupational risks, for example in health workers exposed to ill patients.
- The presence of enlarged lymph glands.

Masculine changes in women

The development of male features in a woman may reflect upsets in the balance between male and female hormones in the body, unless this is clearly a feature of your family or race. If periods are normal,

then a serious underlying hormonal problem is unlikely. However the expectations and acceptability of certain features such as body hair vary enormously between different women and depend to some extent on external factors, such as fashion and also age.

Typical masculine changes are:

- Growth of hair on the face chest, abdomen.
- Balding.
- Deepening voice.
- Disruption of periods.

Probable

◆ Hereditary and racial differences

Racial and family differences in hairiness are well known: for example, both men and women from Mediterranean races tend to be hairier than Nordic peoples. There is no effect on fertility.

Possible

◆ Polycystic ovarian syndrome

See page 308.

◆ Menopause

Some women approaching or going through the menopause notice an increase in facial hair or loss of feminine features.

◆ Hypothyroidism

An under-active gland may often be the reason for masculinisation, as it causes:

- Gruff voice, coarse dry skin.
- Periods become heavy or irregular.

    Additional features of an under-active thyroid gland are:

- Weight gain.

- Slow thought.
- Slow pulse.
- Weakness.
- Constipation.

    The diagnosis is made on the basis of blood tests.

◆ Drugs

Hairiness is a side effect of several widely-used drugs, for instance steroids, used to treat certain arthritic diseases.

Rare

◆ Ovarian tumour

Suspected in a previously healthy woman who develops signs of masculinisation.

    There are no other symptoms of an early tumour, which must be detected by examination and ultrasound investigation.

◆ Cushing's syndrome

There are many causes of this syndrome, which is due to the effects of excessive amounts of steroid hormones either produced in the body or more commonly as a side effect of steroids given to treat other diseases. Among its symptoms are:

- Obese body, but thin limbs.
- Masculine features.
- Easy bruising.
- Excessive production of urine.
- Purple stripes or stretch marks across the hip, and other fat-bearing areas.

Breast disorders

It is wise for women to check their breasts from time to time, aiming to familiarise themselves with how they feel normally so that changes can be spotted early. Remember that the breast is sensitive to hormones present in the body and that these vary with the different phases of the menstrual cycle. The breasts feel slightly different at different times of the month. Any change from the 'normal' feel of the breast tissue should prompt a visit to the doctor. Remember also that the tissues of the breast extend into the armpit, so checks should include that area. Mammography (an X-ray examination of the breast) is used to detect changes before you notice a problem. Such screening programmes are not 100 per cent reliable, and may turn up abnormalities which, on further investigation, prove harmless. However, these false alarms are a price worth paying in order to detect more serious disease such as cancer at an early stage, when treatment is more likely to produce a cure. Further tests include fine needle aspiration cytology (FNAC), where a syringe needle is used to sample cells from the breast. Breast ultrasound may help to clarify or confirm the exact diagnosis. Breast cancer is undoubtedly the most feared and serious cause of symptoms in the breast, but it is not necessarily the most likely cause. The best advice is to seek medical help if you develop any breast symptoms which differ from what you know to be your norm.

Lump in the breast

At some time in their lives most women will feel a lump in one of their breasts. Breasts are frequently lumpy, and some of these lumps are easily felt. In eight out of ten cases, it will be entirely harmless. Where cancer is diagnosed, you should remember that the outlook is much more likely to be good than bad and that most women can look forward to successful treatment with the real possibility of a cure. Breast cancer is one of the most closely studied forms of cancer, but doctors will admit that there is still an enormous amount they do not know about it. Fundamental questions remain unanswered, such as why the cancer starts, how quickly it grows and how best to treat it. Expert opinion about therapy is constantly changing and improving, following the results of treatment trials which are being carried out worldwide.

Probable

♦ **Fibroadenoma**

- Commonest in women between 29 and 40 years old.

- Firm, painless lump.

- Freely mobile: which is why this lump has been described as a 'breast mouse'.

Some women have several of these over many years, but each one should be checked by a doctor and is usually removed. They are not thought to lead to cancer.

◆ Fibrocystic disease

This is a misleading technical term for something that is not really a disease at all.

The breasts are generally lumpy, and within that lumpiness there may be more definite, large lumps which are usually fluid-filled cysts.

- Commonest in women 30 to 50 years of age.
- Lumpiness varies during the menstrual cycle.
- Often pain before a period.
- Often areas of the breast are tender.

Mammography (breast X-ray) is useful for differentiating these lumps from cancer. Many surgeons will drain obvious cysts, using a needle and syringe, and send the contents for detailed analysis. No other treatment is necessarily needed.

◆ Breast abscess

- A painful lump which enlarges over several days.
- Overlying skin is hot and red.
- Fever or flu-like symptoms.
- Sometimes a bloody discharge mixed with milk from the nipple.
- Commonest when breast feeding – usually following an episode of 'mastitis'.

Possible

◆ Breast cancer

You feel a lump; it may be tiny, but you are sure it has appeared recently. Some of the features that would suggest that a lump is likely to be cancerous are:

- A firm, irregular lump.
- Skin over it is dimpled and puckered.
- A newly indrawn nipple, or any nipple changes occurring at the same time.
- Swollen glands felt in armpit.
- Pain in the region of the lump, though the majority of early cancers are painless.
- Bleeding from the nipple.
- Risk factors for developing breast cancer include family history of the disease and increasing age – 80 per cent of cases occur in women over 50.

Tests to confirm the diagnosis include biopsy using fine needle aspiration cytology (FNAC) where a syringe and needle are used to sample cells from the lump, mammography, breast ultrasound and sometimes other scans and blood tests.

Treatment depends on the type of cancer, its size and location (including whether it has spread to other areas), and other important factors such as the age and general health and, most importantly, the preference of the patient. Possible surgical treatments include lumpectomy (removal of the lump), mastectomy (removal of the breast), and exploration and sampling

Reproductive & Sexual Organs

of the lymph glands in the armpit. Surgical reconstruction of the breast may also help with cosmetic and psychological wellbeing. Surgical treatment may be combined with radiotherapy, chemotherapy, and may be followed by a course of medication to modify hormone levels (such as tamoxifen).

Every case is different and the treatment needs to be matched to the needs and preferences of the woman concerned.

◆ Duct papilloma

A lump felt just below the nipple, and associated with a bloody discharge from the nipple. This should always be reported to your doctor.

Rare

◆ Fat necrosis

A hard knock to the breast can damage fat cells, leading to a lump that feels indistinguishable from a cancer.

- The first sign is often bruising visible on the skin.
- A firm lump.
- Does not move freely.
- Skin over it may be dimpled.

The only safe way to deal with this is a biopsy.

◆ Other tumours

It is possible for cancers elsewhere to spread into the breast. The diagnosis will probably only be made on biopsy.

Reproductive & Sexual Organs

Pain in the breast

If pain is widespread and felt in both breasts, it is usually caused by a variation in hormone levels. If it is confined to one area, then you should feel for a localised abnormality, such as a lump or dimpled skin. Breast pain may be no more than a nuisance, but for some women it can be a great problem. Persistent pain should always be discussed with a doctor to establish its cause and whether further tests are needed. Once serious causes have been excluded, there will often be a simple solution such as a change in contraceptive pill, or a recommendation to take evening primrose oil.

Probable

◆ Hormonal variation

- Commonly seen when starting the oral contraceptive pill or HRT.
- Cyclical variation, typically with pre-menstrual tenderness.
- Can be an early symptom of pregnancy.
- Common in late pregnancy or after childbirth, as milk production starts.

◆ Fibrocystic disease

See opposite.

Possible

◆ **Breast cancer**

See page 322.

Most early breast cancers present as painless lumps.

◆ **Breast abscess**

See page 322.

◆ **Pain from the ribs or muscles**

Inflammation of the muscles

between ribs, or where the rib and the breast bone meet.

• One breast affected.

• An injury or strain may be the cause.

• Pain is sharp, and highly localised.

• Pain reproduced by pressing between the ribs, or by pressing on the breastbone.

A harmless symptom that settles over a few weeks.

Breast size

As with any part of the body, there is considerable variation in breast size. Furthermore, the perception or appreciation of breast size is influenced by cultural and popular expectations.

Breast size does not affect the ability to breast feed a child, nor is it related to fertility. Furthermore, it is normal for the two breasts to be slightly different in size and shape.

Probable

◆ **Hereditary**

Breast size is mainly determined by in-built factors, in other words genetic control and expression. Race also plays a part, with Asiatic women generally having smaller breasts. Reasons for breast surgery to increase or decrease breast size or modify breast shape might include: psychological distress, neck and back pains from very heavy breasts, or for cosmetic enhancement.

Possible

◆ **Hormonal**

The contraceptive pill and hormone replacement therapy often cause a slight increase in breast size. Pregnancy, of course, makes the breasts enlarge, as a result of changing hormone levels. Many women notice a slight variation in size during their menstrual cycle.

Rare

◆ **Lymphatic obstruction**

Interference with normal drainage of tissue fluid from the breast via the armpit will lead to one swollen breast.

• Often after radiotherapy to the chest wall, when the arm on that side is very swollen.

• You may feel glands in the armpit: report this immediately.

• Breasts become generally firm. Unfortunately, little can usually be done to cure this problem.

Reproductive & Sexual Organs

Discharge from the nipple

During pregnancy it is normal for a milky fluid to ooze from the breasts. Mothers who breast feed will find not only that suckling causes a discharge of milk, but that even the sound of the baby crying will trigger this response, and again this is entirely normal. Abnormal discharges include milk in the absence of pregnancy, clear fluid, or blood, or yellow/green pus.

Discharges are commonly due to disease of the duct system. This is the network of some 20 channels through which milk flows to the nipple from the milk-producing glands, deep within the breast. Abnormal discharge from the nipple should always prompt a visit to the doctor.

Probable

◆ Hormone disturbance

Milk production is controlled by a hormone, prolactin, secreted by the pituitary gland within the brain. An excess of prolactin causes:

- Discharge of milk from both breasts for months on end.
- Periods become scanty or stop altogether.
- Blood tests will show abnormal levels of prolactin.

The usual reason is a tiny growth in the pituitary gland: this can be controlled with appropriate drugs or surgery.

A few medically prescribed drugs can cause this problem, particularly neuroleptic medication used to treat mental illness.

◆ Breast abscess

See page 322.

Possible

The three following possibilities give similar symptoms, and in all cases will require further investigation, since examination alone is not enough to decide definitely between them.

◆ Duct ectasia

In this condition, enlarged ducts allow the build-up of normal secretions, which then appear as:

- A brown or green discharge.
- Discharge is firm and cheese-like.

◆ Duct papilloma

- A wart-like, benign growth within one of the ducts leading to the nipple.
- A bloody discharge, perhaps just a spot of blood on the bra.
- Sometimes just a clear, yellowish discharge.
- A lump may be felt near the nipple.

◆ Cancer of ducts

- Bloody discharge.
- Possibly a pricking sensation behind the nipple.

Rare

◆ Breast cancer

- Occasionally a breast cancer some distance from the nipple causes bleeding.
- A breast lump is likely.
- Some discomfort is possible.

Reproductive &
Sexual Organs

◆ **Paget's disease of the nipple**

A distinctive condition, most common in older women

- Cracked, dry, red skin around one nipple.

- Oozes blood.
- The nipple becomes distorted.
- This disease is nearly always due to breast cancer.

Retraction or inversion of the nipple

Both nipples normally project a little, becoming flatter when warm or relaxed, and more protuberant if cold, or in response to touch or sexual stimulation. Retracted or inverted nipples appear sunken into the breast.

Probable

◆ **Congenital**

Commonly seen in baby girls who grow up with one or both nipples retracted or inverted, this persists into adulthood and tends to be lifelong.

It is not a sign of disease, but might affect the ability to breast feed.

There are many 'cures' for retracted nipples, but there is little evidence that they work

Possible

◆ **Breast cancer**

The retraction or inversion of a previously normal nipple must be taken as a symptom of breast cancer until proven otherwise. You should search for:

- Lump in the breast.
- Discharge from the nipples.
- Always inform your doctor of any such changes to your nipples.

Symptoms in men

Lumps in the testicles or scrotum

In the same way that women should be encouraged to be aware of and familiar with the normal feel of their breasts, men are advised to familiarise themselves with the normal feel of the contents of the scrotum. This is best done when the muscle contained in the scrotal wall is relaxed, such as in a warm bath. Both testicles should be approximately the same size, with the left one commonly lying

slightly lower than the right. It is possible to feel the epididymis which is a firmish slightly irregular structure wrapped round the back of the testicles and attaching to the spermatic cord above. It is common to find small lumps in the skin of the scrotum; these are usually harmless cysts in the skin or sebaceous glands at the roots of pubic hairs. Any variation in the contents of the scrotum from normal should be reported to a doctor who will examine you and may recommend an ultrasound scan for confirmation of the diagnosis.

Probable

◆ Epididymal cyst

- A harmless swelling, arising from the epididymis.
- The swelling feels separate from the testicle.
- Epididymal cysts may be multiple and present on both sides of the scrotum.

Once confirmed, nothing need be done about a cyst unless it is causing discomfort.

◆ Varicocele

A harmless swelling caused by enlarged varicose veins, 'like a bag of worms' felt above and behind the testicle.

May cause fertility problems if present in both testicles. Sometimes treated surgically.

Possible

◆ Cancer of the testicle

Overall this is a rare tumour, but it is the commonest malignancy affecting men between 15 and 40 years of age. Elderly men are also at risk. A lump in a testicle is cancer until proven otherwise and always requires medical assessment. Typically, cancer of the testicles presents as:

- A firm, painless enlargement of one testicle.
- Depending on the size of the cancer, the scrotum may appear swollen or there may be a sensation of heaviness.

The treatment depends on the precise type of tumour, but carries a very positive outlook, particularly if any changes are spotted early.

Rare

◆ Tuberculosis

Also uncommon, though increasing among the poor and homeless.

- A painless, enlarged testicle.
- May discharge in the same way as an abscess, but without throbbing pain.
- Other features of tuberculosis, such as cough, malaise, sweats, weight loss.

Swollen testicles or scrotum

This means swelling without any obvious lump. For lumps in the testicle or scrotum, see opposite. Swellings may be due to an underlying cancer, and should always be medically examined. Don't delay in reporting to your doctor any changes you notice in your testicles – early treatment has a very significant effect on the likelihood of a complete cure.

Probable

◆ Hydrocele

- An accumulation of fluid around the testicle.
- Tense, swollen testicle.
- Pain may or may not be present.
- If chronic, can be very large.

Reproductive & Sexual Organs

- In children, often accompanies a hernia.
- Not uncommon at, or soon after, birth.

Specialist opinion should be sought, since there may be an underlying cause such as infection or cancer of the testicle.

◆ Orchitis

A general term for a swollen or inflamed testicle.

- Pain builds up over a few hours.
- Scrotum also usually swells with fluid.
- Underlying causes include injury, infection and mumps.

An acutely painful testicle may be twisted (See *Torsion*, opposite), with a risk of future sterility. Urgent medical attention is essential, especially for children.

Possible

◆ Hernia

The bowel bulges through a weakness in the wall of the abdomen, usually in the groin.

- Commonly just a lump in the groin, but may extend into the scrotum.
- In children, commonly extends to the scrotum, which appears to be swollen.
- Swelling may disappear after lying flat.

May require surgical repair, especially in children.

Rare

◆ Filariasis

A parasite which blocks the drainage of tissue fluids, leading to swelling of the affected region.

- Originates in tropical areas only.
- Repeated inflation of the testicles and epididymis.
- After several infections, the scrotum remains permanently swollen.
- Advanced disease needs surgical treatment.

Pain in the testicles

In boys and young men, pain, especially if it is one-sided, equals torsion (see opposite) until proven otherwise. In other adults there is a wider range of possible diagnoses. If a torsion is suspected, medical advice should be sought straight away as an emergency.

Probable

◆ Epididymitis

The epididymis is a structure involved in the transport of sperm from the testicles, and can normally be felt at the back of the testicle. Inflammation or infection usually occurs for no obvious reason, but if there is also discharge from the penis, a doctor must test for STIs. Epididymitis is an unsafe diagnosis to make for a boy before puberty, in whom torsion is far more likely.

- Pain, initially behind testicle, builds up over a few hours.
- There is swelling of the testicle and scrotum, which become exquisitely tender.
- The scrotum feels hot and there may be fever and nausea.

- Sometimes the testicle becomes infected or inflamed – epididymo-orchitis.
- Antibiotic treatment is needed, plus rest, for a couple of weeks.

◆ Torsion

The testicles hang on a cord, which can twist. Other structures near the testicles can also twist, giving a similar condition. Deciding which has happened can often only be done during an operation. Sometimes doppler ultrasound is used to check the blood flow to the testicle, which becomes compromised with a torsion.

Typical features are:

- Sudden, severe pain in one testicle.
- Nausea, vomiting.
- Affected testicle swells and is tender.

An urgent operation is nearly always needed to untwist the testicle, and to anchor it into place in order to prevent recurrence. It is usual to operate on the other testicle also: if one has twisted, the other is likely to do so in the future. Neglected torsion will inevitably lead to death of the affected testicle, with future effects on fertility.

Possible

◆ Injury

- A definite history of injury to the scrotum, such as a kick in the crotch.
- Pain, tenderness, and visible bruising.
- Normal urinary stream and no blood.

Support and time to heal are the only remedies.

◆ Varicocele

See page 327.

◆ Stone

A stone in the urinary system gives rise to:

- Pain of rapid onset and often of great severity, lasting an hour or so.
- Pains recur over days and weeks.
- Appears to radiate from the low back (kidney region) to the testicles, or to the tip of the penis.
- Nausea, vomiting.
- Blood in urine.

Small stones will pass spontaneously, whereas larger ones may need surgical removal.

Rare

◆ Mumps orchitis

Mumps is an increasingly rare disease because of immunisation programmes. A few cases give rise to inflammation of the testicles, called orchitis.

- Mumps causes swellings, like hamster cheeks, just in front of the jaw joint.
- After three to four days one or both testicles may swell.
- Fever, pain.

The risk of orchitis is much less than once thought. Although sterility may follow, it appears that this too is much less of a risk than was once feared.

◆ Pancreatitis

See page 434.

Reproductive &
Sexual Organs

Pain between the legs

Probable

◆ Injury

Injury between the legs may irritate the prostate gland, giving rise to:

- A dull ache between the legs.
- Slight discomfort or difficulty passing urine.
- Blood in the urine, if there has been a severe injury, such as falling astride an object.

Possible

◆ Prostatitis

Prostatitis is an infection or inflammation of the prostate gland. Symptoms include:

- Pain in the saddle area between the anus and scrotum.
- Burning sensation or difficulty when passing urine.

- Urine may appear cloudy and laboratory tests may show infection.
- Sometimes fever, muscle or joint pains.
- May be a recurrent or chronic problem.

This can be an awkward problem to eradicate, often needing extended courses of antibiotics.

Rare

◆ Cancer of the prostate

An advanced cancer may produce the following:

- Ache or pain between legs.
- Pain in the back or pelvis because of spread of the cancer to bones.

More usually, cancer of the prostate is painless, and is found on investigation after:

- Difficulty passing urine, caused by enlargement of the prostate, which obstructs the passage of urine.

Absent testicle

This should be discovered at routine child health checks from birth onwards. A testicle which is not brought down into the scrotum is at risk of decreased fertility and also at greater risk of a malignant change in later life.

Probable

◆ Undescended testicle

- Normal general development.

- Testicle often felt as a lump in the groin.

Three to four per cent of male babies have undescended testicles at birth. Some of these descend spontaneously by the age of one. Medical advice should be sought early to establish the diagnosis and advise on the need for an operation. Surgical treatment reduces the risk of damaged fertility and subsequent testicular cancer.

Reproductive & Sexual Organs

Possible

◆ Retractile testicle

An exaggeration of a normal reflex, which pulls the testicles up into the groin.

- Testicle is present at certain times.
- Cold, and emotion, can cause retraction.
- Usually no treatment is needed for this condition.

Rare

◆ Ectopic testicle

The testicle may lodge itself somewhere in the lower abdomen. It may be felt in the groin, at the base of the penis, or even the upper thigh.

Surgical correction is recommended in order to preserve fertility.

Small testicle

Testicles vary in size and the left testicle usually hangs lower than the right one. Fertility may be normal unless both testicles are very small or defective in their function. Alcoholism and drugs used in treating cancer of the prostate may cause previously normal testicles to decrease in size.

Probable

◆ Previous injury or infection

Likely if:

- Only one testicle is small.
- Previous pain.
- Previous swelling.
- Sometimes occurs in undescended testicles which are surgically brought down into the scrotum, especially if this is done late.

Possible causes include twisted testicles and orchitis. See *Pain in the testicles.*

Possible

◆ Hormone disorders

- Both testicles are small.
- Individual is often very tall.
- Absent or decreased body hair.
- Breast development.
- Infertility.

Hormone testing is needed to pinpoint the root cause.

◆ Genetic disorders

A fascinating, highly complex area, touching on 'intersex' and ambiguous sexual development.

- Testicles and penis may be abnormally formed.
- The individual is likely to be abnormally tall or short.
- Infertility.

Discharge from penis

Whether clear or coloured, discharge from the penis is highly suggestive of a sexually transmitted infection, commonly abbreviated to STI, with non-specific genital infection (NSGI) and gonorrhoea being the most likely causes. Must be seen at a specialist clinic; partner also likely to be infected.

Reproductive &
Sexual Organs

Diseased foreskin

The foreskin is subject to infection, resulting in cracking and scar tissue formation. It may cause pain, interfere with passing urine and make sexual intercourse difficult.

Probable

◆ Balanitis

An infection of the foreskin and adjacent penis.

- Mild pain, itching and redness.
- Discharge around the foreskin, not from the opening of the penis itself.
- Sometimes associated with skin disease, such as seborrhoeic dermatitis or psoriasis.

  Antibiotics, plus salt baths, are the treatment. Diabetes may underlie recurrent balanitis.

◆ Phimosis

Phimosis is an inability to retract the foreskin back from the tip of the penis.

A non-retractile foreskin is normal in boys up to five years old and it is wrong to attempt to do so. It may be abnormal if there is:

- Recurrent balanitis.
- Ballooning of the foreskin on passing urine.

Circumcision or stretching of the foreskin is then advisable.

Possible

◆ Paraphimosis

The foreskin becomes stuck, rolled behind the tip of the penis.

- Pain.
- Swelling of tip of penis prevents unrolling the foreskin back over the tip of the penis.

  This calls for rapid treatment to put the foreskin back in its correct position. Local anaesthetic gels can help a doctor to achieve this, but sometimes surgery is necessary.

Rare

◆ Cancer of the penis

A rarity in the West, but common in some Far Eastern countries.

- It is unusual among circumcised men, the exact reason being unclear.
- Begins as a red area on the tip of the penis, or hidden within the foreskin.
- Grows, ulcerates.
- Discharge, pain, bleeding.

  Treatment is radiotherapy and surgery.

Blood in semen

A fairly common symptom, which looks alarming, but hardly ever has a serious underlying cause. In fact, the reason remains unknown for the vast majority of cases. It is commonest in elderly men. It may be mistaken for bleeding from the vagina after intercourse.

It is sensible to have your genitalia

Reproductive & Sexual Organs

examined, plus a urine check, to ensure that the blood does not come from the bladder. Otherwise, nothing else needs to be done unless the symptom recurs, when an internal check of the bladder and prostate gland may be advisable.

Painful penis

Probable

◆ **Infection**

- Burning pain on passing urine.
- Need to urinate frequently.
- Possibly blood in the urine.
- Urine cloudy or smelly.

These symptoms suggest a urinary tract infection. Such infections, whether in a boy or adult, should always be investigated usually by ultrasound scan or X-ray examination, since underlying physical causes are common.

A discharge suggests sexually transmitted infection (STIs).

◆ **Diseased foreskin**

See opposite.

Possible

◆ **Stone**

See *Kidney stones*, page 171.

Rare

◆ **Peyronie's disease**

See below.

Curved penis

Known medically as chordee. Minor degrees are very common and may cause embarrassment, especially in teenagers. The curvature may be more apparent when the penis is erect.

Extreme curvature may make sexual intercourse difficult.

Probable

◆ **Congenital**

- Noticed at birth.
- The opening for urine (external meatus) may be underneath the penis, not at the end – the medical term is hypospadias.

Delicate surgery to correct these abnormalities makes use of the foreskin, which should therefore not be circumcised.

Possible

◆ **Peyronie's disease**

- A band of firm tissue forms on part of the shaft of the penis.
- In the middle-aged, or older.
- Pain and curvature on erection.
- A firm or nodular area felt on the shaft.
- Treatment is difficult.
- Occasionally it disappears spontaneously.

Rare

♦ **Injury**

Vigorous sexual intercourse or other injury

may fracture the erect penis. Needs early treatment to prevent permanent deformity.

• Sudden pain, bruising and deformity.

Small penis

An objective assessment of size is difficult because of variations at different temperatures, and degrees of erection. Nevertheless, there is some biological and racial variation in size, though this rarely correlates with fertility or sexual performance. Adolescent boys and men beginning sexual activity often present to the doctor worrying that their penis is abnormally small, though examination almost always shows the penis to be within the normal size range. There is less variation in the size of the erect penis amongst men, compared to variation in the non-erect state – in other words most penises end up a similar size when they become erect. Worry about a small penis may be justified in the presence of some

of the following features:

• Absent or small testicles.

• Absence of body hair.

• Excessive height.

• Breast development.

• Obesity.

• Previous injury, torsion of testicles.

In boys, a small penis may appear very small if it is sunk in fat in the groin.

Investigations such as chromosome analysis, hormone profiles and brain scans may be needed. As treatment is possible for boys, cases of true micro-penis are worth reporting to a doctor, sooner rather than later.

Prolonged erection

Also known as priapism. A very painful, prolonged erection in the absence of sexual desire. The tip of the penis may remain soft. Whatever the cause, it needs urgent treatment to avoid long-term damage to the penis.

Probable

♦ **Cause unknown**

Accounting for about three out of five cases; it may follow prolonged sexual activity. Otherwise sound health.

Possible

♦ **Blood disorders**

Blood tests will seek leukaemia or sickle cell disease.

Easy bruising, malaise, large glands suggest leukaemia.

Recurrent joint or abdominal pains suggest sickle cell disease (occurs almost exclusively in men of African racial origin).

Rare

◆ All other causes

A routine search is always made for growths in the pelvis. Drugs affecting erection or damage to the spinal cord are also considered.

Feminization in men

Adult men who start to develop female features need a full hormonal assessment. Female features include loss of body hair, development of breasts, loss of sexual drive, and shrinking testicles and penis.

Probable

◆ Drug effects

Some drugs have oestrogenic (female hormone type) or anti-androgenic (anti male hormone type) side effects.

Common culprits are spironolactone; digoxin and beta blockers used in heart disease; oestrogens and anti-androgens for treating cancer of the prostate and chlorpromazine used to treat mental illness.

Possible

◆ Alcoholism

- A history of heavy, prolonged alcohol consumption or alcohol dependency.
- Impotence.
- Breast development.

- Decreased fertility due to diminished sperm count.
- Tests may show cirrhosis of the liver.
- May reverse or partially reverse if alcohol is avoided.

◆ Genetic problems

Men with genetic problems may be:

- Unusually tall individuals.
- Infertile.
- Problems may be apparent from birth.
- Specialist investigation will identify the diagnosis.

Rare

◆ Tumours

If the above causes are excluded, it is essential to search for cancers in the testicles, lungs, or elsewhere, which may be secreting female hormones. Possible symptoms include:

- Lump in or on a testicle.
- Coughing blood, chest pains, weight loss.

Precocious puberty

Sexual development before the age of nine years is likely to be abnormal. This includes the appearance of body hair, enlarged penis and deepening voice. Cases are rare, but all require specialist investigation.

Reproductive & Sexual Organs

Possible

◆ Hypothalamic disease

This gland in the brain controls many hormones.
  A disorder is likeliest if:

- The boy was normal at birth, and in early childhood.
- Later shows abnormal growth – either too short or too tall.
- Sometimes tumours in this part of the brain cause visual disturbances.

Rare

◆ Testicular tumours

- A lump may be felt.
- There may be a change or swelling in one testicle.

Blood tests may detect abnormally high levels of hormones in the blood.

◆ Adrenal disease

Disease of the adrenal glands, which lie over the kidneys, usually makes a baby very ill within days of birth. Hormone treatment prevents masculine changes appearing during very early childhood.

Symptoms common to men and women

Fertility problems

Low fertility or infertility can be a cause of much heartache to both men and women and can put a relationship under tremendous strain. Furthermore its investigation can be traumatic and difficult and needs to be handled with the utmost sensitivity and skill.
  A young, healthy couple having regular sexual intercourse have about an 85 per cent chance of achieving a pregnancy within a year, a figure which increases to 92 per cent after two years. The remainder may need investigation and assistance. It is important to remember that fertility in women decreases with age and this also applies to the success rates of assisted fertilization techniques. In this respect, men are luckier, as the potency of their sperm shows only a marginal decline with age.

Overall, the cause of low fertility in a couple falls into the following approximate percentage causes:

- Ovulation problems in women: 20 per cent.
- Tubal problems in women: 14 per cent.
- Hostile mucus in women: 6 per cent.
- Endometriosis in women: 6 per cent.
- Sexual difficulties: 6 per cent.
- Male factors: 24 per cent.
- Unexplained: 24 per cent.

Paradoxically, if a couple fall into the unexplained category then statistically they have a 60-70 per cent chance of a pregnancy within three years of investigation, a figure which is higher than where a cause is found.

When considering asking for medical help with fertility, it is always worth checking on general health and lifestyle matters: couples should try not to smoke; keep alcohol intake to a minimum and to optimise diet, exercise and weight. Women should take folic acid supplements to help prevent neural tube defects when a pregnancy occurs.

Female fertility difficulties

Probable

◆ Ovulation problems

This involves hormone imbalance, and would be suspected if there are:

- Absent periods.
- Irregular periods.
- Infrequent periods.
- Very light or very heavy periods.

Ovulation can be monitored by a blood test which looks for a rise in progesterone on day 22 of the cycle, or by using ovulation predictor tests mid cycle, or by means of temperature charts. Ovulation problems may be treated with clomifene or gonadotrophin medications.

◆ Blocked fallopian tubes

These are the tubes through which the eggs travel to the womb. Blocked tubes usually follow repeated pelvic infection causing pelvic inflammatory disease (see page 304), suspected from:

- Recurrent pelvic pain.
- Recurrent, infected vaginal discharges.

- Deep pain on intercourse.

Blocked tubes can be investigated by laparoscopy or X-ray (hysterosalpingogram). Tubal surgery or in vitro fertilisation (IVF) techniques may provide a solution.

◆ Cause unknown

Despite thorough investigation, many cases remain unexplained.

Possible

◆ Endometriosis

See page 304.

◆ General disease

Any serious, general disease can reduce fertility, but should already be obvious.

Rare

◆ Womb abnormalities

Investigations sometimes show a range of unsuspected abnormalities, such as a malformation of the womb which prevents implantation of the egg.

Male fertility difficulties

An early semen analysis is always advisable. It looks for low numbers of sperm, increased numbers of abnormal sperm, or sperm motility problems. Temporary infertility can follow a severe illness, after which it takes a few

Reproductive & Sexual Organs

months for sperm production to recover. The main treatment for male infertility is intracytoplasmic sperm injection (ICSI) where a sperm is recovered from the epididymis or testicle and introduced direct into an egg.

Probable

◆ Unknown cause

Sadly, the majority of cases of male infertility have no identifiable cause.

◆ Damage to testicles

Suggested by:

• Small size, abnormally soft feel.

• History of undescended testicle or testicular surgery.

• History of mumps orchitis.

• History of STIs.

• History of drug use (chemotherapy). Cigarette smoking, alcohol, cannabis

and high temperatures in the area of the scrotum can also decrease sperm production.

Possible

◆ Varicocele

See page 327.

◆ Hormone disorders

A possibility if there is:

• Absent body hair.

• Development of breasts.

Rare

◆ Chromosome disorders

• Unusual height.

• Enlarged breasts.

• Small or absent testicles.

• Absent body hair.

• Abnormally-formed penis.

Lack of interest in sex and reduced libido

Most enduring relationships eventually balance the partners' sexual desires so that neither partner is left feeling frustrated or guilty. The road to that adjustment can be a difficult one. Blame should not enter into this, nor is it ever the fault of one party alone: recognising that there is a problem is the first step to resolving it. Natural variations in a woman's sexual desire occur during the monthly cycle, reaching a peak in mid-cycle (before ovulation) for some women. Major illness and childbirth will usually

decrease sexual desire. Sexual desire and libido also tend to reduce with advancing age.

Probable

◆ Psychological factors

Psychological factors are most likely if you feel that:

• Sex is dirty.

• An aversion to being touched sexually by your partner.

• That things should be better than they are.

Reproductive &
Sexual Organs

- Guilty about your lack of enjoyment of sex.

Psycho-sexual therapy can help this problem. Other counsellors including individual and relationship counsellors can also contribute.

Possible

◆ Adverse sexual experiences

Meaning traumatic events such as painful intercourse, misunderstanding about sexual anatomy and sexual response, fear of falling pregnant. Most important is the memory of early sexual experiences, particularly if either partner was abused. The techniques for dealing with such problems involve explanation, honesty and patience. Gradually exploring your anatomy and sexual response, without initially indulging in sexual intercourse, may be helpful.

Rare

◆ Depression

A decreasing interest in sex in either a man or woman may signal depression. Some other features of depression are:

- Feelings of sadness and low mood.
- Loss of ability to enjoy things.
- Loss of self worth.
- Disturbed sleep.
- Easy crying.
- Thoughts of suicide.
- Slowing of thought.

Depression may respond to psychological treatments (talking therapy) or to antidepressants. Unfortunately, some antidepressants (SSRIs) also adversely effect sexual performance.

Orgasmic failure

Achievement of orgasm is only one part of a successful sexual relationship. Orgasm is a complex physiological process. In men it coincides with ejaculation of sperm, whilst in women the changes are more subtle.

Men may be unable to achieve orgasm for much the same reasons as women.

Some facts about female orgasm:

- It is a real physical and psychological event.
- Stimulation of the clitoris is usually important.

- It is not necessary for enjoyable sex each time.
- It may take longer to achieve for a woman than for a man.
- Women are capable of multiple orgasms: they do not need a resting period, as do most men.

Failure to achieve orgasm may be due to difficulty with the partnership, or because of the techniques used during intercourse. Some people are unable to experience orgasm without masturbation.

It is helpful to share and explore with your partner what forms of stimulation lead to orgasm so that they can be enjoyed together.

Probable

◆ Psychological

This refers to an array of experiences that make a relationship: affection, trust, previous positive experiences. It is common knowledge that uncertainty in these, and other aspects will lead to problems with sex and orgasm.

◆ Poor technique

It is necessary to take anatomy into account. Orgasm usually requires:

• Adequate foreplay.

• Clitoral or penile stimulation.
• Avoidance of pain.
• Proper lubrication.

Possible

◆ Partner's problem

See below. Failure to achieve orgasm in a woman can be a result of a man's:

• Premature ejaculation.
• Impotence.

◆ Drugs

SSRI antidepressants such as fluoxetine have a blocking or delaying effect on orgasm.

Other drugs, such as those used to treat major psychiatric illness, may adversely affect it.

Impotence

Impotence means difficulty in achieving or maintaining a firm erection. It is a common disorder, admitted to far less often than it is experienced. Brief episodes of impotence accompany tiredness and any serious, general ill-health. After ejaculation there is loss of erection, which takes longer and longer to recover with age, perhaps several days by old age. This may cause confusion if the true disorder is premature ejaculation.

Psychological factors are still the most likely reasons for impotence, but it is increasingly clear that physical disorders, especially with advancing age, are more common than once thought, especially problems with blood flow to the penis. This probably reflects an increasing openness towards discussing and investigating sexual activity in the elderly.

A range of treatments is now available, including drugs such as Viagra, and preparations injected or inserted into the penile urethra, or penis itself. Pump devices may also help. See also *Premature ejaculation,* page 342.

Probable

◆ Psychological

Factors here include depression, problems between partners and, more especially, the vicious circle of past impotence causing impotence again. Symptoms strongly suggestive of a psychological cause are:

- Normal erections during sleep, or on awakening.
- Ejaculation during sleep.
- Impotence with one particular partner.
- Sudden onset of impotence.
- Young age.

Therapy will include explanation, exploration of psychological problems, and gradual return to sexual intercourse.

Possible

◆ Diabetes mellitus

Diabetes affects the nerves and blood supply involved in an erection. Undiagnosed diabetes may cause:

- Excessive passage of urine at night and during the day.
- Thirst.

◆ Blood flow problems

An erection is caused by engorgement of the penis's spongy tissues with blood. If the veins carrying this blood supply are leaking, inadequate erection may follow.

Arterial disease can also affect the blood supply, both to the penis, and to the nerves controlling erection. Sophisticated tests of blood flow are available.

◆ Drugs

Many drugs used to treat high blood pressure may cause impotence, as do tranquillizers and heroin. Numerous other drugs may be implicated and this is worth checking.

◆ Alcoholism

Shakespeare sums it up in *Macbeth*: 'It provokes the desire, but takes away the performance'. Chronic alcoholism actually leads to hormonal and neurological changes that make permanent impotence a risk.

◆ Post-operative

Surgery to the bowel, and the prostate gland, runs the risk of damaging the nerves involved in an erection.

Rare

◆ Neurological disease

Of these, the commonest is multiple sclerosis, giving rise to:

- Numbness in various parts of the body.
- Unsteady gait.
- Visual disturbances, transient blindness in one eye.
- Difficulty in controlling passage of urine.
- Anything else damaging the lower spine may cause impotence.

◆ Hormone disorders

There are a wide range of possibilities. A possible cause if the person has:

- Absent or small testicles.
- Lack of body hair.
- Breast development.
- Unusually short or tall stature.
- Extreme obesity.
- Hormone treatment may help such cases.

Reproductive & Sexual Organs

Premature ejaculation

This means ejaculation before the penis enters the vagina, or very soon after entry. While this is not a disease, it can be very troublesome for many men. Considerable time and patience, as well as courage to explore the problem, will be required.

Probable

◆ **Psychological factors**

With experience, sexual relationships expand to include more than intercourse alone, perhaps explaining why premature ejaculation is commonest in young men. Psychological approaches encourage concentration on aspects of sexual behaviour other than intercourse, for example stroking and massaging.

An aid to this is the 'squeeze technique', when the partner, told that ejaculation is near, squeezes around the base of the penis for some seconds. This usually delays progress to orgasm without destroying the erection. Further information should be sought from psychosexual therapists.

Blisters on or around the genitalia

Probable

◆ **Herpes**

The same virus that causes cold sores can cause these blisters on and around the genitalia.

• A few blisters crop up from time to time.

• Intensely painful when they appear, especially on the first occasion.

• May be accompanied by flu-like symptoms.

• Pain and difficulty passing urine in women.

Anti-viral drugs may be helpful.

It is especially important, if you are pregnant, to report any previous or current attacks of herpes to your doctor or midwife.

This enables measures to be taken to diminish the risk of infecting the baby at birth.

Genital lumps, ulcers and sores

Minor infections of the genitalia are very common, and are frequently obvious to an untrained eye. It is important to be alert to early symptoms of STIs, being especially careful if you have many sexual partners.

You owe this not just to yourself but to your sexual partners, too.

Probable

◆ Folliculitis or boils

- Tiny pimples on the skin, or at the base of pubic hairs.
- Tender, rapidly-appearing lumps.
- They come to yellow head.
- Discharge pus and blood, then they disappear.
- Severe cases may require a course of antibiotics.

Frequent or recurrent boils in the genital area can be caused by a skin condition called hydradenitis suppurativa, which is an acne like condition. It also occurs in the armpits. Treatment is long-term antibiotics or other anti-acne medications.

◆ Scabies or crab lice

Scabies mites are too small to see with the naked eye. Crab lice can usually be seen attached to the shafts of pubic hairs. Both bite the skin, causing;

- Itching, with red pimples or burrows in the genital area, or elsewhere on the body.
- Itch worse at night with scabies.
- Scabies commonly bite between the fingers, and on the waist.
- Treatment is with insecticidal shampoos and skin applications, plus careful decontamination of bedding and clothing.
- Partner and other close physical contacts need treatment too.
- Consider possibility of other STIs.

◆ Warts

Fleshy growths a few millimetres in length are fairly common, and as harmless on the genitalia as elsewhere.

- Caused by *Human papilloma virus*, but a different strain to the type associated with cancer of the cervix.
- They respond to simple treatment, but may recur.
- Can be sexually transmitted, so condoms may be helpful.

An altogether different problem is masses of spreading warts: appearing like tiny, branching corals. They are often also found around the back passage. As these may be associated with syphilis, see a specialist in sexually transmitted diseases.

◆ Molluscum contagiosum

- Small pearly lumps a few millimetres in diameter appear in the genital area.
- The lumps have a solid, and a central dimple.
- Caused by a virus.
- Painless unless they become infected.
- Usually disappear spontaneously after a few months, though simple treatment can speed resolution.
- May accompany other STIs.

Possible

◆ Cysts

Women commonly develop Bartholin's or labial cyst.

- Painless swelling in lip of the vagina.
- May cause no other problem.

Reproductive &
Sexual Organs

- If infected, becomes very swollen and tender, sometimes with a fever. Surgical drainage is needed.

◆ AIDS

Suspected in cases of homosexual practices; sexual promiscuity, sex with at-risk partners; or intravenous drug use. Symptoms, apart from the swelling of glands, include:

- Fever.
- Malaise.
- Headaches.
- Mouth ulcers.

Diagnosis requires blood tests over several months. There is now effective treatment, though, as yet, no cure.

Rare

◆ Syphilis

The symptoms of infection with syphilis appear two to four weeks after contact. Either partner may be infected. A painless ulcer appears on the genitals, subsequently turning into firm lump. The ulcer, known as a chancre, may appear in or around the vagina or on the penis, in the mouth, or around the back passage, depending on the nature of the sexual activity. Local lymph nodes enlarge. It heals over several weeks. After a few months, secondary features appear, such as rashes on the palms and soles, joint pains, swollen lymph nodes,

genital warts. Years later, syphilis can rampage through the body, affecting just about every organ and causing dementia. Early disease is cured by penicillin.

◆ Behçet's disease

A combination of:

- Painful ulcers on genitals and in the mouth.
- Red eyes, either conjunctivitis or iritis.
- Symptoms tend to recur.

◆ Tropical venereal diseases

By rare, we mean rare in Europe and the USA. Sexually promiscuous travellers to the tropics are at risk. These diseases are chancroid, lymphogranuloma venerium and granuloma inguinale. They all produce:

- Genital ulcer, within a few days of infection .
- May remain small, or become very large.
- Usually very painful.
- Swollen local lymph glands.

The diagnosis is made on appearance, and results of swabs. Treatment with antibiotics usually leads to a cure.

◆ Cancer

Skin cancer may be the reason for a persistent, ulcerated area on the penis or vagina: see a doctor.

Lumps in the groin

The groin is the region at the top of the thighs, by the side of the genitals in

front of the hip joints. Lumps of the genitals themselves are considered under specific headings elsewhere. Lumps in the groin are very common and are noticed early, it being such a visible part of the body. They are not usually serious.

There are several different structures in the groin and a lump in that region may have many causes. It is usually possible to make a confident diagnosis based on the appearance of the lump.

Probable

◆ Inguinal hernia

An extremely common type of hernia, where the contents of the abdomen bulge through a weakness or defect in its muscle wall. Although typically a problem of adulthood, and made worse by lifting and straining, it may also be seen in children and very young babies. Typical features are:

- A soft bulge in the groin which may be more noticeable on straining.
- Often completely disappears when lying flat.
- A slight aching or dragging sensation is common.

If it becomes painful and firm, a section of bowel may be trapped. If this is the case, seek medical help immediately. Hernias in children should always be treated. Inguinal hernia in adults who are engaged in physical activity or lifting of weights (for example, labourers), can be extremely troublesome. In an elderly person who is not particularly active, repair may not be necessary.

◆ Enlarged lymph nodes

Just like the neck, the groin has groups of lymph glands, whose job is to protect against infection. It is normal to feel a few small glands in the groin, particularly in people of thin build: they are about half a centimetre in size, painless and mobile under your finger. Minor scratches on the legs, or pimples around the groin, will cause these glands to enlarge for a few days, and it is best to keep an eye on these until they shrink again. Glands which remain swollen for longer, which are usually painful or unusually large, need to be thoroughly checked. There are so many possibilities that enlarged glands are treated as a separate topic in *Swollen lymph nodes*, page 449.

Enlarged glands accompanied by any of the following symptoms should be taken seriously:

- Enlarged glands elsewhere, such as neck, armpits.
- Sores on the genitals.
- Bleeding from the back passage.
- Fever, malaise.
- Anaemia.
- Bruising.

Possible

◆ Varicose veins

- Enlarged veins are often seen and felt in the groin.
- Swelling is very soft, easily squeezed by finger pressure.
- A bluish tinge may be noticeable.

Reproductive & Sexual Organs

- Usually varicose veins further down the leg.
- Slight aching after standing .

◆ **Femoral hernia**

A femoral hernia arises from a weakness at the very top of the thigh, and is different from an inguinal hernia. It carries a higher chance of strangulation, when the contents become dangerously trapped. Femoral hernias almost always require surgical treatment.

- Commonest in older women.
- Often appears rapidly as a small tender lump.
- Blockage causes a painful, hard lump, vomiting, and intestinal obstruction.

◆ **Lipoma**

A soft lump, present for many weeks and growing slowly, if at all, is probably a lipoma – a benign fatty tumour.

- Painless.
- Often others elsewhere.

There is no need to remove the lump unless there is any doubt about the diagnosis.

◆ **Undescended testicle**

See page 330.

Rare

◆ **Aneurysm of blood vessel**

The large femoral artery, which carries the blood to the leg, passes near to the surface in the groin. Its wall can weaken and it expands like a balloon, producing:

- A lump, pulsating in time with your heart beat.
- Often tender.
- Can be repaired surgically.

◆ **Tumours and abscesses**

As with lumps anywhere on the body, the possibility of a tumour or an abscess has to be kept in mind. Typically. abscesses are rapidly swelling, painful tender lumps with redness and heat in the overlying skin. They may discharge pus or need surgical drainage.

Tumours may be suggested if there is a hard growing lump attached to surrounding tissues. There may be symptoms from tumours elsewhere, or other symptoms of serious illness such as weight loss.

In either case, seek medical advice straight away.

Loss of pubic hair

Although this is not a common problem, it is alarming. Thinning of the hair is a normal feature of ageing, and it occurs as an expected side effect of chemo-therapy for cancer. Otherwise, it is probably caused by hormone disturbances.

Probable

◆ Alopecia

Alopecia is general term for hair loss of unknown cause occurring in both men and women.

Typical features are:

- Thinning of hair, perhaps with some actual hairless patches.
- In severe cases is there complete, generalized hair loss.
- Loss of eyebrows, armpit hair, and pubic hair.
- Alopecia may resolve spontaneously though some cases persist.

Treatment is difficult and carries a low success rate

◆ Cirrhosis of the liver

- Usually due to alcoholism.
- Hair thins, rather than disappears.
- Small, dilated veins appear on face, chest.
- Red palms.
- Impotence.
- Swollen ankles.
- Nausea, indigestion.
- Easy bruising.

Rare

◆ Addison's disease

A consequence of underactive adrenal glands, causing:

- Profound weakness.
- Dark patches in the mouth, on the gums or on old scars.
- Weight loss.
- Nausea vomiting and stomach cramps.
- Fainting.

The brain and nervous system

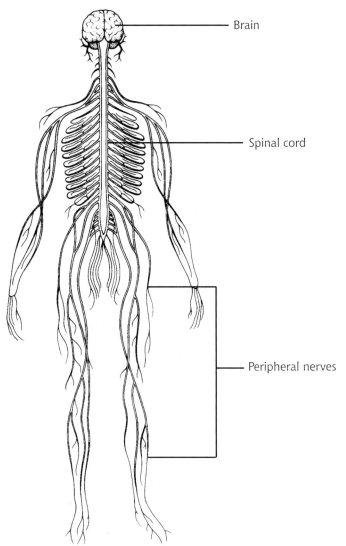

Brain

Spinal cord

Peripheral nerves

Introduction

The brain and the nervous system are unique amongst all the systems and parts of the body considered in this book: they are the physical seat of the psyche and all that makes up thought, personality, who we are and what we feel; *and* they are physically the command and control centres for all the workings of the body. Ultimately, all symptoms are located in the brain which, in turn, controls their perception and expression. Physical processes which affect the brain and nerves may in turn give rise to symptoms: for example, a brain haemorrhage causing a stroke may cause paralysis. Similarly, a person suffering from dissociation (hysteria) may present with an equally debilitating paralysis, but in this case the problem lies within the functioning of the mind and the realms of mental illness. This chapter describes a series of common symptoms which relate to the brain and nervous systems, but not surprisingly, there is some overlap with symptoms in other parts of the book. Topics are arranged alphabetically.

Anxiety

Anxiety can be quite well defined as a state of worry and fear. It is universal and one might correctly identify it as part of the normal human experience. Mild degrees increase the body's readiness to deal with the problems of life, but it becomes abnormal when it is out of proportion to the situation or when one problem or event becomes the focus of severe worry and starts to interfere with daily life (see *Obsessions and phobias*). The symptoms are multiple and include:

- A feeling of tension mingled with apprehension and agitation.
- 'Butterflies' in the stomach.
- Feeling of impending doom.
- Headache.
- Sweating: hands, armpits and forehead are particularly affected.
- Insomnia.

- Palpitations.
- Dry mouth.
- Tremor.

But many other symptoms occur, too, such as over-breathing, impotence, dizzy turns, and restlessness. In children there may be bed wetting, nail biting, thumb sucking, and so on.

Probable

◆ Anxiety state

Worry comes naturally to human beings, to some more naturally than to others; heredity plays a part. Every society has its own anxieties: the worry of choosing perfectly matched table decorations does not, on the face of it compare with the worry of a sabre-toothed tiger intent on repossessing your cave. But who are we to judge? Childhood experiences, repressed sexual urges, the depersonalization of modern society: all are theoretically reasonable explanations of anxiety, suggested by some of the wisest minds, one thing is certain: there is more and more of it about.

Diagnosing anxiety is usually straightforward, based on the symptoms given above; sympathetic discussion will usually reveal an underlying cause of stress. Physical symptoms as alarming as breathlessness may need investigating before the individual can accept the symptom is psychological in origin. Treatment ranges from drugs for acute, disabling anxiety to explanation via counselling or psychotherapy – for instance cognitive behavioural therapy (CBT).

Possible

◆ Other psychological disease or mental illness

Possible when anxiety appears:

- In previously stable personality.
- Without an obvious source of stress.
- With other disturbance of mood, thought, or concentration.
- Accompanied by bizarre behaviour or beliefs.
- Accompanied by severe memory problems or disorientation.

Possibilities which are dealt with separately, and should be followed up, include *Depression*, *Dementia*, and *Schizophrenia*.

◆ Overactive thyroid gland

Gives all the symptoms of anxiety, but there are suggestive additional features:

- Fine tremor.
- Weight loss.
- Increased appetite.
- Intolerance to heat.
- Rapid pulse.
- Bulging eyes.
- Swelling in the neck.

The condition is easily confirmed by a blood test.

◆ Drug and alcohol effects

Drugs such as amphetamine, cocaine and crack cocaine commonly trigger anxiety. Similarly, withdrawal from many abused drugs (for instance heroin and benzodiazepine tranquillisers) and from alcohol in alcoholics may cause:

- Coarse tremor.
- Anxiety.
- Sweating.
- Hallucinations.

There may be other features of drug abuse such as:

- Neglected appearance.
- Needle marks on limbs.
- Social disintegration, crime, unemployment.

Specialized clinics are available to help with these problems.

Rare

◆ Low blood sugar

Usually occurs in a person with diabetes on treatment with tablets or insulin.

The symptoms appear rapidly and consist of:

- Light-headedness.
- Sweating.
- Hunger.
- Drowsiness.

The condition is readily confirmed by finger prick testing of blood glucose levels, and reverses quickly with glucose and carbohydrate supplements.

◆ Phaeochromocytoma

A very rare tumour which produces hormones that cause high blood pressure. The level of hormone can rapidly increase, causing:

- Sudden anxiety, sweating, palpitations.
- Pallor or flushing.
- Headache.
- When an attack is in progress, blood pressure will be very high.

Coma

Coma is a precise medical term meaning a state of unrousability and unresponsiveness to stimuli. At its most severe there is:

- No response to pain.
- No movement.
- No speech.

Stupor is less severe: the individual can be roused by painful stimuli. The causes are the same. There are many stages in between the two, such as sleepiness and confusion and there maybe some delirium, too.

Cases of coma require urgent hospital admission to treat and support vital body functions and in order to search for the many possible causes. You will be providing extremely useful information to the hospital if you can report on:

- A history of diabetes; any drowsiness and confusion in the preceding hours.
- Drug and alcohol abuse; evidence of such as bottles, syringes.

- Epilepsy with details of previous fits and of medication.
- A head injury in the previous few weeks.
- Previous stroke; treatment for high blood pressure.
- Depression and suicidal intent: empty pill containers.

Probable

◆ Stroke

- Usually in the elderly.
- Sudden collapse.
- One-sided paralysis.
- Loss of speech.

A very sudden severe headache at the back of the head accompanied by vomiting and followed rapidly by loss of consciousness suggests a particular type of stroke called a *Subarachnoid haemorrhage* (see page 377).

The Brain & Nervous System

◆ **Drugs or alcohol**

Diagnosis tends to depend on knowledge of the person's habits and other pointers, such as the smell of alcohol. Opiate drug abuse is a strong possibility if there are:

• Needle marks (red marks on the arms or thickened, hard veins).

• Pinpoint-sized pupils.

• Shallow breathing.

Deliberate overdose of prescription drugs as a suicide attempt may be suggested by:

• A history of depression or mental illness.

• Recent major life event or loss.

• Finding a suicide note or empty medication packets.

◆ **Injury**

A head injury is the commonest injury causing coma, usually following an accident. The diagnosis will be obvious. Recovery depends on the degree of brain trauma. Stupor or coma occurring a few weeks after a serious head injury may be due to blood clot on the brain (subdural haematoma – see page 356) resulting from that injury. This condition is commoner in the elderly, alcoholics, or those taking anticoagulants. Surgical removal of the blood clot usually allows full recovery.

◆ **Metabolic disease**

Most probably diabetes, liver or kidney failure, usually already known about.

• Hypoglycaemia (low blood sugar) is suggested initially by light-headedness, hunger, shakiness and confusion followed by increasing drowsiness and unconsciousness.

• Hyperglycaemia (high blood sugar) is often accompanied by another illness or missed insulin injections and suggested by: thirst, vomiting, deep heavy breathing, increased or reduced urine output followed by increasing drowsiness and unconsciousness.

• Liver failure may be suggested by a history of previous alcoholism or other liver diseases and there may be jaundice or ascites (filling of the abdominal cavity with fluid).

• Kidney failure may be suggested by an alteration or loss of urine output, though frequently the diagnosis only comes to light after a blood test.

Treatment is aimed at correcting the metabolic disturbance, for example giving sugar to the diabetic patient with hypoglycaemia.

◆ **Epilepsy**

After a severe convulsion someone suffering from epilepsy may be comatose for a few minutes or longer.

Possible

◆ **Infection**

Although any severe infection may cause coma through shock, meningitis is the most likely, especially in babies. It should be suspected in any infant showing otherwise unexplained:

- Irritability.
- Increasing drowsiness.
- Purple rash on body.
- In a baby, a bulging soft spot on the skull.

In larger children, teenagers and adults, there may also be:

- Severe headache.
- Neck stiffness.
- Aversion to bright lights.
- Vomiting.

Meningitis is a life-threatening emergency. Take the individual to hospital without delay.

◆ Heart attack

Coma following:

- Severe chest pain.

- Breathlessness.
- Sweating and blue lips.
- May have known risk factors – high blood pressure or cholesterol, smoker, family history, diabetes.

Rare

◆ Hypothermia

A profound drop in body temperature, most common in the elderly, in winter, following a fall or a stroke.

◆ Other causes

A book could be written about the other causes of coma, since it can be the final scenario of any serious upset to the body's working. Rare causes can only be diagnosed after investigations, blood tests and medical examination.

Lack of concentration

Peoples' attention span is very variable and depends on factors such as mood, conditions of work and stress. There is rarely any serious reason for this symptom. Children have much shorter attention space than adults, as measured scientifically by the "but you've only just had an ice cream" test.

Probable

◆ Tiredness

- May affect adults and children.
- Normally sound health and adequate concentration.
- Obvious lack of rest or overwork.

- Concentration returns after rest.
- May be accompanied by insomnia or disturbed sleep.

◆ Anxiety

See page 349.

◆ Depression

See page 363.

◆ Drugs and alcohol

Alcohol intoxication produces obvious problems with concentration and behaviour. Likewise, chronic alcoholism may damage the brain, leading to cognitive impairment and concentration difficulties.

Many prescription drugs – such as tranquillisers – reduce concentration; similarly drugs of abuse such as cocaine and heroin produce the same effect.

Possible

◆ Attention deficit hyperactivity disorder (ADHD) and attention deficit disorder (ADD)

Symptoms start in early childhood, progress through adolescence and may persist into early adulthood. Typical features include:

* Constantly on the go.

* Constant movements and restlessness.
* Behind or in trouble at school.
* Impulsive or inconsiderate behaviour.
* Disobedience and lack of discipline.
* Familial tendency.

Treatment is usually undertaken with the help of specialist services and may include the use of psychostimulant drugs such as methylphenidate, behavioural therapy, and special educational input.

Confusion

Confusion is a combination of disorientation and emotional upset. Gradual onset of confusion over weeks and months is most likely to occur in the elderly and may be part of the natural aging process or degenerative brain disorders (see also *Dementia*). Sudden confusion at any age may have an immediate underlying medical cause and needs urgent investigation. It may be accompanied by drowsiness or altered consciousness, agitation, delusions or hallucinations (see also *Delirium*, page 371).

Probable

◆ Senile confusion

Seen in the elderly or very elderly. At its worst, it develops into dementia (page 360), but for many elderly people confusion is just a nuisance.

Features that suggest senile confusion are:

* Memory for recent events becomes poor. Confusion follows and the individual may become disorientated in time and place.
* General health normal for age.
* No confusion or problems with familiar tasks and journeys.
* Can cope by using notes, lists.
* Social functioning unaffected or mildly impaired.
* Deterioration occurs only gradually, but major changes in lifestyle, for example, a holiday, may bring it on.

Possible

◆ Abnormal blood sugar levels with diabetes

* Hypoglycaemia (low blood sugar) is

The Brain & Nervous System

suggested initially by light headedness, hunger, shakiness and confusion followed by increasing drowsiness and unconsciousness.

- Hyperglycaemia (high blood sugar) is often accompanied by another illness or missed insulin injections and suggested by: thirst, vomiting, deep heavy breathing, increased or reduced urine output followed by increasing drowsiness confusion and unconsciousness.

The condition is confirmed by measuring blood sugar levels. Diabetic patients should be taught how to recognise and treat hypo and hyperglycaemia and to seek medical advice when it occurs.

◆ Drugs or alcohol

This diagnosis tends to rely on knowledge of a previous history of drug abuse or alcoholism. In alcoholics, an acute state of confusion may accompany alcohol withdrawal and needs urgent medical attention. Many prescription drugs (such as sleeping tablets), especially when used in the elderly patient, may potentially cause confusion.

◆ Heart failure

Confusion as a symptom of heart failure is most likely to affect the elderly, especially those with a known history of heart disease, high blood pressure or diabetes. Suggested by:

- Shortness of breath on exercise.
- Swollen ankles.
- Breathlessness on lying flat in bed.
- Recent chest pain could indicate a

heart attack or angina which may accompany, or be associated with, heart failure.

◆ Infections

In the elderly (and children), any infection may worsen a tendency to confusion. There may or may not be a fever. Common infections may present as:

- Cough and phlegm with a chest infection or pneumonia.
- Need to pass urine frequently suggests a bladder infection.

Combination of: confusion, headache, neck stiffness and aversion to light suggests meningitis, needing emergency hospital care.

◆ Minor stroke

- Sudden confusion.
- Sudden slurring of speech or difficulty finding words.
- Face may droop on one side.
- Possibly loss of function or sensation in an arm and leg.

Recovery from such minor strokes is often rapid. Always see a doctor for further assessment.

◆ Respiratory failure

- Most likely in someone with chronic bronchitis or emphysema, usually a smoker.
- Long history of breathlessness, cough and phlegm.
- A chest infection may be the trigger.
- Blue lips and tongue.
- Warm hands.
- Needs hospital treatment.

◆ **Hypothermia**

Confusion is a common early symptom of low body temperature.

Usually affects the elderly living alone during winter months.

◆ **Underactive thyroid gland**

See page 320.

◆ **Metabolic failure**

This includes liver and kidney disease.

• Liver disease suggested by previous history of alcoholism; jaundice; easy bruising; red palms; swollen ankles.

• Kidney disease suggested by either very high or very low urine output; anaemia; malaise; yellow tinge to skin.

Usually diagnosed on a blood test.

◆ **Subdural haematoma**

This is a collection of blood adjacent to the tissues wrapping of the brain. Occurs following a head injury and later results in pressure on the brain. This condition is commoner in the elderly, alcoholics, or those taking anticoagulants. Small clots may resolve spontaneously while larger ones require neurosurgery to remove them – usually with good recovery.

• Symptoms emerge over several weeks following a history of head injury or fall.

• A fluctuating degree of confusion and abnormality of behaviour.

• One-sided weakness of arm and leg may develop.

• Diagnosed by CT or MRI scan.

Convulsions

The features of a convulsion, also known as a fit or epileptic attack, are:

• Possibly a warning of an impending attack, called an aura; it may be a feeling, a visual disturbance, a smell, a headache.

• The individual may cry out, then collapse unconscious.

• Remains stiff; may turn blue around the lips for about 30 seconds.

• Arms and legs then begin to jerk in a coordinated manner.

• Possibly incontinence of urine, frothing at mouth, cheek or tongue biting.

• Afterwards, drowsiness, confusion,

before return to normal.

Not all convulsions are as dramatic. One form of convulsion is no more than a brief absence of consciousness, which may be misinterpreted as a blank look. A convulsion is different from a simple faint, where there is no aura, no incontinence, no shaking of limbs. Investigations are needed if there is any doubt.

Probable

◆ **Epilepsy**

Epilepsy is caused by abnormal electrical discharges in the brain. Most cases are of unknown origin, but it can result from previous brain injury, for instance a stroke or a head injury. Alternatively, a structural abnormality may be causing it, such as a brain tumour or an anomaly in the cerebral blood vessels. Anyone having a fit for the first time needs careful medical assessment which would include blood tests, a MRI or CT scan of the brain, and an electroencephalogram (a recording of the electrical brain activity). Some patients with epilepsy are advised to avoid situations which would be dangerous if they had a fit, such as climbing ladders, driving, swimming or using hazardous machinery. Treatment usually involves long-term medication with anticonvulsant drugs, though some people manage without if the condition improves.

◆ Febrile fit

Febrile fits occur in children between the ages of six months and five years. They are fairly common, occurring in some 10 per cent of all children, and do not mean that the child will grow up to become epileptic. Parents observing their child having a first fit frequently fear that death is occurring or imminent, though this is not the case. A child having a febrile fit for the first time needs immediate medical attention: often admission to hospital will be advised where the cause of the fever will be sought. Usually this turns out to be a minor respiratory or viral infection, though meningitis is a rare possible cause. Children who have recurrent febrile fits can be managed at home, as long as the parents know how to give an anticonvulsant if the fit becomes prolonged. Most febrile fits can be prevented by giving paracetamol or ibuprofen at the first sign of a fever. This works by reducing body temperature; exposing and cooling the skin also helps. Typical symptoms associated with a febrile convulsion are:

- Child is feverish, typically with a cold or ear infection.
- The fit usually occurs early on in the fever, as the temperature rises.
- Sudden stiffness, rolling of eyes, breathing stops and the child may turn blue.
- Then, coordinated jerking, of limbs and possibly incontinence.
- May last five to ten minutes.
- Child recovers and becomes responsive, but remains drowsy for a few hours.

In children below six months or older than five years, it is not safe to make a diagnosis of febrile fits and other causes must be considered by a professional.

Possible

◆ Alcohol related

Convulsions are usually precipitated if someone with problematic drinking or alcoholism suddenly abstains from drink. They may be accompanied by withdrawal shakes or hallucinations. Long-term treatment should be aimed at addressing the problem drinking or alcoholism. Alcoholics are as likely as anyone else to develop true epilepsy, so the usual full assessment should be made.

The Brain & Nervous System

◆ **Head injury**

A convulsion happening after a head injury should always be assessed in hospital as significant brain injury may have occurred.

◆ **Stroke**

A convulsion can sometimes accompany a stroke. Hospital assessment is mandatory.

◆ **Meningitis**

An infection around the brain possible at all ages, but an especial worry in childhood.

◆ **Metabolic disorder**

This usually means breakdown in the function of the kidneys or liver and should be detected on routine investigation of epilepsy. Low blood sugar (hypoglycaemia) in diabetes is a possible cause of a convulsion.

Rare

◆ **Eclampsia of pregnancy**

A risk of later pregnancy or following birth: the blood pressure suddenly rises too high and the mother has a convulsion. The situation should nearly always be avoidable by routine antenatal checks aimed at identifying pre-eclampsia, the condition which precedes it. Warning symptoms suggesting pre-eclampsia are:

• Fingers and feet swell rapidly.

• Sudden weight gain.

• Headache, flashing lights.

• Irritability.

• Abdominal or chest pain.

• Tests will show high blood pressure, protein in the urine, and abnormal blood biochemistry.

This is an emergency, calling for urgent specialist assessment.

Treatment is aimed at safely delivering the baby at the earliest opportunity, whilst monitoring the mother for the complications of high blood pressure and the other bodily disturbances associated with the condition.

Delirium

Delirium is characterised by the rapid appearance of confusion, restlessness, hallucinations, incoherent speech and thought. It is often worst at night. The confusion may fluctuate, with severe symptoms interspersed with relatively normal phases. The causes are those given under *Confusion*, but with an added urgency because of the greater risk of serious underlying illness, and with a higher chance of an infection being the cause. The elderly are likely to become delirious during an otherwise moderately serious illness. In children, delirium frequently accompanies a feverish illness and should be treated by bringing the temperature down, though it is wise to seek medical advice.

If there is any suspicion of:

- Headache.
- Aversion to light.
- Neck stiffness.

Meningitis may be the cause, and immediate medical attention is needed.

Delusions

There is no reliable definition of a delusion: conventionally, it is a belief which appears unfounded in reality – reality as judged by a reasonable group of people sharing the same cultural background. The difficulty defining what constitutes a delusion gives scope for gross abuse of the term. It has, indeed, been a convenient way of labelling as mentally ill those who have held such shocking beliefs as liberty, democracy and freedom. Nevertheless, there are individuals who hold beliefs that are so bizarre that they are taken as prime signs of mental illness. The unshakeable conviction, for instance, that you are Napoleon Bonaparte; or that if your left knee itches your wife is being unfaithful. The deluded person may then act on that belief, so that what appears to be a motiveless action proves to have been the logical outcome of a delusion. With appropriate caveats, psychiatrists therefore take delusions seriously.

Probable

◆ Schizophrenia

This is a common mental illness in which the sufferer experiences a psychotic distortion of thinking and perception. The illness damages the thought processes which give a normal person their sense of individuality, personality and self direction. About one per cent of the population suffers from this condition. A 'schizoid state' is a less serious condition and describes individuals who have an abnormal set of emotional responses and relationships with others, and are frequently loners. Schizophrenia is not the 'split personality' of popular myth, in fact the derivation of the word means 'shattered mind' – a description which very aptly describes the disorder. Most specialists believe that schizophrenia is the result an abnormality of brain chemistry. Treatment based on this view is quite successful and may enable good social integration and functioning. Onset typically occurs in early adulthood and may endure long-term. Specialist assessment and treatment with ongoing medication is usually advisable. Families and carers also need support. Typical symptoms include:

- Delusions, ranging from single ideas to whole networks of belief about the nature of reality. Typically there is complete lack of insight that the thoughts or delusions might be abnormal.
- Hallucinations – often hearing voices.
- Paranoia.

The Brain & Nervous System

- Fragmentation in the train of thoughts, with bizarre or incoherent speech.
- Mood is often flat and emotionless.
- Apathy, self-neglect.
- Odd or abnormal behaviour or movement.

Possible

◆ Early dementia

See *Dementia*, below. In the early stages, memory loss may result in giving delusional explanations for events, whose cause the individual has forgotten: for example, believing that a mislaid handbag has been stolen.

◆ Depression

Those with severe depression may come to hold delusions about their own health or that of their families – for example, they may believe themselves or a loved one has an incurable disease. Delusions may also convince the sufferer they are so worthless that suicide seems a logical option. Treatment with antidepressants and other measures is effective and may be life saving.

Dementia

With dementia there is a general deterioration of intellectual capacity, together with impairment of memory. Dementia becomes more common with age. About 20 per cent of those over 80 suffer from it to some degree. Once established, the condition inevitably deteriorates, though the progression occurs at very variable rates.

Symptoms include:

- Memory loss – an early symptom particularly of recent events or conversations. Long-term memories are initially preserved.
- Disorientation – unable to identify correct current location and time.
- Slow thinking, muddled thought and increasing confusion.
- Personality change.
- Self-neglect and loss of initiative.
- Depression and anxiety accompany early awareness of deterioration.
- Disturbed behaviour.
- Delusions and hallucinations.
- Eventually incontinence, weight loss, and bedridden state.

Despite this picture, the individual appears fully conscious, with no drowsiness. Medical advice should be sought so that the cause of the dementia can be established. Investigations may include psychometric testing of mental state, physical examination, blood tests, and CT scanning.

Treatment depends on the cause of the dementia and presenting symptoms. Drug treatment may partially relieve some of the symptoms or slow progression, though the results may be disappointing. Social support and care are equally important to the sufferer and their carer or family, who often shoulder much of the burden.

The Brain & Nervous System

Probable

◆ Alzheimer's disease

This is the commonest cause of dementia accounting for 65 per cent of cases. The symptoms are documented above.

◆ Vascular dementia (multi-infarct dementia)

This type of dementia accounts for a further 25 per cent of cases. Essentially it consists of damage to the brain, resulting from multiple tiny strokes. Symptoms are recorded above but also include:

- Onset sometimes sudden.
- Stepwise deterioration (corresponding to the occurrence of the multiple small strokes).
- Often accompanied by a history of high blood pressure, other vascular disease, or other types of stroke.

Treatment of high blood pressure or the causes of the mini strokes may help.

Possible

◆ Drug effects

Might be suspected if:

- Dementia appears rapidly and fluctuates.
- The individual is on multiple treatments: especially common with tranquillizers and drugs to treat Parkinson's disease.
- Condition improves when the offending drug is stopped.

◆ Alcoholism

Gives rise to a distinct form of dementia, due to lack of B vitamins.

- Profound loss of memory for recent events.
- A tendency to make up excuses to cover up for memory loss.
- Disorders of eye movements, for instance jerking.
- Unsteady gait.

This condition is treatable with high-dose vitamin supplements.

◆ Lewy-body dementia

This type of dementia includes the following specific additional features:

- Pronounced 'fluctuation' in alertness and attention, such as frequent drowsiness, lethargy, lengthy periods of time spent staring into space, or disorganized speech.
- Recurrent visual hallucinations.
- Symptoms mimicking Parkinson's disease, such as rigidity and the loss of spontaneous movement.
- May also cause depression.

◆ HIV/AIDS

A symptom of AIDS in HIV positive individuals.

- Commonest in countries where HIV is widespread and where medical resources are scanty.
- May present with psychiatric symptoms and personality change, initially.
- Clumsiness and difficulty walking are common accompaniments.

Dementia of this type is largely preventable with antiviral (HAART) treatment given in the earlier stages of

HIV disease. If it occurs, the dementia can improve dramatically with HAART treatment.

Rare

◆ Huntington's chorea

- Family history (this disease has a known inheritance).
- Involuntary coarse movements and tremor of limbs may be the first symptom.
- Begins in the 30s or 40s.
- Physical and mental deterioration is progressive and inevitable.

◆ Hypothyroidism

See page 320. Treatment with thyroid hormone will reverse this condition.

◆ Hydrocephalus

An uncommon condition of increased pressure and volume of fluid within the brain, usually found when a CT or MRI scan of the brain is done. Additional symptoms include:

- The degree of confusion fluctuates.
- Urinary incontinence.
- Unsteady gait.
- Clumsiness.

  Treatments are available.

◆ Liver and kidney disease

Should be detected on routine screening. See under *Metabolic failure*, page 352.

◆ Meningioma

A very slowly-growing brain tumour.

Apart from dementia, dependent on its position, it may cause:

- Epilepsy.
- Weakness of an arm or leg.
- Progressive headache.
- Loss of sense of smell.

  Diagnosis will be confirmed by a brain scan.

◆ Brain haematoma

A blood clot on the brain, following a head injury. A possible cause of dementia of rapid onset.

See *Subdural haematoma*, page 356.

◆ Vitamin B12 deficiency

Pernicious anaemia.

- Tingling in the hands and feet.

  Another rare, but treatable cause of dementia.

◆ Creutzfeldt-Jakob disease (CJD) or variant CJD

This is the human equivalent of BSE (mad cow disease).

May be accompanied by fits, paralysis, or visual problems.

◆ Syphilis

In its final stages, many years after first infection, syphilis can cause dementia, plus:

- Unsteady gait.
- Drooping eyelids.
- Delusions, often of grandeur.
- Small, irregular pupils.

  Blood tests will confirm the diagnosis and antibiotic treatment can then halt, though not reverse, the condition.

The Brain & Nervous System

Depression

When is it an illness? And when is it a natural response to life's trials? Nearly everyone experiences feelings of depression and unhappiness at some point in their lives. This becomes a problem when it is prolonged, severe or starts to interfere with normal functioning. Everyone has a duty to be aware of depression as a significant illness in its own right. Growing out of unhappiness, or perhaps just from long-term 'knocks', 'clinical depression' goes beyond unhappiness and carries the real risk of suicide. Mood, appearance and speech are usually enough to make a firm diagnosis of severe depression. The symptoms, not all of which may be present, are familiar to all and include:

- Low mood, sadness, tearfulness, feelings of despair and hopelessness.
- Often worse in the morning and improving through the day.
- Inability to enjoy things.
- Lack of energy and poor concentration.
- Feelings of anxiety.
- Negative thoughts about the future.
- Slowing down of thought, speech and movement.
- Feelings of guilt.
- Poor sleep, with early morning wakening.
- Loss of appetite and weight.
- Self-disgust, low self-esteem, sense of failure.

- Suicidal thoughts.
- Loss of sexual desire, or impotence.
- Preoccupation or worry about the presence of a physical illness.
- Lack of energy and constant exhaustion.
- Difficulty making decisions.
- Feeling that you're forgetful.
- Loss of identity.
- Loneliness, even when around others.

Telling a depressed person to pull themselves together is as useless as telling someone with appendicitis to snap out of it. The elderly deserve particular attention, as does anyone who has attempted suicide; also women experiencing severe depression after childbirth. Treatments range from counselling to anti-depressants to hospital admission for electro-convulsive therapy. Exercise and alternative or complementary therapies are also useful.

People suffering from depression frequently believe they will never get better; in fact quite the reverse is usually true. Other causes of depression to be considered are:

Possible

◆ Other physical disease

Depression is an extremely common accompaniment to significant physical illness, for instance: cancer, heart disease, stroke, and diabetes. Often this is overlooked in the quest to look after the physical body. So much more can be gained by simultaneously treating the psyche.

◆ **Post-viral syndrome and chronic fatigue syndrome (CFS)**

• Usually follows a physical illness with aches, pains.

• Profound weakness and tiredness are common.

• Muscle aching.

• Unrefreshing sleep.

• Impaired memory and concentration.

• Mild depression common.

The cause of post-viral syndrome and CFS is not understood. There are no precise tests to diagnose or monitor the condition. Treatment is difficult, though it often improves with time. A programme of gradually increasing graded activity and exercise may help, as does psychological support and sometimes antidepressant medication.

Complementary or alternative therapies are widespread.

◆ **Early dementia**

See *Dementia*, page 360. In the late middle aged or elderly.

◆ **Early schizophrenia**

See page 359.

Rare

◆ **Hypothyroidism**

A severely under-active thyroid gland may give rise to a state simulating depression. Some other hormone disorders may do likewise.

◆ **Parkinson's disease**

• In the elderly.

• Tremor of hands.

• Stiff, shuffling gait.

• Impassive appearance.

This can be helped by drugs.

Dizziness

Dizziness is a common symptom, but rather difficult to define since it can mean different things. For some, it appears to be an inability to concentrate, with feelings of light-headedness; for others, it is true vertigo with giddiness. You will find that your doctor will try hard to pin down just what you mean by dizziness.

Dizziness with vertigo

There is giddiness, unsteadiness and the room spins when you turn your head. Vertigo is the illusion of movement. A person with true vertigo will be able to tell you which way the room is moving.

Probable

◆ **Labyrinthitis**

A harmless disorder of the inner ear giving rise to:

- Abrupt onset of giddiness.
- Worse when turning head or changing position suddenly.
- No pain or ringing in ear.
- Lying flat, you feel completely well

Though alarming, the symptoms fade over a few days, sometimes with the help of anti-nausea drugs. It may be caused by a viral infection.

◆ Benign positional vertigo

A condition caused by movement of matter within the fluid in the inner ear. Sudden vertigo lasting 30 seconds or more is provoked by head turning. Usually self limiting within a few months but sometimes treated by a special repositioning technique (Epley head manoeuvres) done by a doctor.

Possible

◆ Mèniére's syndrome

A gradual process of degeneration in the ear. Symptoms include:

- Ringing in the ear (tinnitus) is an early feature.
- Gradually worsening deafness.
- Can effect one or both ears.
- Sudden attacks of vertigo, in which the above symptoms worsen for a few minutes.

Treatments include drugs, and devices to mask the tinnitus.

Rare

◆ Disease of the brain or spinal cord

Although highly unlikely as a cause of a few episodes of sudden dizziness, there are several such diseases – for example multiple sclerosis – which can cause dizziness in combination with:

- Unsteady gait.
- Tingling or numbness of hands or feet.
- Visual disturbances such as double vision.
- Weakness of an arm or leg.

A neurologist's opinion will be needed.

Dizziness without vertigo

The crucial clues are: in what circumstances the dizziness occurs; at what time of day; for how long; how often; and how you feel before and afterwards.

Probable

◆ Cause unknown

This accounts for a great majority of cases. A safe conclusion as long as:

- You are otherwise well.

- Attacks of dizziness are not prolonged or recurrent.

A medical check-up may be reassuring: investigations are not needed.

◆ Emotional factors

Here dizziness is used to mean:

- Inability to concentrate.
- A 'band' around the head.
- Muddled thinking.

The Brain & Nervous System

- Difficulty in making decisions.

Try to review what in your life is giving rise to unusual degrees of stress and worry.

Possible

◆ Anaemia

- Pallor.
- Tiredness.
- Breathlessness.
- A light-headed feeling when you stand up.

Unless the cause of the anaemia is obvious, for instance, very heavy periods, a prudent doctor will probably recommend some investigations.

◆ Low blood pressure

- Dizziness when you stand up.
- Passes off after a few seconds.

This is common in the elderly, whose circulation is less efficient at making the rather complex adjustments for standing up. Occasionally, it is because treatment for high blood pressure has been over-effective and sometimes medication must be changed. It is also common in pregnancy. Another increasingly recognised cause is vaso-vagal syndrome, where emotion causes low blood pressure. Specialised tests are now available, such as tilt-table tests.

◆ Low blood sugar

Most common in people with diabetes, especially if a meal is missed.

- Rapid onset.
- Difficulty concentrating.

- Irritability.
- Sweating.
- Symptoms are quickly relieved by eating.

Rare

◆ Heart and circulatory problems

These can really only be confirmed by medical examination or hospital tests. They become commoner with age, and pointers include:

- Palpitations.
- A pulse rate that feels unusually fast, unusually slow or irregular.
- Breathlessness.
- Chest pains.
- Dizziness when looking up.

Symptoms of minor stroke, with temporary limb weakness, disturbed speech or vision.

The underlying problem may be abnormal heart rhythms or narrowed valves of the heart: conditions which can be treated. Most likely, arteries to the brain have become 'furred up'.

◆ Polycythaemia

The opposite of anaemia, in which there is an over-concentration of blood. Commonest in those with chronic lung problems such as bronchitis and emphysema.

- A red complexion.
- Headaches.
- Itchiness of skin.

Treatment depends on the underlying cause.

◆ Temporal lobe epilepsy

Difficult to diagnose if dizziness is the only reported feature.

Other symptoms may include:

• A warning sensation (an aura) preceding the dizziness.

• Associated drowsiness.

Drowsiness

Drowsiness caused simply by lack of sleep or by excess alcohol is not covered here. Drowsiness in someone otherwise expected to be alert is an important symptom, and in children unusual drowsiness is a warning symptom which always needs medical assessment.

Probable

◆ Drug effects

• Most likely in the elderly.

• Commonly those on sleeping tablets, or sedative medication.

• Drowsiness clears as the day goes on.

The dosage of medication may need adjustment, or shorter-acting drugs may be appropriate.

◆ Infection

Drowsiness commonly accompanies the early stages of many illnesses, especially viral ones. There may also be:

• Fever.

• Aching eyes.

• The infection soon shows itself typically, as a cough, sore throat or flu-like illness.

• More serious infections need medical attention.

Possible

◆ Obstructive sleep apnoea

During sleep, the muscles at the back of the mouth and upper airway relax and breathing becomes obstructed. During this obstruction, which lasts for periods of more than 10 seconds each time, there is no breathing (apnoea); this pattern recurs many times per hour. The oxygen levels in the blood fall causing the sufferer to wake briefly (often unconsciously) with a sudden loud snore or breath, followed by further sleep and the cycle repeats. The consequence is that sleep quality is very poor. Common features include:

• Frequently drops off to sleep in the day.

• Daytime fatigue.

• Spouse or partner notices snoring or episodes of apnoea.

• Much commoner in the overweight, especially those with large collar size.

• May accompany chronic bronchitis, emphysema, or heart disease.

Treatment involves weight reduction, stopping smoking, and various devices to reposition the jaw and airway. In severe cases, pressurised air delivered through a mask at night (CPAP devices) can help to keep the airway open.

The Brain & Nervous System

◆ **Encephalitis**

A non-specific irritation of the brain, commonly caused by viral infections, but which may accompany meningitis.

• Severe, persistent drowsiness.

• Confusion.

• Headache.

• Bright lights hurt the eyes.

• As it worsens, convulsions, coma, paralysis of limbs.

If you suspect encephalitis in a child, get medical advice at once; adults should also see a doctor unless the above combination of symptoms is very mild.

◆ **Head injury**

Drowsiness occurring after a blow to the head may signify bleeding within the skull. Other warning signs are:

• Confusion.

• Nausea and vomiting.

• Loss of use of a limb.

• Double vision.

• Slow pulse.

Urgent hospital assessment is needed.

Rare

◆ **Brain tumour**

Brain tumours really are rare and when they do occur they have usually spread to the brain from a tumour elsewhere, typically the lung or breast.

The features of a brain tumour are:

• Consistent and progressively worsening headache, especially on waking and easing through the day.

• Change of personality.

• Double vision.

• Later, paralysis of one side of the body – symptoms like a stroke.

Treatment depends on the type of tumour and its location.

◆ **Narcolepsy**

• Sudden sleepiness, totally out of the blue.

• For a while, the individual cannot be roused.

• This unusual illness tends to run in families.

It is treated with stimulant drugs.

Emotional instability

Feelings of emotion are part of the normal human experience. The range of such feelings is enormous and their expression, likewise, is diverse and variable. Cultural factors play an important part here. Emotional instability typically becomes a problem when it occurs in somebody who has not previously suffered from it, or when it appears to be out of context with the person's situation. Likewise, it becomes a problem when it interferes with normal social and psychological functioning. Symptoms that might indicate that there is an underlying problem include:

- Changes in personality.
- Persistent irritability.
- Mood swings.
- Inappropriate behaviour.
- Poor judgement with loss of insight.

In some highly-strung people, apparent emotional instability is merely an exaggeration of the normal. They have abrupt swings of mood, often intensified by alcohol. They are not 'ill' as long as:

- Emotional states do not interfere with work, social and domestic life.
- The individual retains insight into his or her personality.
- General health and thought processes appear normal – for instance, no delusions.

However trying such people may be, they are often successful and creative. That leaves relatively few underlying causes of emotional instability:

Probable

◆ Anxiety

Anyone, whatever their previous personality, will become emotional under conditions of stress and tension. They will be aware of the change and they will retain insight into their personality.

See *Anxiety* and *Anxiety state*, page 349.

Possible

◆ Mental illness

When emotional instability really does appear to exceed the norm, psychiatrists will look for:

- Delusions.
- Hallucinations.
- Loss of insight into behaviour.
- Severe depression.
- Manic, irresponsible behaviour.

Underlying diagnoses include bipolar disorder, severe depression and schizophrenia.

◆ Menopause

See page 318.

◆ After childbirth

Feeling 'The Blues' shortly after childbirth is very common and usually settles with time. This differs from post-natal depression, which is more serious and usually requires professional support or treatment.

◆ Early dementia

See page 360.

◆ After a stroke

Mood swings or frequent and immediate weeping are common after a stroke, particularly in the elderly or in those types of strokes which affect the base of the brain.

Rare

◆ Brain tumour

See opposite.

◆ Brain disease

Numerous conditions can affect emotional control and are covered under *Dementia*.

The Brain & Nervous System

Fainting

A momentary interruption in the flow of blood to the brain will cause light-headedness; a longer pause is very likely to become a faint. Serious causes are unusual, unless fainting is recurrent or abrupt.

Probable

◆ Harmless causes

The great majority of causes are trivial: standing too long in the heat, missing a meal, over-tiredness. Fainting is common in pregnancy, after emotional shock and in reaction to severe pain.

• Recovery occurs within moments.

• No convulsions or incontinence.

• Lying down and raising the legs helps with recovery.

Possible

◆ Low blood pressure

See page 366.

• Recurrent light-headedness on standing.

• Most likely if you have diabetes, or if you take drugs which affect or control your blood pressure.

Rare

◆ Heart problems

Worth considering if there is:

• Faintness on exertion.

• Palpitations.

• Slow, rapid or irregular pulse rates.

Most of the heart problems that will lead to fainting are treatable.

◆ Bleeding

Faintness, in combination with injury or pain, may be a symptom of serious blood loss.

• Sweating.

• Pallor.

• Thirst.

Sometimes a small cut can produce the same effect, possibly through psychological triggering. Careful examination will reveal the source of bleeding. If you suspect internal bleeding, for example, after a car accident, seek medical help immediately.

◆ Epilepsy

See page 356.

◆ Minor stroke

Suggested also by temporary loss of speech, or of the use of a limb.

Hallucinations

A sensory experience without any basis in reality: a vision, a sound, a sensation. Dreams are 'normal' hallucinations. Likewise, many normal people (including children), in the twilight state before sleep begins, see things that aren't there. These are described as hypnagogic hallucinations. Another common hallucination phenomenon occurs following bereavement; typically the bereaved person reports hearing or seeing a loved one who has recently died. This is normal and does not signify any sort of mental illness. Other hallucinations occurring in clear consciousness can be symptoms of a psychiatric disorder, and appropriate medical help should be sought.

Possible

◆ Delirium

See page 358.

◆ Schizophrenia

See page 359.

◆ Depression

Very severe depression may give rise to hallucinations, for instance of abusive, mocking voices.

Rare

◆ Temporal lobe epilepsy

Hallucinations of smell and taste are commonest, and may present with other features such as convulsions – see page 367.

Hyperactivity

Typically a childhood problem (in adults, see *Mania*, page 374) combining:

- Constantly on the go.
- Frequent movements and restlessness.
- Behind or in trouble at school.
- Impulsive or inconsiderate behaviour.
- Disobedience and lack of discipline.
- Familial tendency.

Possible

◆ Normal child

Some parents have a low tolerance for normal childhood behaviour. Thirty seconds' exposure in a crowded surgery usually makes or (literally) breaks this diagnosis.

◆ Attention deficit hyperactivity disorder (ADHD)

See page 354.

◆ Psychological conflict

A possible diagnosis where the close family displays:

- Emotional conflict.
- Alcoholism.
- Mental illness.

Rare

◆ Food allergy

A controversial diagnosis, which may be supported by experimenting with exclusion diets.

◆ Minimal brain damage

Most likely if there is also:

- Clumsiness, difficulty in completing simple manual tasks.
- Severe learning difficulties.

  Such children often need special schooling. This syndrome is new and not fully defined. Not all doctors agree on its cause, or how best to manage affected individuals.

The Brain &
Nervous System

Hysteria and dissociation

The popular definition of hysteria is wild, reckless, exaggerated behaviour. The (more precise) medical definition is: symptoms that have no physical basis, which appear to arise without a conscious desire to deceive. The term hysteria has a somewhat pejorative feel to it and the condition is now more properly known as dissociation. It can be difficult, if not impossible, to prove that the behaviour is not motivated by a need to deceive.

Dissociation symptoms include amnesia, blindness, paralysis of a limb, lack of speech and difficulty swallowing. Women, usually between the ages of 30 and 50, are more commonly affected than men.

Probable

◆ Psychological factors

This diagnosis has some validity when physical disease has been excluded and is likely if:

- There is demonstrable psychological bonus from the behaviour: typically, attention or enhanced status.

- The sufferer is indifferent to symptoms a 'normal' person would find devastating – say, blindness.

- Sometimes follows a known trauma, for instance soldiers in World War One exposed to the horrors of trench warfare.

Treatment is extremely difficult. It requires the sufferer to recognise that the costs of his or her behaviour outweigh the short term psychological gain. In most cases recovery occurs within a year or so.

Possible

◆ Undetected physical disease

About 5 per cent of people diagnosed with dissociation are subsequently found to have an actual physical disorder. This emphasises the need for very careful physical assessment before arriving at the diagnosis.

Rare

◆ Brain disease

Dissociation may be an early symptom of dementia or other brain disorder. If symptoms specific to these diseases accompany the condition, seek medical advice. See *Dementia*, page 360.

Insomnia

Sleep is still a mystery; that we all need it is certain, but how much is astonishingly variable. Imagined insomnia is often a mismatch between how much sleep someone thinks they need and how much their body really needs. It is often worth asking the individual's partner how much sleep they are getting.

Probable

◆ Temporary disturbance of sleep patterns

Worries, pain, and life's stresses all cause insomnia which frequently persists once these problems have passed. Stimulants such as coffee and alcohol may be to blame, as may day-time snoozes. A cause is usually obvious – after a little reflection. Associated symptoms include:

- Day-time drowsiness.
- Sleep eventually comes – because you are exhausted.

Logically, the cause of the insomnia should be addressed, for example, trying to sort out the cause of the stress. If this is not possible, then other measures may help. For instance, it is best to not go to bed until you feel tired, avoid stimulants such as caffeine and try to follow a set routine leading to bed that produces suitable relaxation. Exercise may also help. Sleeping tablets have a role, but only in the short-term treatment of insomnia. Long haul air travel, where time zones are crossed, may present short term problems. Judicious use of sleeping tablets and melatonin can help here.

Possible

◆ Reduced need for sleep

For many people, 'eight hours sleep and a daily bowel movement' is Life's Golden Rule. Some individuals often cannot accept that they need far less of either, and the rules of the institutions where they may find themselves may reinforce this opinion. The fact is that plenty of people function perfectly normally with, say four to six hours sleep. Symptoms suggesting reduced need for sleep are:

- No obvious worries.
- No day-time drowsiness.

People with reduced need for sleep do well to accept that they have gained extra hours in their day; that nature is telling them to do the ironing at 3.00 am and to leave the extra daylight hours for better things.

◆ Depression

Insomnia is an important symptom of depression – see *Depression*, page 363.

Irritability

Greater than normal anger and hostility. No one need be in any doubt about normal irritability: it is a simple response to the 'F' words of workaday life:

- Fatigue.
- Frustration.

- Being fed-up.

Hunger and lack of sleep often makes irritability worse.

The more sinister causes of irritability are:

Possible

◆ Anxiety state

See page 349.
    Irritability out of proportion to circumstances.

◆ Drugs and alcohol

Drug and alcohol intoxication both lead to irritability and unreasonable behaviour.

Rare

◆ Early dementia

See page 360.

◆ Head injury

An injury severe enough to cause unconsciousness is frequently followed by:

• Irritability.

• Difficulty in concentrating.

• Swings of moods.

◆ Overactive thyroid

See page 319.

◆ Meningitis

See page 388.

Mania and Hypomania

Mania is the opposite of depression. Typical symptoms include:

• Euphoria and elevated mood.

• Irritability.

• Distractibility and poor concentration.

• Hyperactivity.

• Insomnia.

• Ideas spilling out, but barely connected.

• Grandiose thoughts.

• Rapid speech.

• Nervous, jittery activity.

• Poor judgement, with loss of insight.

• Hallucinations.

    Full-blown cases of mania are rare. Hypomania, which is much commoner, has the same symptoms, but is less severe.

Probable

◆ Bipolar disorder

This disorder (also known as manic depression) consists of alternating periods of high (manic) and low mood (depression). It is a long-term condition, typically starting before the age of 25. Characterised by:

• Recurrent mania.

• Recurrent depression.

• A combination of both.

• Sometimes there is a family history of the condition.

    Treatment of the highs and lows are with sedatives and antidepressants, respectively. Most sufferers with severe recurrent symptoms benefit from mood stabilisers, such as lithium.

◆ Drugs

Amphetamines or cocaine may precipitate mania.

Prescription drugs such as steroids and antidepressants can also be responsible.

◆ Emotional stress

A severe anxiety state may mimic a hypomanic state, though typically there is preservation of insight, and self neglect is rare.

The source of the anxiety is often obvious.

Possible

◆ Schizoaffective disorder

Sometimes there is a blurring of symptoms between the major mental disorders involving psychosis. This overlap between say schizophrenia and mania is sometimes referred to as schizoaffective disorder. See also under *Schizophrenia*, page 359.

◆ Overactive thyroid gland

See page319.

◆ Dementia

Mania arises from the loss of inhibition. A distressing combination. See *Dementia*.

Poor memory

It is common to have an excellent memory for some types of information, for instance, names, but a poor memory for others, such as phone numbers.

◆ Normal ageing process

Every day, 10,000 of our brain cells die, more than 250 million over a 70-year lifetime. A dense web of additional cells and rich interconnections mask the effects of this loss; but eventually it catches up with us, and we notice our memories worsening. This normal process rarely produces more than passing irritation, differing from dementia in this respect. Typical symptoms include

- Memory for long-past events remains good.
- Difficulty in learning new tasks.
- Personality generally unchanged.

◆ Dementia

See *Dementia*, page 360.

◆ Anxiety

Interferes with concentration and memory. See *Anxiety*, page 349.

◆ Head injury

Following a head injury there may be loss of memory for the time around the trauma. Later on there may be difficulty with concentration and poor memory retention.

◆ Stroke

Sudden loss of memory together with:

- Loss of use of a limb.
- Interference with speech.

There is often recovery from a minor stroke over several months. See *Confusion*.

◆ Psychological trauma and dissociation

Severe psychological trauma can result in distortion or blocking of memory. One example is post traumatic stress disorder. *See also Hysteria and dissociation*, page 372.

Mental impairment

A general lack of intellectual capacity, as shown by:

• Poor learning ability.

• Difficulty in coping with complex situations.

• Poor language skills.

• Clumsiness.

Past illness or injury may be to blame, but many cases remain unexplained.

Probable

◆ Cerebral palsy

Cerebral palsy refers to a group of disorders that involve loss of movement or loss of other nerve function. Often the cause is unknown, though it may involve a lack of oxygen resulting in brain damage around the time of birth. Many cerebral palsy sufferers have no mental impairment and merely suffer from movement or speech difficulties, though it can be part of the overall picture consisting of:

• Seizures.

• Muscle contractions.

• Difficulty sucking or feeding.

• Delayed development of motor skills, such as reaching, sitting, rolling, crawling, walking, and so on.

• Mental impairment and learning disability.

• Speech problems.

• Visual problems.

• Hearing problems.

• Spasticity.

• Joint contractures that slowly get worse.

• Limited range of motion.

◆ Congenital

A similar picture to that of cerebral palsy, above, but with specific features, giving a recognised condition such as Down's syndrome.

◆ Stroke

A reason for sudden deterioration in a previously normal intellect.

Possible

◆ Dementia

See page 360.

◆ Head injury

Has much the same effect as a stroke.

Rare

◆ Degenerative disorders of the nervous system

This can happen in several ways. Possible if:

• Intellect was previously normal.

• Gradual deterioration of thought processes.

• Associated tremors, weakness, paralysis and epilepsy.

Diagnosis is for a specialist.

◆ Vitamin deficiencies

Affects the growing child and is a tragic cause of impaired intellect in undeveloped countries.

- Poor growth.
- Swollen belly, poor bone formation.
- Loss of hair, patchy pigmentation of skin.

Vitamin deficiencies are also found in alcoholics.

◆ **Metabolic disorders**

Such as liver and kidney disease.

Paralysis, rapid onset

Usually the inability to use an arm or leg, but less commonly affecting muscles of the eyes, swallowing and breathing. The manner of onset gives a clue to the cause. Urgent medical attention is always needed.

Probable

◆ **Stroke**

This is by far the most likely cause. The mechanism is an interference to the blood flow to the brain, usually from a blood vessel blocked with a clot. This is called a thrombosis where a clot forms within the brain circulation, or an embolism where a clot travels from outside of the head typically the heart or arteries in the neck. Alternatively, a vessel bursts causing a haemorrhage in the brain. Characteristic features and symptoms are:

- Normally in the middle-aged or elderly.
- Often a history of high blood pressure, high cholesterol, smoking or diabetes.
- Paralysis affects one side of the body and face.
- Speech is slurred or lost.

- Confusion of variable degree, even coma.

Medical attention must be sought urgently. Investigations are initially designed to locate and define the cause of the stroke, usually by CT scanning. If a haemorrhage can be excluded, then drugs may be given to dissolve the clot. This is known as thrombolysis, though it can only be usefully done within six hours of the onset of the stroke. Otherwise, treatment consists of aspirin plus attention to underlying causes, such as high blood pressure or heart disease.

A stroke caused by an embolism may be treated with an anticoagulant drug (warfarin). Good nursing care, intensive physiotherapy and occupational therapy are also crucial. In many cases, a good return of function is achieved. Occasionally, investigations show up a brain tumour or abscess.

◆ **Subarachnoid haemorrhage**

A special type of stoke, caused by a bleeding blood vessel on the surface of the brain.

Relatively common in those aged 55-60, but possible at any age.

- Sudden, severe headache, 'like being hit on the back of the head'.

The Brain & Nervous System

- Vomiting.
- Collapse, neck stiffness, aversion to light.
- Sometimes coma and sudden death.

Surgical intervention is sometimes necessary to stop bleeding from the vessel and to prevent further occurrences.

◆ Injury

A severe blow to the head. Probably coma and one-sided paralysis.

Possible

◆ Arterial disease

Sudden paralysis of one leg, less

commonly an arm, may be due to blockage of an artery with a blood clot (arterial embolus). Symptoms would include:

- Sudden pain in the affected limb.
- Sudden pallor of the limb, developing into blueness.
- The limb is extremely cold and looks lifeless.

To save the limb, the obstruction must be rapidly removed.

Rare

◆ Hysteria and dissociation

See page 372.

Paralysis, slow onset

Probable

◆ Compression of a nerve

Common sites are the neck, affecting the arms; or a slipped disc in the back, affecting a leg or foot.

- Persistent pain and tingling confined to one part of one limb.
- Partial weakness of the limb.
- Health otherwise sound.

Investigations will show a reason for the compression and exclude general disease of the nervous system. Treatment depends on the cause, for example, a slipped disc in the back may be treated by physiotherapy or chiropractic manipulation, or occasionally by surgery.

Possible

◆ Multiple sclerosis

A slow, degenerative disease of young to middle-aged adults.

- Often begins with a sudden loss of vision in one eye.
- Numb patches, tingling, weakness of limbs, clumsiness.
- Symptoms come and go over months and years.
- Characteristically, relapses occur with subsequent incomplete improvement.
- Bladder symptoms and infections are common.

The outlook is very variable, often with years of relatively good health. An unfortunate minority become severely disabled.

◆ Brain tumour

- Slow, progressive weakness of one side of the body.
- Headache.
- Change of personality.

The slow progression makes diagnosis difficult, but MRI or CT brain scans readily confirm the diagnosis.

◆ Vitamin B12 deficiency

- Pallor.
- Tingling of hands and feet.
- Smooth, sore tongue.
- Stiff, weak legs.

The commonest cause is pernicious anaemia (see page 448), easily treated with injections of Vitamin B12.

Rare

◆ Guillain-Barré syndrome

A rare inflammation of the peripheral nerves that may follow a minor infection.

- Initially, tingling in the hands and feet.
- The condition worsens and paralysis of the limbs appears (may evolve over a few hours to as long as a few weeks).
- May spread to involve muscles of swallowing and breathing.

This serious condition needs intensive nursing care and sometimes assistance with breathing and feeding in an intensive care unit. Although recovery may take months, sufferers often recover completely or with only minor disability.

◆ Motor neurone disease

An exceptionally rare, tragic disease causing deterioration of muscle function in middle age.

- Begins with loss of bulk of the muscles of the hands.
- Muscle-wasting spreads more generally, with resulting paralysis.
- Widespread twitching of the muscles.
- Mental function remains intact.
  There is no known cure.

◆ Poliomyelitis

Now almost eradicated, thanks to immunisation programmes. Symptoms include:

- Mild, viral symptoms of sore throat, diarrhoea, muscle aches.
- Then symptoms of meningitis.
- Then increasing muscle ache.
- Followed by paralysis, especially of leg and shoulder muscles.
- Recovery can take a year; residual paralysis is common.

Change of personality

Probable

◆ Psychological disorder(s)

It is hardly surprising that psychological factors underlie most changes of personality, since personality is the sum of our emotional state, mood and intellectual outlook, and reflects our

The Brain & Nervous System

upbringing and experiences. Any psychological disease can affect personality. Noticeable features include.

• Anxiety.

• Emotional instability.

• Irritability.

• Aggression or passivity.

• Delusional thought.

• Self-neglect.

These symptoms have to be judged against the back ground of:

• General health.

• Relationships.

• Pressures at work and at home.

• Age.

• Drug and alcohol consumption.

The symptoms are covered elsewhere in this section under individual headings. Stress and minor anxiety states will most often be to blame.

Possible

◆ Alcohol or drug abuse

Usually a self-evident diagnosis, suggested by:

• Self-neglect.

• Tremor, emotional instability.

• Drunken or drug-intoxicated behaviour.

• Needle marks or drug-taking equipment evident.

• Smell of alcohol at inappropriate times.

• Social, employment and criminal problems.

◆ Head injury

Personality change after severe head trauma is common, together with:

• Irritability.

• Poor memory.

◆ Stroke

See page 377. The resulting brain damage can cause erratic behaviour, irritability and emotional instability.

Rare

◆ Brain tumour

Although a rare reason for personality change, doctors bear it in mind if rapid change in personality is combined with other symptoms of a brain tumour – see page 379. Tumours affecting the frontal lobe typically cause personality change.

Obsessions and phobias

Meaning morbid fears or a recurrent train of thought. Mild obsessions are common: for example, fear of spiders, or checking you have locked the back door three times before going on holiday. Severe forms can dominate your life: for example agoraphobia, fear of experiencing a difficult or embarrassing situation from which you cannot escape. Probably these symptoms reflect an inner insecurity, though often there is no obvious cause. Obsessions and phobias feed on themselves: what you have avoided in the past, you fear to meet in the future. Suffers commonly develop avoidance behaviour. Psychological treatment and medication can prove very effective.

Probable

◆ Psychological factors

In this situation, external factors cause stress, which leads to exaggerated feelings. These then become an obsession or phobia. Rest of personality and thought is normal. The individual retains insight into the problem but feels powerless to control it.

It is only when the particular phobia starts to make life unnecessarily difficult or impossible that you need professional help.

Possible

◆ Schizophrenia

See page 359.

Shock

In medical language, 'shock' means a massive and rapid fall in blood pressure with its accompanying effects. It a very serious condition that requires rapid treatment. This is totally different from the layman's use of the term in which shock is the emotional reaction to a serious psychological blow, such as awful news or witnessing a serious accident. Nonetheless, the symptom is considered here in the context of the brain and nervous system because shock can appear to be a nervous reaction – indeed, the nervous system is in part responsible for its occurrence.

Anyone thought to be in 'medical' as opposed to emotional shock needs emergency help as quickly as possible.

See also *Bluish skin*, and *Collapse with shock or coma*, page 435.

Critical features of medical shock are the rapid appearance of:

* Collapse.

* Sweating.

* Pallor.

* Weak rapid pulse.

* Confusion.

Probable

◆ Blood loss

The source may be obvious, for example, after a stab wound; less obvious sources are:

* Bleeding into the stomach – may vomit fresh blood or altered blood, looking like coffee grounds.

* Black, tarry–looking bowel motions following a bleed into the gut.

* Ruptured ectopic pregnancy (see page 312)

* Severe chest or abdominal pain going through to the back with ruptured aortic aneurysm – (see *Aortic aneurysm*, page 153).

The Brain & Nervous System

◆ Heart attack

A combination of:

- Chest pain.
- Collapse.
- Breathlessness.

See page 213.

Possible

◆ Serious infection

Danger arises when infection spread into the bloodstream. Commonest in babies or the elderly.

- Usually a pre-existing illness, commonly of the chest or of the skin.
- Fever, sweats and rigors.
- Rapid collapse.
- Purple spots may appear on the skin.

◆ Dehydration

Extreme loss of fluid from the body, for instance from severe diarrhoea and vomiting, eventually causes:

- Thirst.
- Restlessness.
- Dry mouth, lax skin.
- Reduced output of urine.

Those especially at risk are babies and diabetics.

Rare

◆ Allergic shock

Medical term: anaphylaxis.

This is an unpredictable reaction to, say, bee sting, an injection, or some foods.

- Face and lips swell within minutes.
- Breathing rapidly becomes wheezy.
- Collapse, possibly within a few minutes.

Those who know that they are at risk should carry an adrenaline injection which they can administer themselves. This can be lifesaving.

Features following emotional shock from a severe 'fright reaction' include:

- Pallor.
- Numbness of thought.
- Difficulty in concentrating.
- Life seems trivial.
- Nothing matters except the event.
- Tearfulness.
- Feelings of guilt.
- Loss of confidence.

Continuous support from relatives and friends is important. Talking about the event and crying aloud are helpful and necessary.

'General' symptoms

Introduction

The following pages contain 'general' symptoms, including looking pale or anaemic; fever; weight gain; and weight loss. They are, of course, the ones which are not easily assigned to other, more specific, sections of the book.

Low birth weight baby

Defined as less than 5lb (2.5 kg) birth weight or very low birth weight – less than 1.5kg. Generally the smaller the baby the more risk of problems which include:

- Breathing problems immediately after birth.
- Difficulty feeding.
- Jaundice.
- Bleeding in the brain.
- Heart problems (patent ductus).
- Bowel problems (necrotising enterocolitis).
- Eye problems.

There are two main reasons for babies being born with low birth weight – premature birth, i.e. birth before 37 weeks gestation (about two thirds of cases), and small-for-dates babies, whose growth has become restricted despite normal gestation (about one third of cases). Sometimes both causes co-exist. Routine antenatal care aims to detect and to control problems in the mother, such as high blood pressure or smoking, which might result in a premature or a low birth weight baby. Estimates of fetal growth can be made by measuring the enlargement of the womb (fundal height measurement), or serial ultrasound scanning to directly measure fetal dimensions.

Low birth weight babies often need sophisticated monitoring and support after birth in special care baby units (SCBU). Frequently, the reason for low birth weight is unknown and the baby goes on to develop into a normal child.

No one can be certain of the long-term consequences of low birth weight, but there is some evidence that babies born small can remain smaller than average at least up to puberty, and sometimes into adult life. There may be an association with the development of type 2 diabetes in later life.

Probable

◆ Prematurity

That is, a baby born before 37 weeks gestation, for any reason. Sometimes doctors find it difficult to judge whether a baby is premature or has a low birth weight. The diagnosis depends on the overall appearance and behaviour of the baby.

◆ Socio-economic disadvantage

The birth weight of a baby is linked to the mother's standard of living, presumably reflecting her general nutrition and self-care during pregnancy.

◆ Smoking, alcohol and illicit drugs

Babies born to mothers who smoke are, on average, about 0.5lb (0.25 kg) lighter than babies of mothers of similar social class who are non-smokers. Similarly, alcohol and illicit drugs can cause problems

Possible

◆ Multiple pregnancy

Twin pregnancies tend to produce smaller babies and are more at risk of premature birth.

◆ Maternal illness in pregnancy

The most common in developed countries is high blood pressure (pre-eclampsia). Other possibilities are heart, lung, or kidney disease. Worldwide, severe malnutrition is the major scourge.

◆ Abnormalities of the baby

Many congenital abnormalities and genetic defects cause low birth weight.

◆ Inadequate maternal weight gain

Women who gain less than the normal 25-35lbs in pregnancy have a higher risk.

Rare

◆ Infection in the mother during pregnancy

Genital infections in the mother, such as chlamydia, can cause premature birth. Rubella, which is completely preventable through immunisation, can harm the baby.

Other maternal infections such as cytomegalovirus, toxoplasmosis, and chickenpox are also dangerous.

Baby or child unable to put on weight or to grow adequately

The medical term for this symptom is failure to thrive, and it applies to babies and young children who fail to reach the accepted milestones of growth and development for their age. Growth can be readily assessed by measuring height and weight and comparing them to the expected norms on a chart.

It is especially significant if a previously normally growing child fails to put on weight at the expected rate. The search would be on for physical reasons, but it is well recognized that emotional neglect can also contribute to failure to thrive.

Probable

◆ Feeding problems

No neglect is implied, but simple problems such as:

- Breast feeding difficulties.
- Bottle feeds prepared or given incorrectly.
- An over-rigid feeding schedule.
- The baby rapidly catches up once the problem is identified.

Possible

◆ Vomiting

All babies vomit, some more than others. It is usually a passing feature and the baby's weight soon catches up.

Gastro-oesophageal reflux is common in small babies and may result in repeated vomiting.

Pyloric stenosis is a rare reason for persistent vomiting. It is caused by a blockage in the stomach outlet and relieved by a minor operation:

- Much commoner in boys than girls.
- Vomiting begins after the first few weeks of life typically at 6 weeks of age.

'General' Symptoms

- The baby feeds normally then vomits forcefully – so-called projectile vomiting.
- The baby is ravenous.

◆ Malabsorption

The child has a normal intake of food, yet fails to grow. Suspicious symptoms would include:

- Chronic diarrhoea, especially with bulky, greasy, smelly stools.
- Recurrent chest infections.

The commonest causes of malabsorption in developed countries are *Cystic fibrosis* and *Coeliac disease* (see page 137).

◆ Infection

Repeated infection over time slows down growth. The most common culprit is a urinary infection, causing fevers and abdominal pain. However, urinary infections may cause no symptoms at all, other than poor growth. Recurrent chest infections and gastrointestinal infections are other causes. They need to be individually investigated.

◆ Anaemia

Anaemia can be a symptom or a cause of failure to thrive. The commonest cause is not enough iron in the diet.

◆ Low birth weight

Severely premature babies, with low birth weight, may not to grow as well as normal babies at first. Babies born small, but on

time, can be expected to grow at a normal rate, although they may remain smaller then other children.

◆ Neglect

This includes emotional neglect, as well as food deprivation.

- A withdrawn, unresponsive child.
- Fearful of strangers.
- Other signs of neglect such as injuries, bruising, dirtiness.

◆ Cow's milk (lactose) intolerance or allergy

Symptoms include:

- Persistent diarrhoea.
- Sometimes skin problems or wheeze.

Resolves with elimination of lactose in diet – substitution of cow's milk formula with soya milk.

Rare

◆ Hypothyroidism

This should be avoided by early heel-prick blood testing for the condition and, if identified, is easily treatable. If it goes undetected, symptoms could include:

- Prolonged jaundice in the days after birth.
- A lethargic baby, tending to constipation and poor feeding.
- Later delay in development, and learning disability.

Birth abnormality plus failure to grow

If the causes of failure to grow as above have been excluded, malformation

might be suspected. Specialists will test for: interference with swallowing, perhaps due to a cleft palate; cerebral palsy; heart disease; a Chromosomal abnormality; or (rare), a metabolic disorder or kidney failure. See relevant sections for further details.

Distressed or crying baby

First, know your child. All mothers know that a child will cry in different ways, depending on whether he or she is hungry, angry or in pain. Daily experience of your child qualifies you to recognize when the child is crying in an unusual way. When this happens, check through the common causes below.

Remember also that a usually placid baby or child can become irritable in response to your own mood, or even to the way you handle him or her.

Probable

◆ **Hunger or thirst**
- Due for a feed.
- Roots for the breast or bottle.
- Sucks eagerly and settles when fed.

◆ **Discomfort**
- A dirty nappy.
- Too hot – look for flushed appearance and sweating.
- Too cold: blue hands, cold to the touch.
- Noise, bright lights, smoke.

◆ **Desire for comfort**
- Excited when you appear.
- Crying stops when cuddled, recurs when put down.

Possible

◆ **Colic**
- After a feed or in the evening.
- Draws up legs, whimpers.
- Relieved by winding or, in the case of evening colic, the problem simply stops after a few weeks.

◆ **Infection**
- Snuffles, a cold or a cough.
- Other signs of infection: fever, off feeds, vomiting or diarrhoea, increased sleepiness, flushed appearance or rash.

◆ **Pain**
- Rubbing ear; teething.
- More of a scream than a cry.
- Only briefly relieved by comforting.
- May respond to simple painkillers such as paracetamol.

◆ **Injury**

Usually a fall or accident that has been witnessed or heard by a parent. Sometimes, if the accident occurs out of sight, the only sign may be a cut or a bruise.

More serious injuries may cause fractures – look for swelling of limbs or joints and the child 'not using' the injured part.

'General' Symptoms

Rare

◆ Meningitis

A serious infection of the brain and its coverings; meningitis can appear in hours in a previously well baby or child. It is rare, but potentially so serious that anxiety is understandable. Difficult to diagnose in very young babies: much depends on how ill the child looks. Because of the difficulty of diagnosis, see a doctor immediately if you suspect meningitis. The child may well need admission to hospital for investigation.

- The baby or child is initially irritable.
- Increasingly drowsy, lethargic.
- Vomiting.
- Soft spot of skull may be bulging.
- High-pitched, animal cry.
- Fine purple skin rash.

Short stature in children

This is generally defined as height which is in the lowest 3 per cent of the population for age. Although parents worry about it, regular measurements at three-monthly intervals will show whether a child is small, but growing at a normal rate, in which case the child is almost certainly short because he or she is made that way.

Probable

◆ Family pattern

Short parents have children who will be short, although genetic mechanisms ensure that, on average, the children end up taller than the parents. There are formulae, based on parental height, which can help to predict the final height of a child.

◆ Constitutional growth delay

A term used to describe children who are small for their age but who have a normal growth rate. Also known as 'Late Bloomers' these children often have:

- A close relative who displayed growth delay.
- In girls, periods may start at a later age.
- Growth which may continue longer.
- Adult height may not be reached until after the age of 18.
- Eventual height in keeping with size of rest of family.

Possible

◆ Chronic disease

Any long-term disease will stunt growth. Common culprits are kidney disease, heart disease, and respiratory disease.

◆ Malnutrition

Worldwide this is much the commonest cause, associated with poverty and socio-economic factors.

◆ Chromosomal or genetic disorder

Common disorders are Down's syndrome, with characteristic flat face;

Achondroplasia

Another example of a genetic disorder is Achondroplasia in which there is an alteration of body proportions – typically:

• Very short limbs.

• Head and trunk normal size.

◆ **Hypothyroidism**

An underactive thyroid gland. See page 386.

Rare

◆ **Growth hormone deficiency**

This unusual condition is now treatable by giving injections of the missing hormone.

• The child is normal, but grows slowly.

• Tendency to be overweight around the waist.

large hands; fold of skin on inner part of eyeball and other abnormalities. Another is Turner's syndrome; two symptoms of this condition are:

• Webbed neck.

• Infertility in later life.

Bruising

A bruise is an area of skin discoloration which occurs when small blood vessels break and leak their contents into the soft tissue beneath the skin. Medical attention should be sought if the size of the bruise is large or disproportionate to the supposed cause. See also *Bleeding – spontaneous and general*, page 398.

Probable

◆ **Accident or trauma**

Bruises on exposed areas, such as shins or elbows, which come and go.

◆ **Drug side effect**

Typically seen after minor or trivial trauma in people taking anticoagulants, such as warfarin. Aspirin has a similar but weaker effect.

Possible

◆ **Senile purpura**

Purple bruise-like marks occurring without obvious trauma, commonly seen in elderly people on arms and backs of hands. These need no treatment and are not dangerous.

◆ **Blood disorder**

Severe anaemias and serious blood disorders.

• Purple spots or patches appear on skin.

• Spontaneous bleeding from gums, nose.

• Rapid onset in an already ill person.

'General' Symptoms

A blood test is essential and should be taken as soon as possible.

◆ Physical abuse

Suggested in particular if there is a history of family difficulties.

* Multiple bruises of varying ages, some old, some fresh.

* Inadequate explanation.

* Appearance of neglect – dirty, ill-fed.

* Bruising around ankles or wrists.

* The characteristic bruising of bite marks is not unusual on abused children.

Rare

◆ Scurvy

Caused by lack of Vitamin C.

Pale appearance (pallor) – slow onset

Some people are naturally pale, so the best way to check for pallor is to look at the areas where blood flows close to the surface, for example beneath the fingernails and under the eyelids. Pallor alone, even if the cause can be narrowed down to anaemia, invariably requires medical assessment and detailed investigation. This section refers to pallor coming on over weeks or months.

Probable

◆ Anaemia

See also *Looking pale and anaemic*, page 392.

General features include:

* Tiredness; being easily fatigued.

* Breathlessness – gradual onset.

* Dizziness, especially on standing up

In addition, there may be symptoms suggesting the underlying cause, such as:

* Weight loss.

* Self-neglect.

* Sores on skin and bruising.

* Heavy periods.

* Jaundice.

It is essential to determine the cause of the anaemia in order to treat it fully.

Possible

◆ Hypothyroidism

An under-active thyroid gland causes a slow-down in all aspects of body function over several months. As well as pallor, which is due both to a mild anaemia and to changes in the skin, you may notice:

* Sensitivity to the cold.

* Gruff voice, coarse skin, thinning hair.

* Constipation, slowness of thought.

This condition is readily treatable by taking thyroid tablets once the diagnosis has been established by a doctor.

Rare

◆ Hypopituitarism

A failure of the pituitary gland in the brain, crucial to controlling many hormones – the body's 'chemical messengers'. Pallor can be a striking feature of this condition, plus other symptoms, such as:

- Hypothyroidism, as above.
- In women, periods cease; loss of sexual drive.

- Reduction of pubic and underarm hair.
- Lack of stamina.

This condition requires specialist medical assessment and management.

Pale appearance (pallor) – rapid onset

This section refers to pallor coming on over days, hours or minutes. Unless the individual has simply fainted, this may well signify a problem which requires urgent medical attention.

The likeliest reason is blood loss.

Probable

◆ Fainting

The many well-recognized causes of fainting include missing a meal; emotional shock; prolonged standing; excessive heat; pregnancy.

- Otherwise sound health.
- Initial light-headedness, sweating, dizziness.
- Collapse to ground or on to furniture.
- Cold, clammy skin; thin, slow pulse.

It is essential to leave someone who has fainted lying flat until they recover, which generally takes just a few minutes.

◆ Internal bleeding

Often there is a previous history of abdominal discomfort. The blood loss may be obvious:

- Bloody or black stools.
- Vomit containing blood or with specks looking like coffee grounds.
- Excessive vaginal bleeding, especially after a delayed period.
- Blood in urine.

Early symptoms are similar to those of anaemia but of more rapid onset. As blood loss increases there will be:

- Severe giddiness or faintness.
- A feeling of being cold, plus cold, clammy extremities.
- Low urine output.
- Rapid breathing.
- Eventually, drowsiness and unconsciousness.

There will probably be pointers to the cause of the bleeding. Previous dyspepsia (indigestion) suggests a duodenal or gastric problem. Bowel disturbance may signify inflammation of the bowel, a tumour or a perforation (hole) in the intestine.

Aspirin and other anti-arthritic drugs can also cause bleeding into the stomach or gut. Previous alcoholism may suggest bleeding oesophageal veins (varices).

'General' Symptoms

Possible

◆ Hypoglycaemia

A problem for diabetics, especially those on insulin, who must learn to recognize the early symptoms:

• Hunger, irritability, light-headedness, progressing to:

• Sweating, confusion, slurring of speech, unconsciousness.

Taking glucose or glucagon gives relief in minutes.

◆ Heart rhythm disorder

Very rapid, slow or irregular heart rhythms mean that blood is pumped around the body with reduced efficiency. Commonest in the 50-plus age group.

• You may be aware of a thumping or a fluttering in your chest.

• Onset is usually abrupt; symptoms often end abruptly, too.

• Pallor, breathlessness, dizziness.

◆ Gastric upset

The early stages of a severe attack of gastroenteritis may be ushered in with:

• Nausea, vomiting, sweating, griping abdominal discomfort.

• Pallor.

• Diarrhoea follows within a few hours.

◆ Heart attack

Pallor will probably not be the only, or even the main, symptom. The classic picture is:

• Crushing pain in the central chest going into the left arm or neck, arising suddenly.

• Breathlessness, sweating, pallor.

Heart attacks, especially in the elderly, may not be so clear-cut, causing just pallor, fatigue and breathlessness. Always seek urgent medical help.

Rare

◆ Acute blood disorder

Including leukaemia and any breakdown in the blood's clotting mechanism. Commonest in children and young adults.

Suggested by:

• Pallor.

• Nose bleeds, bleeding gums, blood in bowel or urine.

• Spontaneous bruising.

Medical assessment is essential.

Looking pale or anaemic

The red blood cells in the body last on average 90 days. They are in constant production, whilst those cells coming to the end of their lives are broken down and their constituents recycled. When the number of red blood cells fall below the necessary level (either through inadequate production or excessive loss); or if haemoglobin, the oxygen-carrier in red blood cells, is omehow impaired or reduced, anaemia develops. This results in:

- Paleness or pallor – an important sign of anaemia, but often a misleading one, since many people are naturally pale. Best judged by looking at parts of the body where the blood runs close to the surface, typically the under-surface of the eyelids or under the fingernails and confirmed by a blood test.

- Feeling tired much of the time.

- Fatigue on exertion.

- Faintness (in severe cases).

- Breathlessness.

There are a vast range of possible causes or anaemia, but in practice a blood test, together with the patient's history and an examination, usually help narrow down the possibilities and help with the diagnosis.

Probable

◆ Menstrual blood loss

The 70 to 80 ml of blood lost in normal menstruation is replaced by the body within a day or two. If more blood is lost then anaemia becomes a possibility. This is suggested if periods are:

- Very heavy with clots.

- Very frequent.

- Prolonged, or there is bleeding between periods.

- If you have a poor diet.

◆ Pregnancy

Anaemia in pregnancy should be detected by routine blood tests. In fact, it is so common in pregnancy that some degree of anaemia is considered normal. Iron supplements are not always given to pregnant women: your doctor will advise you if it is necessary. If it is needed iron is commonly given together with folic acid – another important vitamin for blood production. Further blood loss occurs during birth and may require treatment with iron.

◆ Poor diet

That is, a diet deficient in iron or in the vitamins needed to make haemoglobin. The elderly, alcoholics or those on low incomes are at risk. Similarly, people with restricted diets, such as vegans, can become anaemic. The chief source of iron in the diet is red meat; green vegetables contain lesser amounts.

Possible

◆ Cancer or other chronic disease

Anaemia is unlikely to be the only symptom, except in the case of cancers causing internal bleeding (mainly cancer of the colon). Likewise, with chronic diseases such as kidney failure or rheumatoid arthritis.

Management is generally a question of controlling the underlying disease and giving drugs to improve blood production. Occasionally a blood transfusion is helpful.

◆ Chronic bleeding

Caused by disease, such as a bleeding peptic ulcer, or by drugs, of which aspirin, anti-inflammatory agents, and steroids are the commonest culprits. Also, don't underestimate the effect of chronically bleeding haemorrhoids. Symptoms of chronic bleeding include:

- Passage of bloody or black stools.

- Blood in vomit.

- Excessive or prolonged menstrual bleeding (see page 393).

- Features of underlying disease, weight loss, loss of appetite, alteration of bowel habit.

◆ Thalassaemia and sickle disease

Both of these conditions are genetically inherited disorders of haemoglobin production – the oxygen carrying protein in blood. Thalassaemia is commonest amongst people of Mediterranean extraction, whilst sickle disease affects people of African descent. A mild form of these conditions – sickle or thalassaemia trait causes no problems; whilst the severe form of each disease can result in major debility.

Rare

◆ Pernicious anaemia

Caused by lack of Vitamin B12, due to failure to absorb the vitamin.

- Gradual onset, sometimes leading to very low levels of haemoglobin.

- Often, a family history.

- Sore, smooth tongue.

- Tingling, numbness of limbs.

- Unsteady walk.

◆ Worm infestations

For example, hookworm; unlikely in developed countries, but common causes of anaemia in tropical countries. Detected from stool samples.

Looking pale or anaemic plus skin problems

Rashes, sores and skin changes can be a feature of anaemia, but usually only if the anaemia is especially severe, or if it is one of the rarer types which are a side effect of some other underlying disease. Full medical evaluation is advised.

Probable

◆ Iron deficiency anaemia

General features of anaemia, plus:

- Painful cracked skin at corners of mouth.

- Sore smooth tongue.

Common causes include poor dietary intake of iron or abnormal blood loss from the gut or female genital system.

Possible

◆ Pernicious anaemia

Can cause a sore, smooth tongue. See above.

Rare

◆ Drug side effect

Any drug which causes anaemia may also cause skin rashes, blotches, bruises and a sore mouth.

'General' Symptoms

▶ Auto-immune disease

range of diseases in which the body ttacks its own components resulting in general effects of malaise, rashes, joint pains. A butterfly-shaped rash across the cheeks is characteristic of Systemic lupus erythematosis (SLE).

Looking pale or anaemic, plus losing weight

his is a worrying combination, specially in the middle-aged and lderly. There is the possibility of underlying disease causing internal bleeding or possibly affecting the ability of the body to absorb the food, iron and vitamins needed to make red blood cells. In children, the combination is more likely to suggest poor food intake or a malabsorption condition. Medical advice should always be sought.

Probable

▶ Neglect

ypically self-neglect, with a diet so poor that individuals are literally starving themselves. In developed countries, it is usually only seen in those who are either very poor, living alone, or too frail to provide adequately for themselves. It is sometimes found in alcoholics and, drug abusers, and people suffering from depression or dementia. In children, there may be other signs of neglect by their guardians, such as:

- Unexplained bruising.
- Dirty appearance.
- Withdrawn behaviour.
  No food in the house.

◆ Malabsorption

The term covers a range of conditions which undermine the digestive tract's ability to absorb nutrients. The possibilities are wide and what is probable in children is rare in adults. Some clues which suggest malabsorption as the underlying cause of anaemia and weight loss are:

- Gradual appearance of symptoms.
- Change in bowel habit, with persistent, loose stools or diarrhoea. Sometimes the stools float and are difficult to flush away.
- An apparently adequate intake of food.
- Appetite healthy until later stages of the illness.
- Co-existing, recurrent chest infections in patients with cystic fibrosis.

Possible

◆ Bowel cancer

Bowel cancer is common. In the United States, routine, annual bowel examinations are increasingly used to test for cancer. A simpler screening test consists of a stool examination to detect the presence of hidden blood, which if

'General' Symptoms

positive is followed by a more detailed examination of the bowel (by colonoscopy, barium X-rays, or CT scanning). A family history of bowel cancer means that you run a significantly increased risk of developing the condition. This common cancer has an excellent outlook if diagnosed sufficiently early. Besides anaemia and weight loss, the other warning signs are:

- Persistent change of bowel habit from the normal known pattern for the individual in question. Alternating diarrhoea and constipation is often a suspicious pattern.
- Blood in stools
- Mucus or slime from back passage.
- A feeling of not completely emptying the bowel.

◆ Inflammatory bowel disease

The term covers either ulcerative colitis or Crohn's disease.

- Diarrhoea, often with blood.
- Weight loss.
- Abdominal pain.

◆ Chronic disease

Several chronic diseases, such as tuberculosis or long-term infection, can cause this combination of symptoms. HIV/AIDS is another possibility. The nature of the underlying disease will require full investigation. Seek help from your doctor.

◆ Stomach cancer

Again, the earlier this is diagnosed, the better the outlook. In addition to weight loss and sometimes anaemia, symptoms include:

- Indigestion and acidity as a new symptom in middle – or old – age.
- Loss of appetite.
- Persistent pains in upper abdomen.
- Vomiting of blood or passage of black motions.

◆ Anorexia nervosa

Although associated with young women, it is sometimes seen in men. Those with anorexia are often good athletes or high achievers at school.

The signs are:

- Obsession with body image: the individual is convinced that she is obese.
- Appearance may vary from very slim to outright starved.
- In women, monthly periods cease.
- An excess of fine body hair may appear.
- Bouts of binge eating (bulimia).
- Excessive exercising.
- Self-induced vomiting or laxative abuse.

Rare

◆ Chronic myeloid leukaemia

A disease of gradual onset in middle age, which may present with anaemia and weight loss.

May also cause:

- Susceptibility to infections.
- Bruising or bleeding.
- Enlarged spleen.

Diagnosis made on blood tests.

Bluish skin (cyanosis)

Otherwise known as cyanosis: a bluish-purple colouring, visible especially where blood flows close to the surface, for example the lips, the tongue and under the fingernails. It arises when blood becomes deoxygenated – unable to discharge waste carbon dioxide, or to take on fresh oxygen from the lungs. Fingers commonly show cyanosis in cold weather due to sluggish blood flow. In more serious cases, the lips and tongue also become blue.

Probable

◆ Temporarily poor circulation

Common at any age:

- Results from a drop in temperature.
- A slight degree of cyanosis, confined to fingers and toes, which feel cold and numb.
- Disappears rapidly on warming the limb.
- Worse in winter, better in summer.

Sometimes seen in Raynaud's syndrome, where there is spasm of the blood vessels in the fingers, temporarily reducing circulation. Raynaud's may also produce whiteness in the fingers.

Occasionally, a blood clot may block the circulation to part of a limb, usually the lower leg or toes. This gives a quite different set of symptoms, typically found in an elderly person with pre-existing circulatory disease or an irregular heartbeat (atrial fibrillation).

- Sudden onset of pain, coldness, numbness and paralysis of the limb.

- Limb may at first look pale, cyanosis setting in over a few hours.
- This is an emergency: seek urgent medical help at once.

Possible

◆ Chronic obstructive pulmonary disease (COPD)

Chiefly caused by chronic bronchitis and emphysema in smokers, these lung diseases cause persistent cough with phlegm, wheeze and breathlessness. It is only after many years of disease that cyanosis becomes a regular feature, by which time the sufferer has long suffered breathlessness on the slightest exertion.

- Cyanosed nail beds, tongue and lips.
- Hands and feet can feel surprisingly warm. Caused by high concentrations of carbon dioxide in the blood.

There are a number of other rare lung diseases which cause cyanosis.

◆ Heart failure

Mild heart failure, caused usually by diseased coronary arteries, does not cause cyanosis. It is readily and effectively treatable. Only in severe cases is cyanosis a prominent symptom, together with:

- Constant breathlessness.
- Swollen legs.
- Breathlessness on lying flat.
- Coughing frothy fluid.

There may be coexistent COPD (see above) a condition called cor pulmonale, or disease of the heart valves.

'General' Symptoms

◆ Lung infections and asthma

Severe pneumonia or asthma can produce cyanosis – this is a very grave sign, indicating life-threatening illness.

Similarly, a child with symptoms of croup or epiglottitis (See pages 195 and 211) who becomes blue is in serious danger of suffocation – call an ambulance or doctor at once.

Rare

◆ Congenital heart disease (children)

Following conception, the human embryo's heart and great blood vessels develop via a complex process open to error at all points, and it is remarkable that so few serious congenital heart conditions occur. If they do, the result may be a 'blue' or cyanosed baby, in whom the blood is not pumped properly through the lungs. Symptoms show at or very soon after birth.

- Breathlessness on feeding.
- The baby fails to gain weight normally during the first few weeks and months of life.
- Dizziness, headache and fatigue.
- Thromboses (blood clots).

◆ Drug overdose

Suspected in an otherwise well young person who is:

- Unconscious.
- Breathing reduced to a point at which cyanosis appears.
- Pinpoint pupils suggest a heroin or opiate overdose.

◆ Inhaled foreign body

The rapid appearance of cyanosis in someone who is suddenly breathless suggests an immediate obstruction to airflow.

In children it may be caused by inhaling a small object or item of food such as a peanut.

- Typically occurs when eating steak or similar chunky food, or in children,nuts.
- Clutching at the throat, trying to gasp; clearly very distressed.
- Collapse.

The Heimlich manoeuvre (abdominal thrusts) is a useful first aid procedure designed to relieve such obstructions. See page 219.

Bleeding – spontaneous and general

Everyone experiences surprise bleeding from time to time: a nosebleed or perhaps bleeding from the back passage. Follow up these symptoms in detail under the relevant sections for the part of the body involved.

Covered here is spontaneous bleeding from the gums or the nose; blood in the urine, in stools and from the vagina. It will almost certainly be accompanied by widespread bruising. The symptoms point to a general breakdown of the blood clotting process. Lesser degrees of all the causes listed below will give rise to prolonged clotting time after an injury, or easy bruising.

Probable

◆ Anticoagulant treatment

The drug warfarin is widely used for certain heart disorders, and also for thrombosis in a limb. Regular blood tests help to check that the dose is correct, at a therapeutic dose blood takes longer to clot and spontaneous bleeding is more likely, but in overdosage bleeding can be catastrophic. See your doctor immediately if you begin bleeding unexpectedly while taking warfarin. Nosebleeds can be the first sign of excessive dosage.

◆ Thrombocytopaenia

A general term for a reduction in the numbers of platelets in the bloodstream. Platelets are crucial to blood clotting, so if they are in short supply, widespread bleeding or bruising occurs. Many serious general illnesses can cause thrombocytopenia, the cause usually being obvious after just a few investigations, for example:

- Aplastic anaemia, with rapid appearance of weakness, pallor and malaise.
- Childhood leukaemia, as with aplastic anaemia, but also sore throat.
- Adult leukaemias: a slower onset than childhood leukaemias, enlarged lymph nodes, sweats.
- Bone cancers, with pain, malaise, weight loss.

Thrombocytopenia can also be drug-induced. There is also a benign form, affecting children, which cures itself spontaneously. Treatment is aimed at the underlying cause, if known.

Possible

◆ Haemophilia

A bleeding disorder caused by a genetically-controlled deficiency in the blood factors necessary in the normal clotting mechanism.

It is found almost exclusively in males.

- A family history is common: two-thirds of cases are hereditary.
- Early symptoms are prolonged bleeding from, say, a small cut; spontaneous bruising; or bleeding into joints, giving joint pain and swelling.

◆ Severe infection

Many serious infectious diseases cause chaos in the blood clotting system. These include septicaemia (blood poisoning), malaria and typhoid fever.

- Sweats and chills while the patient is also;
- Generally very ill.

Rare

◆ Scurvy

Results from a diet lacking Vitamin C, which is contained in fresh fruit and vegetables. So the problem is usually one of the elderly or malnourished.

- Chronic feeling of being ill.
- Bleeding, especially from between the teeth.
- Sore gums, loose teeth.
- Easy bruising.

Readily treated by Vitamin C supplements.

'General' Symptoms

Tallness

Meaning (for a given age) height greater than that of the tallest 3 per cent of the population. Only rarely is tallness due to disease.

Probable

◆ Natural tendency

Tall parents have tall children. There are formulae which can predict a child's height, based on the heights of the parents.

◆ Early puberty

The complex hormonal changes of an early puberty can make a child leap up in height. As puberty progresses, growth slows, so the child who was unusually tall with an early puberty may eventually finish smaller than his or her peers. The familiar signs of puberty are:

* Growth of body hair around genitalia, armpits.
* Breast development.
* Deepening voice.

Rare

◆ Hyperthyroidism

This will enhance growth in childhood.
See page 319.

◆ Genetic abnormality

* The commonest (it affects one in 500 males) is Klinefelter's syndrome.
* Tall and thin with a female body shape, small testicles and breast development.
* Usually infertile.

◆ Excess growth hormone

In children, this causes excessive height and size. In adults it causes acromegaly with progressively coarse, heavy features.

* Enlargement of hands and feet.
* Protrusion of lower jaw.
* Possibly heavy sweating and diabetic symptoms.

◆ Marfan's syndrome

This interesting hereditary condition affects about two people per 100,000. It causes:

* Long, thin bones, spider-like fingers and toes.
* An unusually high arch to the palate.
* Heart valve problems, which may cause breathlessness.
* Visual disturbance through dislocation of the lens of the eye.

Body swollen with excess fluid

Three categories of disorder cause generalized body swelling with excess fluid – known as oedema: heart failure, kidney disease and low protein states.

The mechanics of swelling are complex. Because fluid sinks to the lowest level of the body the early signs are swollen ankles or a puffy face in the morning.

This is easy to test for in the ankles by applying gentle pressure with a finger tip to the swollen ankle – when the finger is removed an indentation remains, confirming the presence of oedema. As more fluid accumulates, swelling spreads up the legs and builds up inside the abdomen and chest.

Probable

◆ Pre-menstrual swelling

Hormone changes in the few days before a period cause a mild degree of fluid retention:

- A regular pattern each month; health otherwise normal.
- Breasts, abdomen, ankles all become slightly enlarged.
- Weight gain of a few pounds.
- Disappears within days of the period beginning.

◆ Heart failure

A common cause of persistent swelling of the legs in later life.

- Often high blood pressure, angina or other heart disease.
- At first, swelling of ankles, tiredness.
- Later, breathlessness on exertion, or when lying down (causing inability to lie down).
- Paroxysms of breathlessness at night, coughing frothy sputum.

Modern drugs can usually provide effective treatment, although the swelling may not clear completely.

Possible

◆ Liver disease

One of the liver's many functions is to make proteins. These circulate in the blood stream, and if their levels fall, oedema follows.

- Often a history of alcohol abuse, hepatitis, drugs toxic to the liver.
- Easy bruising, blood-stained vomit.
- Tiredness, loss of sexual drive, clubbed fingers.
- Tiny, spider-like red veins on face, upper body.
- Red palms.
- Swelling of the abdomen, with fluid.
- Jaundice is a late symptom, as is confusion, coma.

◆ Pre-eclampsia

A condition causing oedema, high blood pressure and loss of protein in the urine in pregnant women. See page 358.

◆ Malnutrition

Globally, this is a major cause of oedema in children:

- Swollen abdomen.
- Patchy pigmentation of body.
- Apathy, coarse skin, lack of resistance to infection.

◆ Malabsorption

A possibility in those with chronic bowel disease, for example coeliac disease or ulcerative colitis – which interfere with absorption of nutrients.

Some general symptoms include:

- Failure to thrive (children); diarrhoea, smelly, greasy stools.
- Bleeding from bowel.
- Chronic abdominal pain.
- Recurrent, severe chest infections.
- Clubbing of finger nails.

◆ Glomerulonephritis and nephrotic syndrome

Glomerulonephritis is actually a group of diseases, all of which involve some degree of inflammation of the kidneys. This can cause oedema, partly due to loss of protein in the urine and partly due to failure to excrete sufficient urine. Nephrotic syndrome, which may de due to glomerulonephritis, refers to the oedematous state of the body, in combination with loss of protein in the urine.

In children, glomerulonephritis and nephrotic syndrome present with:

- Sudden onset, often after a minor throat infection.
- Low urine output.

- Blood in urine.
- Puffiness, especially of the face.

The outlook for recovery is good. In adults it tends to present more slowly, with:

- Progressive swelling of the legs.

Assessment involves blood tests and biopsy of the kidney, after which the outlook can be judged, depending on the type of glomerulonephritis. Often the outlook is good, with full recovery, though some cases progress to kidney failure.

Rare

◆ Thiamine deficiency

Otherwise called beri-beri.

Thiamine is found in whole-grain cereals including rice, and in liver. In developed countries, the deficiency is likely only through severe deprivation, as thiamine is routinely added to many manufactured foods.

- Early symptoms are tender calves and vague weakness.
- Then swelling of legs, palpitations.
- Eventually, general swelling, exhaustion, rapid pulse.

Swollen part of the body

Probable

◆ Injury

Tissue swelling is the normal reaction to any modest injury, together with reddened, warm skin.

◆ Infection

Including insect bites and minor cuts.

- Throbbing pain, redness.
- Swelling of local lymph glands.
- Pus may be visible.

◆ Dependent oedema

Older people who are inactive frequently notice this, one of the commonest reasons for a mild degree of ankle swelling. No need for treatment unless it is a nuisance. Care should be taken to distinguish this condition from other causes of oedema (see above) requiring medical treatment. It is best to ask a doctor to help with this distinction.

With dependent oedema:

- General health good.
- Swelling lessens if activity is increased.

Possible

◆ Deep vein thrombosis (DVT)

Sudden swelling of a limb, nearly always a leg, suggests thrombosis. It occurs when clotted blood obstructs a vein. Risk factors include the contraceptive pill, long-haul air travel, and certain blood disorders.

- Acute onset of pain in calf.
- Swelling and warmth of calf.

If confirmed, needs anticoagulants to reduce the risk of a pulmonary embolus. See page 210.

◆ Allergy

In reaction to an insect bite or injection.

- Limb swells dramatically in a few seconds.

- Swelling may spread to body, lips and throat.
- At worst, difficulty breathing, collapse.

◆ Lymphatic obstruction

Also known as lymphoedema. Results from interference with the lymphatic channels, which drain away tissue fluid. Commonest after surgery in the groin or armpit – typically to treat breast cancer. In rare cases it can be congenital.

- Gross swelling of limb.
- Swelling becomes hard; does not easily indent when pressed.

Rare

◆ Cancer

Suspected in otherwise unexplained swelling of a limb. Long bones are the likeliest sites.

- Persistent pain, tenderness.
- Enlarged local lymph nodes.

Cancer may also obstruct the drainage of lymphatic fluid or blood from a limb: for example, pelvic cancers may cause swelling in the legs.

◆ Filariasis

A tropical worm infestation capable of causing massive swelling of limbs (elephantiasis).

'General' Symptoms

Weight loss – progressive

Persistent, progressive weight loss ranks as one of the major symptoms of disease. People with weight loss usually seek help at an early stage, when other

features of disease may not be prominent.

Obtaining the individual's full background story usually reveals other symptoms, for example, abdominal pain, and these may lead to tentative diagnosis. The following are some of the possibilities for which there are few other symptoms to point the way. Many of these possibilities are considered in more detail elsewhere in the book.

Possible

◆ Diabetes

In young adults and children, the onset of diabetes tends to be dramatic: rapid weight loss is prominent, alongside thirst and excessive urine output.
See page 446.

◆ Anxiety and depression

Modest, slow weight loss could reasonably be put down to anxiety or depression in the absence of other symptoms, and where there is no other clear cause for concern.
However, it is prudent to exclude physical causes of weight loss first.

◆ Chronic infection

This includes chronic abscesses and chronic chest conditions, such as cystic fibrosis.
See page 208.

◆ Anorexia nervosa

Excessive dieting, usually in young women who have a distorted image of their true size.
See page 396.

◆ Overactive thyroid

Weight loss alone is unusual, unless the accompanying tremor and sweating have been overlooked. The full picture is described on page 319.

◆ Tuberculosis

The poor, alcoholics and people from underdeveloped countries might have this serious but curable infection.
See page 427.

◆ Cancer – general

Laymen and doctors think of cancer to explain weight loss in the 40-plus age group. It is by no means the only explanation, yet it remains true that, occasionally, an advanced cancer, which has spread around the body, produces only vague symptoms until a late stage. So, be aware of your body: report to your doctor any unusual changes such as bleeding, swellings, weight loss, pain or prolonged cough.

◆ HIV/AIDS

Needs to be considered in any case of vague ill-health, weight loss, fevers and cough.
HIV/AIDS is widespread in certain parts of the world. Transmitted by sexual contact or blood-to-blood contact.

Rare

◆ Malabsorption

This causes weight loss by preventing the absorption of food.
Associated symptoms are:

- Difficulty in swallowing.
- Anaemia.
- Recurrent abdominal pains, intermittent diarrhoea, greasy stools.
- Bleeding into stools.

'General' Symptoms

Underlying causes include cancer of the oesophagus, which causes very rapid weight loss, ulcerative colitis, Crohn's disease, coeliac disease and chronic pancreatitis.

◆ Parasite infection

Not a usual cause of weight loss except in Third World countries where it is very common. Diagnosis is confirmed by stool tests.

◆ Kidney disease

At the early stage of causing weight loss, this needs to be confirmed by blood tests. See page 352.

◆ Pyloric stenosis

A childhood condition: part of the intestine is obstructed, causing profuse vomiting and rapid weight loss a few weeks after birth. See page 134.

Occasionally seen in adults with stomach cancer.

Losing weight, plus jaundice

This combination points to disease of the liver and related parts of the digestive system. Appearance in adults must trigger a careful search for a primary cancer, which may have spread to involve the liver, for example bowel cancer. The jaundice results from obstruction to bile flow from the liver.

The primary cancer is likely to have shown itself already, with symptoms such as:

• Weight loss.

• Pain.

• Swelling.

• Unusual bleeding.

Probable

◆ Cancer of the pancreas

The pancreas lies at the back of the abdomen, partly surrounding the bile duct. The tumour blocks the bile duct, producing jaundice.

• Initially, vague upper abdominal pain.

• Weight loss.

• Painless jaundice.

◆ Secondary cancer of liver

Cancers of many kinds can spread around the body from their original site. The liver is a common secondary site.

Possible

◆ Cancer of stomach

See *Stomach disease*, page 154.

◆ Primary cancer of liver

A complication of liver cirrhosis in an alcoholic, or hepatitis B (or C) infection

◆ Pernicious anaemia

The combination of anaemia and a yellow tinge to the skin gives an impression of jaundice.

The diagnosis is based on blood tests. See page 448. Treatment reverses symptoms.

'General' Symptoms

Rare

◆ Cancer of gall bladder

A disease of the elderly, causing symptoms similar to gall stones.

- Recurrent pains in the right upper abdomen and Jaundice.

Posture appears stiff and hunched

Probable

◆ Ageing and osteoporosis

With age, bone density is lost and there is shrinkage of the discs between the vertebrae – the bones which link together to form the spine. Rapid thinning of bone, or osteoporosis, takes place, leaving the vertebrae somewhat delicate and liable to collapse.

- Posture becomes hunched over several years.
- Collapse of a vertebra causes a sudden change of posture plus pain.

Osteoporosis is treatable with bisphosphonate drugs, calcium and Vitamin D supplements, or other medication. Some bone repair can take place with these treatments, but lost height and deformity persist.

Possible

◆ Ankylosing spondylitis

A disease that begins in early adult life, especially affecting men. Over many years, the normal joints and ligaments of the spine are replaced by inflexible bone. A blood test for the tissue type HLA B27 is generally positive.

- Initially just back pain, and morning stiffness of the spine.

Paget's disease

- The back becomes increasingly rigid, with a stooped posture.
- Eventually, spine movements are severely restricted.

The stooped posture, though not totally avoidable, need not be as severe a problem as in the past, thanks to improvements in treatment.

◆ Kyphoscoliosis

This is twisting of the spine, often starting during the teenage years for no apparent reason. Treatable surgically.

◆ **Parkinson's disease**

See page 409. A neurological disease rarely present before the age of 50. The main symptoms are:

* Tremor of the hands at rest.
* Stooped, inflexible posture.
* Shuffling gait.
* Immobile facial expression.

◆ **Paget's disease**

A disorder of bone formation, quite common in a mild form in later life and frequently causing no symptoms.

* Pain in bones.
* Legs becomes bowed, back stoops;

head may enlarge (hat size may increase).

* Deafness.

Advanced cases are generally easy to recognize, but usually X-rays and blood tests are needed to confirm the diagnosis. More information, see below.

Rare

◆ **Tuberculosis (TB) of the spine**

This used to be common. The infection destroys bone.

* Increasing pain and stiffness in part of the spine.
* Other features of TB such as malaise, weight loss, cough, night sweats.

Looking old before your time

Possible

◆ **Smoking**

This is known to accelerate lining of the face and coarsening of the skin.

◆ **Underactive thyroid**

See page 320. This common condition makes the skin thicken and coarsen.

◆ **Sun damage**

In hot, sunny climates, such as that of

Australasia, sun damage is the most common cause of a prematurely aged appearance.

Rare

◆ **Hereditary causes**

With one exceptionally rare condition, progeria, growth ceases by about three years of age, and the child becomes mentally retarded, bald and develops a beaked nose.

Body size, shrinking

Probable

◆ **Osteoporosis**

See page 259.

Rare

◆ **Paget's disease**

Also known as osteitis deformans.

'General' Symptoms

Abnormal turnover of bone causing thickening and deformity, particularly of the skull, and the long bones. The bone, despite appearing thicker, is weaker than normal. The disease affects men and women equally, but rarely affects people from Asia, Africa or the Middle East. It normally appears after the age of 40. Although often symptom free, there may be:

- Bony deformities. The skull may appear large; often, only one bone is affected.

- Fractures.

- Kyphosis (see page 270) causing apparent height loss.

- Heart failure, due to increased workload on heart.

- Vision and hearing deteriorate as deformed bone damages nerves.

Diseased bone can, very rarely, develop into a malignant bone tumour – osteosarcoma.

Diagnosis is confirmed by blood tests.

Trembling or shaking

Probable

◆ Normal variation

How steady are your hands? Everyone has tremor to a greater or lesser degree.

- Mostly causes no interference with delicate manual activities.

- Worsened by anxiety, alcohol, stimulants such as coffee, some illicit drugs.

◆ Benign essential tremor

An exaggerated form of normal tremor and an embarrassment rather than a disease.

◆ Hereditary

- Slow tremor, affecting upper limbs and head.

- Gradually worsens with age.

Possible

◆ Overactive thyroid

See page 319.

An over-active thyroid gland causes an exaggeration of normal tremor.

◆ Parkinson's disease

Trembling movements of the thumb and forefinger:

- An early symptom is loss of normal swinging of arms when walking.

- Limbs held rigid, slowing of all movements.

- Tremor at rest, diminishing on activity.

- Immobile, 'mask-like' facial appearance.

- Handwriting becomes increasingly small.

- Dribbling.

There are now many useful treatments for this common disorder.

◆ Drug side effect

Some drugs, especially major tranquillizers used in the treatment of mental illness, cause tremor.

Rare

◆ Brain disease

Brain tumours, strokes, multiple sclerosis and head injuries may all cause tremors. Associated symptoms might include:

* Paralysis of one side of the body
* Progressive headache, blurring of vision.
* Change of personality.
* Deterioration of memory, slurring of speech.
* Noticeable flicking movements of eyes.
* Difficulty in walking.

Twitching

Uncontrollable, short-lived muscle jerks. The gulf between the common twitches and those with a serious cause is so wide that there should rarely be any reason to suspect disease in the absence of other symptoms.

Probable

◆ Habit or nervous tic

Blinking and similar grimaces, normal in everyone to a degree, which sometimes become excessive. Deserves sympathy even in grubby, twitching schoolboys, in whom it disappears gradually.

* Typically young boys or nervous adults.
* Frequency increases under stress.

No satisfactory treatment and, please remember, sufferers really cannot help it.

◆ Spasmodic torticollis

Recurrent jerking of the neck to one side

* A disorder of the middle-aged.

The individual is otherwise perfectly well.

* Treatment with botulinum toxin (Botox) helps.

Possible

◆ Benign fibrillation or fasiculation

A part of a muscle that twitches spontaneously; the thigh or around the eye are common sites, probably because it is easily noticed.

* Other muscles unaffected.
* Muscle strength normal.
* Disappears after a few days.
* Tiredness is a common cause.

◆ Epilepsy

Spasmodic jerking of limbs is a feature of most forms of epilepsy:

* Same limb is affected each time.
* Brief warning before the jerking episode starts.
* May progress to a generalized fit, with loss of consciousness, incontinence, foaming at mouth. There is usually very little doubt that epilepsy is the cause.

Rare

◆ Chorea

Irregular involuntary flailing movements of limbs. Rheumatic fever was once a common cause. Other neurological conditions with twitching as a feature include Huntington's chorea:

- A strong family history.
- Disintegration of personality in middle-age
- Eventually dementia, epilepsy, paralysis.

◆ Tourette syndrome

A disorder with a reputation out of all proportion to its rarity.

- Onset in adolescence.
- Multiple tics.
- Abrupt swearing or obscenities, grunting.
- Echoing other people's words.

◆ Motor neurone disease

Exceptionally rare, tragic disease causing deterioration of muscle function in middle-age.

- Begins with loss of bulk of muscles in hands.
- Muscle-wasting spreads generally.
- Widespread twitching of muscles may be seen.
- Mental function remains intact.
- Eventually, paralysis.

◆ Kidney failure

A late symptom in someone already known to have kidney disease:

- Nausea, vomiting.
- Twitching of muscles.
- Clouded consciousness.
- Spontaneous bleeding.
- Low urine output.

Fever: introduction

Just why the body produces fever in response to illness is still not fully understood. Presumably it helps in some way to fight illness, but exactly how is still surprisingly controversial. Since ancient times, fever has been recognized as a key signal that someone is unwell.

Fevers tell us much about the illness itself: not only is it important to take account of its severity, but also of its variation during the day, and over the course of the illness. Modern medicine offers diagnosis and treatment of most prolonged fevers, replacing the long, anxious period of observation until the fever breaks.

When to start worrying?

With the decline of serious infections, at least in developed countries, the onset of fever should not cause alarm. In the very young and in the elderly fever still calls for a careful assessment of health; but in older children and for much of adult life a day or two of raised temperature will usually be the prelude to one of the minor illnesses considered in the following pages. Of course, there are more sinister causes, but they are rare, and fever alone is unlikely to raise even the professional's suspicions. Before worrying about serious disease, look at the individual's overall condition, assessing:

- Risk factors for unusual disease, for example, foreign travel, poor sanitation, epidemics.
- Rapid onset of a high fever – greater than 40°C.

- Severe headache or delirium.
- Pain.
- Night sweats.
- A rapid pulse or fast breathing, remembering that:
- Pulse rate rises by about ten beats per minute for every °C rise in temperature.
- A baby's normal pulse rate is about 120 per minute, even at one year of age.

Taking temperature

An adult's normal temperature is conventionally taken to be 37°C, based on a mouth reading. You may have a temperature half a degree either way and be perfectly well. In children, temperature can be measured under the armpit, in which case 36.5°C is the norm.

Take into account:

- Mouth breathers, whose mouth

temperature is lower than normal.

- The amount of clothing worn may raise or lower temperature.
- Warm or cold drinks alter temperature in the mouth for about 15 minutes.
- Feeling the brow offers comfort, but is not very reliable, especially if there is a low-level fever, with sweat on the forehead that cools the skin.

Fever: the possibilities

To list all the hundreds of possible reasons for fever would simply be confusing. Instead, we look, on the following pages, at fevers of different durations. We believe that this is how you will usually meet the problem. The possibilities listed are those expected in a developed country. There is a separate section (see page 419) on tropical diseases. We remind you again that fever in the very young and very old

demands special attention, and that in any case, concern about a person's overall condition means you must get professional advice, even if the fever itself is minor.

Fever, the first 48 hours, page 412.

Fever, 3 to 14 days, page 414.

Fever, lasting two weeks or more, page 416.

Fever, recurrent attacks, page 418.

Fever, in or after visiting the tropics, page 419.

Fever – the first 48 hours

See also *Fever, introduction,* page 410. Along with the fever there will be some combination of chills, muscular aches, sweating, a mild headache and fatigue.

Probable

◆ Viral illness

Including the build-up to a common cold or 'flu.

• Mild sore throat.

• Headache and muscle and joint aches.

• Symptoms oscillate between mild and irritating within hours.

• Sniffing and sneezing begins after a couple of days.

• Or the illness fades away leaving you, and your doctor, none the wiser.

◆ Ear infection

Very common in children, sometimes with no other symptoms

• Typically, the child already has a cold.

• Abrupt onset of pain in ear.

• Babies just begin crying and will not settle, even with comforting. They may shake their head, or rub an ear.

• Occasionally progresses to a burst ear drum, causing a green or yellow, possibly bloodstained discharge for a few days.

  Healing over a couple of weeks is the norm. Painkillers will help the symptoms. The role of antibiotics is controversial.

Mumps

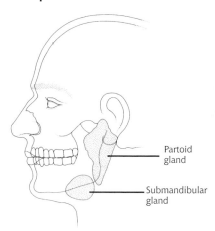

Partoid gland

Submandibular gland

◆ Tonsillitis

The picture presented is usually unmistakeable:

• Pain in the throat, worse on swallowing.

• Swollen neck glands.

• Nasal twang to speech.

• Breath smells foul.

• White spots on the tonsils.

◆ Chest infection

Again, the picture is usually clear:

• Cough.

• Phlegm.

• Shortness of breath or wheeze.

• Chest pain when breathing deeply.

◆ Urinary infection

Common in women, unusual in men.

• Pain or burning sensation when passing urine.

'General' Symptoms

- A need to pass urine frequently.
- Aching over the kidneys or bladder.
- In severe cases, rigors, blood in the urine.

In babies, there may be no symptoms other than fever and irritability, hence the need to test urine in a feverish infant.

Possible

◆ Chickenpox

A viral illness causing small fluid or pus filled blisters over the body, in the mouth and in the scalp. Usually occurs in epidemics. Incubates for about 11-21 days after contact with another carrier.

- Itchy rash appears within 48 hours of fever.
- Rash lasts for two or three weeks.
- The rash consists of spots, which tend to appear in crops and soon become blisters; they dry out and become scabs. Usually a mild, though miserable, illness calling for plenty of care and attention.

Rare

◆ Rubella (German measles)

Mild in itself but notorious because of the risk it poses to the developing baby if the mother catches it during early pregnancy. For this reason there are public health immunisation programmes which have made this disease very infrequent.

- A fine, red-brown rash appearing after 24-48 hours of fever.
- Rash with no particular pattern to its

spread appears all at once.
- Swollen tender glands at the back of the skull.
- In adults, commonly accompanied by mild arthritis lasting for some weeks.

◆ Mumps

An infection of the salivary glands. The incubation period is two to three weeks. Like Rubella, mumps is very infrequent due to immunisation programmes.

- Non-specific fever and chills for 24-48 hours.
- Then the salivary glands enlarge at the angles of the jaw and just in front of the ears.
- The illness settles in five to ten days.

Complications can include pain in the testicles and the abdomen or deafness, but these are rare.

◆ Scarlet fever (Scarlatina)

- Onset is sudden with high fever, sore throat or tonsillitis.
- A very fine generalized red rash after 24-48 hours.
- The rash spares the area around the mouth, giving it a contrasting, white appearance.
- Furred tongue goes from whitish to raw over a few days.

Scarlet fever was once much feared because it could cause rheumatic fever and glomerulonephritis (see page 95). These complications are now extremely rare. However, penicillin is

'General' Symptoms

still necessary if scarlet fever is diagnosed.

◆ Meningitis

Mentioned here as a reminder that it should be considered in any feverish child, especially if the child shows:

- Drowsiness.
- Stiff neck.

- A wish to avoid bright lights.
- Sudden appearance of a fine purple rash.
- And, in a baby, a bulging soft spot (fontanelle) on the top of the head.

  If suspected, this is a medical emergency.

Fever – 3 to 14 days

See also *Fever, introduction*, page 410. Minor viral illness is still likely to underlie this symptom, just as with fever lasting 48 hours. However, the need to consider less common illnesses arises.

Probable

◆ Viral illness

No rash, no progression, and no other symptoms apart from sweats, aches and generally feeling unwell. But although the cause is probably a virus, it is prudent to review the diagnosis every few days, considering the possibility of any of the following:

Possible

◆ Glandular fever

- Bad sore throat or tonsillitis.
- Enlarged lymph glands.
- Sometimes abdominal pain or jaundice with inflammation of the liver or spleen.
- Fatigue persisting for weeks or months.

  A blood test will confirm the diagnosis.

◆ Pneumonia

Certain forms of pneumonia are known for causing fever alone, without the other, more dramatic symptoms of pneumonia.

- Slight cough.
- Feeling vaguely unwell; fatigue, night sweats.
- A chest X-ray confirms the diagnosis and treatment is straightforward.

◆ Abdominal infection

Suspect this if fever starts soon after abdominal surgery, or after abdominal pain. Prolonged fever can signal an abscess in any of the abdominal organs, the commoner ones being:

- The appendix, preceded by a few days of pain, which may start centrally but then settles low down on the right.
- The large intestine: pain in the left lower side, possibly bleeding from the back passage, intermittent diarrhoea.
- Infected ovaries or fallopian tubes:

lower abdominal pain, vaginal discharge.

- Gall bladder infection, typically with pain in the upper abdomen on the right side, usually in the presence of gallstones.

◆ Infectious hepatitis

Caused by several different viruses – hepatitis A, B, or C being the usual culprits. Hepatitis B and the less common hepatitis C are the dangerous forms which can lead to long term liver complications – the virus is spread by shared needles used for intravenous drug abuse and unprotected sexual intercourse. Hepatitis B can also be passed from mother to baby in pregnancy. The incubation period of hepatitis A is a few weeks, and of hepatitis B a few months. Both hepatitis A and B are preventable by immunisation.

- Fever, chills, joint pains, back aches; generally feeling unwell for a week.

- Jaundice – yellowish discolouration of the skin – first spotted in the whites of the eyes; then the skin turns yellow.

- Darkening of urine, light stool colour.

◆ Roseola

A fairly common, harmless viral illness which can fool doctors into suspecting measles.

- High fever for three to four days; the child is snuffly.

- A pinkish rash appears over the body.

- The fever stops, and the child perks up.

Rare

◆ Measles

'Measles is misery' sums up this childhood illness, which is very infrequent now due to immunisation programmes.

There is an incubation period of 10 to 14 days from being infected by another carrier.

- A miserable, snuffly, coughing child with bloodshot eyes who wants to avoid bright lights.

- Delirium at night is common.

- White spots may be seen in the mouth by the back teeth.

- A blotchy red rash appears after four days of fever, spreading downwards, from face via chest to the limbs.

- The child continues feverish for several more days as the illness subsides.

Measles is a serious problem in underdeveloped countries, but in developed countries its complications, such as pneumonia or encephalitis, are rare.

◆ Typhoid or paratyphoid fever

Infections spread via food and water in conditions of poor sanitation. Profuse diarrhoea is a major feature.

- Fever, gradually rising to a peak over a couple of weeks.

- Cough, headache, limb pains.

- After a week, a non-itchy rash appears on the stomach, chest and lower back. In typhoid, it is sparse and rapidly fading; in paratyphoid, more widespread.

'General' Symptoms

- Diarrhoea begins after a week or so, becoming profuse.

  Typhoid is still a very serious illness, despite modern antibiotic treatment. Paratyphoid, though less serious, is nevertheless very unpleasant.

  Immunization is recommended for travel to many parts of the world.

◆ Septicaemia

This means infection spreading in the blood stream. It is usually a rapidly developing illness causing chills and collapse.

◆ Endocarditis

See page 427. An infection of the valves of the heart, causing chronic illness including fever, anaemia and clubbed finger nails.

Fever lasting two weeks or more

See also *Fever, introduction*. By now, fever is a diagnostic challenge. It is likely that someone who is ill as well as feverish for as long as this would be admitted to hospital for investigation.

However, in some people, fever shows itself only with the feeling of being vaguely unwell (malaise) together with night sweats and other symptoms pointing to nothing in particular.

Causes now include not only infections, but also rheumatic diseases, connective tissue disease, cancers and drug side effects. But remember that many of the illnesses noted in *Fever, 3 to 14 days*, could still be suspected, along with the following:

Probable

◆ Chronic infection

This is still the likeliest reason for prolonged fever. Recent surgery, together with abdominal pain, could be pointers. Less common causes might include:

- Prostatitis in men, pain between the legs, burning urine.

- Osteomyelitis: pain and tenderness in a bone; usually in children. The long bones, typically of the leg, are most commonly involved.

- Bronchiectasis causing persistent cough, sweats, possibly breathlessness, finger clubbing.

◆ Tuberculosis

A significant possibility, causing chronic illness, weakness and infection.

- A low-grade fever.

- Weight loss.

- Cough.

- Night sweats.

- Possibly bloodstained sputum.

Possible

◆ Ulcerative colitis

A chronic inflammation of the bowel. The early symptoms can be limited to:

- Persistent diarrhoea.

- Low-grade fever.

- Vague malaise.

'General' Symptoms

Once suspicion is aroused, this illness can be rapidly confirmed and treated.

◆ Cancer, leukaemia

Fever otherwise unexplained and lasting for months brings these to mind. There may well be other suspicious symptoms, such as:

- Weight loss.
- Unusual pains.
- Unusual bleeding from bowel, bladder, vagina, stomach.
- Chronic cough.

These symptoms may allow the cancer to be tracked down. Blood tests will screen for leukaemia. Cancer of the kidney is one tumour well known to cause persistent fever.

◆ Hodgkin's disease and other lymphomas

These are malignant disease of the lymphatic tissues. Hodgkin's disease mostly affects young adults. The treatment is usually chemotherapy and radiotherapy – in the case of Hodgkin's disease, the chances of a cure are good.

- Persistently swollen, painless glands in the neck, groin or armpits.
- Night sweats.
- Anaemia.

◆ HIV/AIDS

HIV acquired through sexual or blood contact can produce a 'flu-like illness early on (days or weeks after contact). This occurs as the body sero-converts – the point at which anti HIV antibodies develop in the blood and are shown by the HIV antibody blood test becoming positive. Months or years after sero-conversion, an untreated sufferer develops impaired immunity which may present as odd, opportunistic infections or malignancies.

Symptoms of opportunistic infection include fever with:

- Diarrhoea.
- Enlargement of lymph nodes.
- Cough.
- Headache or confusion.
- Thrush in the mouth.
- Rashes.
- Loss of weight.

Many other symptoms are possible. Tell your doctor if you think you might be at risk of HIV infection.

◆ Rheumatoid arthritis

Usually there will be joint pain, swelling and deformity. Persistent fever and vague malaise can continue for several weeks.

See page 261.

◆ Systemic lupus erythematosis (SLE)

One of a group of connective tissue disorders in which the body reacts against its own tissues It can be a very vague illness at first. Commonest in women aged between 30 and 50.

- Rashes, joint pains, malaise.
- A butterfly rash across the cheeks is typical.

Early diagnosis is important to prevent progression to the kidneys or the brain.

'General' Symptoms

Rare

◆ Syphilis

Characteristically, six to 12 weeks after the initial infection, syphilis causes:

- A rash over hands and feet, including the palms and soles.
- Malaise, fever, enlarged lymph nodes; aching joints.
- Wart-like swellings around genitalia and back passage.

Readily treatable.

◆ Drug side effect

When all else fails, drugs may be suspected as the cause of a persistent fever.

◆ Brucellosis

A disease spread through cow's and goat's milk, and therefore a risk for workers in the dairy industry.

- Gradual onset, with fevers, joint pains, cough, anorexia, night sweats.
- Bouts of fever every few days or every few weeks.
- Often cures itself.

Fever – recurrent attacks

See *Fever, introduction*. Apart from brucellosis, most of these infections are somewhat unusual in developed countries. Their symptoms return after a period of apparent recovery. This is in contrast to the far more conventional pattern of infections in which there is fever by day or by night, whose disappearance can be taken as a reliable sign of recovery.

Possible

◆ Malaria

See page 422. Anyone who has returned from abroad, who has been in an area where malaria is present, and who develops a high temperature and chills should be suspected of having this dangerous illness, particularly if they have not been taking anti-malaria tablets. Depending on the type of malaria, the episodes of fever and

shaking return every three or four days.

- The fever may recur some months after foreign travel.

◆ Brucellosis

See above. It gives rise to bouts of fever for days at a time, which appear to settle, only to recur after weeks or months.

◆ Typhoid

See page 415. A feverish illness causing severe diarrhoea, spread through poor sanitation or contaminated water, or food – mainly shellfish products. The illness takes three to four weeks to run its course.

Rare

Meaning rare in developed countries. Elsewhere these are fairly common diseases, but they pose a relatively small risk for tourists. Enquire locally about areas where these diseases might be a hazard. If you develop a feverish illness soon after returning from a danger area, report it to a doctor without delay, being ready with details of where you have been.

◆ Dengue fever

A mosquito-borne infection of south-east Asia and Africa.

- Begins with sudden fever, aches and rash.
- Severe pains in back and bones are particularly characteristic.
- Improvement over about a week.
- Relapse after another few days, with a more widespread rash.
- Recovery takes several weeks.

◆ Relapsing fever

Spread by ticks. Common in Africa, India, South America and parts of the Mediterranean.

- Abrupt high fever and confusion lasting for about a week.
- Then apparent recovery, followed by relapse after another week or so.

- Several further relapses may occur.
- Effective treatment exists.

◆ Trypanosomiasis

Sleeping sickness. Different forms exist in Africa and South America. Treatment, started early, is quite effective. After an insect bite there is typically:

- Painful swelling at the site of the bite.
- Then relapsing fevers, enlarged lymph nodes.
- Eventually, after months or years, lethargy, continuous mild confusion, headaches, drowsiness.

◆ Yellow fever

Especially prevalent in Africa, Central and South America. There is no specific treatment for this serious illness, but vaccination is effective.

- Abrupt fever, rigors, jaundice.
- Signs of improvement by the fourth/fifth day.
- Relapse during the next week with more fever, jaundice.

Fever after visiting the tropics

Tropical disease should always be considered in someone who becomes feverish soon after returning from a Third World country or, indeed, certain developed countries where they are a known risk. The following are the commoner examples, rather than an exhaustive catalogue, of these many dangerous diseases. If suspected, seek help urgently: you will probably be sent to a specialist centre.

Protective measures and vaccinations exist for many of these diseases and anyone likely to be at risk should see their doctor to arrange these before travelling. Some of the measures require time to become effective.

The most likely tropical disease is

'General' Symptoms

malaria, common in Africa, India, and the Far East. Symptoms include high fever, drenching sweats and rigors. see page 418.

Among the rarities are:

◆ Plague

Far East, Africa, India, South America. It is a flea-borne illness, with dramatic onset, high fever, delirium and tender, swollen lymph nodes (glands) in the groin.

◆ Relapsing fever

South America, Africa, India, Near East. Sudden high fever, rigors, delirium. Liver and spleen enlarge.

◆ Sleeping sickness

Tropical Africa. Spread by the tse-tse fly. At first fever, enlarged lymph nodes, anaemia. Later (months, years), drowsiness, tremors, fits.

◆ Typhus fever

A term covering several diseases, named for the areas where they are found, for example, Rocky Mountain spotted fever. Fever increasing over several days, with headache, red eyes, rash, delirium.

◆ Yellow fever

Africa, especially West Africa, and South America. Fever with rigors and jaundice. Effective vaccination exists.

Abnormally low temperature

Defined as a fall in 'core' body temperature to below about 35°C when measured via the rectum (rear passage). Technical term: hypothermia. Below about 32°C, there will be drowsiness, apathy, coma and eventually death.

Those at risk are the elderly without adequate heating and the new-born. Cold new-born babies do not shiver: they become lethargic, with cold limbs.

Hypothermia is an emergency, requiring immediate warmth and warm fluids. Severe hypothermia requires gradual, carefully monitored re-warming. Rapid heating up can be dangerous.

Probable

◆ Exposure to cold

• Shivering, feeling cold.

• Then apathy, slurred speech, difficulty in concentrating.

• Finally confusion, coma.

Remember, babies cannot control their temperatures as adults do. They are at risk in low temperatures, unless kept warm.

The elderly

Elderly people who suddenly become confused in the winter may be suffering from hypothermia. It is not advisable to give alcohol to an elderly person whom you suspect is suffering from hypothermia. It may worsen their condition.

'General' Symptoms

Possible

◆ Excess alcohol

By dilating blood vessels, alcohol increases heat loss. Add confusion (if not unconsciousness) following a heavy drinking bout, plus cold conditions, and there is potential for serious danger.

Rare

◆ Underactive thyroid

A grossly underactive thyroid gland can cause severe hypothermia. It is rare nowadays for this degree of underactivity not to be noticed.

◆ Drug side effect

Anti-depressants and tranquillizers can make temperature drop. Usually this is a trivial effect, unless the drugs are taken in overdose or combined with self-neglect, alcohol and exposure to the elements.

Shivers or chills plus fever and headache

In adults, this combination of symptoms, in a mild form, is not unusual and is often the earliest sign of a viral illness. In children this is by far the most likely reason, but other possibilities need to be considered, especially if the headache seems to be the major feature.

Probable

◆ Common cold

See page 423.

◆ Influenza

See *Viral illness*, page 412.

Possible

◆ Chest infection

These three symptoms in combination can be a feature of severe chest infections.

◆ Infection elsewhere

Any infection in the body may give this combination of symptoms. Parts of the body which might give rise to them when infected range from joints, through internal organs, to the skin. Consider whether you have any other noticeable symptoms and look those up too.

Rare

The possibilities below are the rarities that someone in a developed country might occasionally encounter.

◆ Meningitis

An infection of the brain and surrounding tissues. Meningitis is mainly a disease of childhood. The condition is checked for as a matter of routine if a baby appears to be seriously ill.

- The illness may develop rapidly over a few hours.

- Light hurts the eyes.

- Pain or stiffness in the neck on trying to lift the head.

- Nausea and vomiting.

'General' Symptoms

- Drowsiness, delirium or coma.

Meningitis in the very young can occur in outbreaks, and on the face of it can seem identical to a simple viral illness. So, if you hear of meningitis in your locality, be on the look-out for:

- Excessive irritability, or worsening of an existing condition.
- Temperature rises higher than expected.
- Pain on being moved about.
- Inability to feed or drink adequately.
- Fine purple rash.

Always seek help or advice at an early stage. If later still in doubt, check again with your doctor. If suspected, immediate medical attention is required.

◆ Weil's disease

Rats spread this disease by infecting lakes, canals, sewers and mines. Swimmers, sailors and canoeists should be aware of this, as should sewage workers, miners or anyone working in a rat-infested area.

- Rapid onset of fever, headache and backache.
- Red eyes.
- A mild degree of jaundice is usual.
- Spontaneous bleeding from mouth or nose may occur.

◆ Malaria

Caused by a parasite spread by mosquitoes. A major risk in the tropics, where mosquitoes enjoy long periods of warmth and humidity. Modern air travel means that malaria can spread to anywhere in the world, so the possibility is worth considering in someone recently returned from Africa, Asia or India, even if they have been taking anti-malaria tablets.

- Attacks every two or three days.
- Attack begins with an hour or two of severe shivering and headache.
- High temperature starts as shivering finishes, and lasts for several hours.
- Heavy sweating.
- In between attacks, the infected person may feel quite well.

If malaria is suspected, seek medical help urgently.

◆ Other tropical disease

If someone recently returned from the tropics becomes ill with high fever, it is safest to suspect tropical disease first. Which one it is will depend on where they have been staying, and on the features of their illness. Seek medical help urgently.

◆ Typhus

A general term for a variety of diseases spread by fleas and lice. Found not only in the Third World, but also in parts of America ('Rocky Mountain spotty fever') and in Britain (Lyme disease).

- Illness develops over seven to 14 days.
- Tenderness and redness of the eyes is typical.
- A rash eventually appears.
- Joints may be painful.

The illness varies from mild to severe, depending on the cause.

'General' Symptoms

A cold?

Runny nose, itching eyes and aching across the face? Statistics say that you will suffer from this miserable, though trivial, illness two or three times a year. It is usually caused by an infection of the upper respiratory tract, which includes nose, larynx and pharynx. Hence the medical term for a common cold – upper respiratory tract infection, or 'URTI'. Any of more than 100 different viruses may be responsible. However, a cold might be more than just a cold if the symptoms are recurrent or persistent.

Probable

◆ Common cold

A Nobel Prize awaits the medical researcher who finds a cure for this condition.

- Begins with a sore or raw throat.
- Increasingly runny nose and sneezing with clear mucus.
- Mucus may turn yellow or green.
- Two or three days of loss of smell and taste.
- Occasionally progresses to a chest infection.
- The illness runs its course over five to seven days, usually requiring no more than fluids, rest and warmth.

   Antibiotics not needed unless complicated by a chest infection.

Possible

◆ Hay fever

An allergic reaction of the lining of the nose in response to pollens, grass and other irritants.

Upper respiratory tract

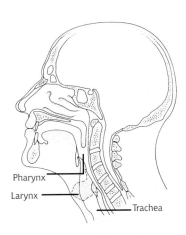

Pharynx
Larynx
Trachea

- Sneezing in specific places or at certain times of year.
- Persistent sniff and blocked nose.
- Tickly feeling in throat and palate.
- Itching, watery eyes.
- Sufferers frequently also have eczema or asthma.

◆ Allergic rhinitis

A general term which includes hay fever and perennial rhinitis – 'allergic' runny or streaming nose

- Reactions as for hay fever, but:
- Provoked by certain environments occurring throughout the year.

◆ Sinusitis

- Persisting common cold symptoms.
- Passage of large quantities of yellow or green mucus through nose or dripping

'General' Symptoms

down back of the throat, sometimes bloodstained.

- Aching across face, above and below the eyes, especially on leaning forward.
- Nasal tone of voice.

◆ Nasal polyps

Common in people who suffer from allergic rhinitis.

- Visible as fleshy gray lumps inside the nostrils, easily removed surgically but they frequently recur.
- Constant feeling of blocked nose.
- A persistent sniff with clear nasal discharge.

◆ Foreign body in the nose

Peculiar to small children for whom small, round objects and body openings have a compelling interest.

- Persistent infected discharge from one nostril.
- Discharge may be blood streaked.
- The foreign body, typically a bead, is often visible.

Rare

◆ Head injury complication

Leakage of cerebrospinal fluid, the liquid which surrounds the brain, might be suspected if, after a head injury, there is a persistent, clear watery discharge from the nose.

◆ Nasal tumour

- Persistent, one-sided bloody or foul-smelling discharge.

Sweating

Sweating is one of the body's ways of balancing heat loss against heat gain – an unglamorous, but nonetheless sophisticated mechanism. Normally, it goes on as a background activity with barely noticeable perspiration. Even apparently heavy sweating may not be abnormal if it is serving to regulate temperature.

Probable

◆ Exercise

It is of course normal that one should sweat when taking vigorous exercise. If you haven't taken any for a long time, and you are also overweight, you may be unpleasantly surprised at how much sweat you produce – but it is normal.

- Perspiration from brow, armpits and back.
- Clearly related to increased levels of exertion.
- Diminishes over a few minutes once exercise is stopped.

◆ Fever

Most fevers are accompanied by sweating. There will be the familiar symptoms of feverish illness such as:

- Aching muscles, headache, malaise, shivering.
- Commonly progressing to a sore throat, cough, earache.

General Symptoms

Sweating as part of a feverish illness is less noticeable in the very old and the very young, whose temperature control mechanisms are less efficient than those of adults.

◆ Stress

Or anxiety, which can be described as a long-term form of stress.

- Sweaty palms, but dry mouth.
- Rapid heartbeat.
- Tension in neck muscles and across forehead.
- Those who are prone to chronic anxiety may suffer chronic sweating.

Possible

◆ Excess alcohol

Strong drink dilates the blood vessels, and this often causes sweating across the brow.

◆ Pain

Any severe pain causes sweating through nervous reflexes that also cause:

- Pallor, restlessness.
- Rapid pulse.
- Collapse – in severe cases.

Thus sweating would be expected in any of the conditions causing *Collapse* (see page 430), including heart attacks

and severe abdominal pain. But if there has been so much blood loss that the circulation is beginning to fail, clamminess replaces sweating.

Rare

◆ Drug related

Reactions due to abrupt withdrawal from alcohol or narcotic drugs cause sweating plus:

- Restlessness, muscle pains, drowsiness.
- Runny nose, dilated pupils, abdominal pains (narcotics).
- Tremor, disorientation, hallucinations (alcohol withdrawal).

Several other drugs, including antidepressants, can cause unusual sweating and need to be considered in otherwise unexplained cases.

◆Tuberculosis

Frequent night sweats may well be the first indicator of this serious infection. You should seek a doctor's advice as soon as possible.

◆ HIV/AIDS

Sweating is a common symptom in AIDS, sometimes in association with AIDS-related opportunistic infections.

'General' Symptoms

Heavy sweating

Covered here are causes of sweating other than infectious diseases, for which see *Fever*, pages 410.

Probable

◆ Natural tendency

In other words, the way you are

made. Though frequently just a nuisance, it becomes a significant problem if it ruins clothes, causes unpleasant body odour or interferes with manual activities such as draughtsmanship. The problem starts after puberty.

• Hands, armpits or feet pour sweat.

• Symptoms tend to be unrelated to exertion, temperature.

Several effective roll-on and lotion treatments are available. As a last resort, it is possible to cut the nerves near the spinal cord which control sweating of the hands or feet.

Possible

◆ Overactive thyroid

See page 319. The thyroid gland could be described as the body's thermostat. Overactivity 'turns up' all aspects of body function. Profuse sweating plus:

• Hyperactivity, jitteriness.

• Prominent, staring eyes.

• Weight loss, hunger, diarrhoea.

• Trembling hands.

◆ Menopause

Even before periods cease, women may be aware of flushes and sweating. Blamed, perhaps unfairly, for a wide range of middle-age symptoms.

• Usually in the 40 to 55 age range.

• Periods become infrequent, then cease.

• Associated with increased wrinkling

(loss of elasticity) of skin, irritability or mild depression.

• Hot flushes.

• Sudden sweats at any time, especially at night.

• Tiredness, headache, palpitations.

Rare

◆ Carcinoid syndrome

Another hormone disorder caused by a hormone-secreting tumour in the intestine or liver. The full picture may take years to develop.

• Bouts of profuse watery diarrhoea with excessive bowel sounds.

• Facial flushing and sweating, especially after alcohol.

• Asthma.

◆ Phaeochromocytoma

A tumour, which may occur near the kidneys, though not exclusively. Causes high blood pressure and sudden, severe bursts of anxiety. It is curable, and though relatively rare, doctors quite often run tests for it if there is:

• High blood pressure, sometimes highly variable.

• Abrupt episodes of headache, sweating, pallor, palpitations.

Tracking the tumour down can be like detective work. Removed by surgery.

◆ Acromegaly

See page 95.

'General' Symptoms

Night sweats

If this goes on for a few days in an otherwise well person, don't worry. It is, however, a different matter if the symptoms are prolonged, especially if there has been recent illness, surgery or debility. Possibilities revolve around infectious diseases or collections of pus in the body.

Probable

◆ Flu-like illness

- Muscle aches.
- Mild headache.
- Sweating can be profuse.
- After a few days, symptoms die away, with the possible emergence of a sore throat, cough or similar mild illness.

Possible

◆ Abscess

An abscess is a collection of pus; it can form anywhere in the body and can cause a variety of symptoms. Most commonly pain at the site of the abscess should help localise the problem. Recent surgery can sometimes be followed by abscess formation near the operation. Blood tests, ultrasound or CT scanning may give further information. Treatment consists of surgical drainage of the infection and antibiotics.

◆ Subphrenic abscess

A collection of pus underneath the diaphragm. Could be a possibility after abdominal surgery or peritonitis. There may be no more than non-specific features, such as:

- Malaise, sweats, anaemia.
- Recurrent fever.
- Shoulder tip pain is a more tell-tale sign, caused by irritation of the diaphragm.

Treatment involves drainage and intensive antibiotic therapy.

◆ Endocarditis

Infection of the valves of the heart. There is usually a previous history of heart valve problems. May occur after minor surgery or dental procedures – hence the need for at-risk patients with known valve problems to take prophylactic antibiotics before dental or surgical treatment. Onset can be gradual, with:

- Anaemia.
- Malaise, recurrent sweats.
- Eventually, clubbed finger nails, enlarged spleen.
- Splinter-like marks under the finger nails.

Treatment with intravenous antibiotics takes several weeks, with monitoring of the heart valves by echocardiography.

Rare

◆ Tuberculosis

Although previously a disease of underdeveloped countries, low-income

'General' Symptoms

groups and alcoholics, tuberculosis is on the increase again after many years. All ages and all income groups can be affected.

• Cough, which may be blood stained.

• General malaise, weight loss, debility.

Modern treatments cure the disease if continued over several months.

◆ **Brucellosis**

See 418.

◆ **Hodgkin's disease**

See 449.

◆ **HIV/AIDS**

See 417.

Tiredness

This symptom is so common one might consider it normal. When tiredness becomes a burden, or does not have a simple explanation, then medical advice can be helpful. In most cases, no serious medical cause is found.

Causes include:

Probable

◆ **Overexertion**

A few remarkable people never need relief from constant pressure and stress and can make do with short periods of sleep. But even they usually have some compensatory mechanism. The rest of us suffer from fatigue, which commonly goes with:

• Irritability.

• Tense feelings in neck and head.

• Diminished enthusiasm for life.

◆ **Anxiety**

One expert has described this universal symptom as 'fear spread thin.' As well as the symptoms given above for overexertion:

• Palpitations, muscle tremors.

• Sweating.

• A constant fear that something unpleasant is going to happen.

At worst, anxiety is a truly disabling disorder needing treatment with a combination of psychological counselling and medication.

Possible

◆ **Anaemia**

See page 202.

◆ **Pregnancy and childbirth**

The birth and the physical process of looking after a newborn baby will challenge even the strongest parent. There is some comfort in knowing that night feeding usually ceases after a few weeks or months. Tiredness associated with early pregnancy can be a puzzle, since it can predate the first missed period, when diagnosis is easy. Other signs of early pregnancy include:

• Tender breasts.

• Desire to pass urine frequently.

◆ Viral infection and post-viral fatigue

Common viral infections such as colds or 'flu typically cause a feeling of tiredness or weakness. Usually this will resolve as the illness subsides. Sometimes tiredness persists longer. Glandular fever caused by the Epstein-Barr virus is well known for causing a prolonged period of tiredness – sometimes lasting weeks or months.

Psychological support and an undemanding lifestyle are the best advice that doctors can offer at present.

◆ Depression

(See page 363.) Commonest in adult life, appearing over several weeks.

- Low mood.
- No enjoyment of anything, lack of motivation.
- Sleep disturbance.
- Changes in body weight.
- Poor concentration.

◆ Diabetes

Fatigue can be an early symptom of diabetes when there are no other obvious features. As diabetes is such a common disease, anyone with unusual fatigue should be tested for it. For more details, see page 447.

◆ Underactive thyroid

A disease of middle and later life, progressing so slowly that even the close family may not spot anything wrong, sometimes putting the symptoms down to ageing.

- The skin becomes dry and rough.
- You 'feel the cold'.
- Your voice becomes gruff, your features coarse.
- Weight gain, constipation, slow speech, slow thought.

It is important to recognize this combination of symptoms because the disorder is so easily treated.

◆ Overactive thyroid

Surprisingly, an overactive thyroid gland can also cause tiredness. This is usually a rather dramatic disease appearing over a few weeks with:

- Nervousness, fine tremor of the hands.
- Sweating, weight loss, increased appetite.
- Muscle ache.
- Staring eyes.
- Diarrhoea.
- Rapid heart rate or palpitations.

Again, treated easily.

Rare

◆ Heart disease

In heart failure, especially in the elderly, fatigue may be the only early symptom. Look also for:

- Breathlessness on mild effort, and when lying flat.
- Swollen ankles.

◆ Cancer

Fatigue is worrying if found together

'General' Symptoms

with other symptoms suggesting cancer, such as:

- Weight loss, loss of appetite.
- Unusual pains.
- Unusual swellings.
- Blood in phlegm, vomit, urine, motions or from the vagina (see under individual entries for these symptoms).

◆ Malnutrition

Common worldwide, but rare in the developed world. The fatigue is due to lack of vitamins, protein and energy sources. In the developed countries, may be seen in those with malabsorption (see page 395) or alcoholics who eat poorly.

◆ Kidney disease

Tiredness can be a symptom of kidney failure, usually diagnosed on a blood test.

◆ Neurological disease

Diagnosis is a matter for specialists, since early changes are subtle and non-specific. Neurological disease might be suspected if there is:

- Progressive weakness of a group of muscles.
- Tingling, numbness or tremors of limbs.
- Unsteady gait.
- Fatigue is a common symptom in multiple sclerosis.

◆ Other

Severe, unexplained fatigue also raises the possibility of two rare disorders: adrenal insufficiency; and myaesthenia gravis, a disease of gradual onset in which muscles seem to work normally but rapidly tire, with exceptional weakness. Drooping eyelids are typical.

Feeling weak or feeble

Weakness is such an unspecific symptom that few medical textbooks even recognise it as a topic in its own right. Nonetheless, people often go to their doctors saying that they feel weak, and expecting the doctor to discover associated symptoms that will point to a diagnosis. Usually, no medical cause is found and the

explanation lies in an imbalance between the physical and psychological capabilities of our bodies and the expectations of modern life. Sometimes there will be a medical explanation.

The possibilities are broadly similar to the causes listed under *Tiredness* page 428.

Collapse

The term collapse means different things to different people. Common to most is the picture of a person, who was either

upright or capable of being upright, suddenly lying in a heap on the ground. Prostration is another term for the same thing. Often there is a transient disturbance of consciousness. Broadly speaking, the causes of collapse depend on the age of the sufferer (with some degree of overlap) – below we summarise them in three groups: young adult up to 40 years; middle age 40-60 years; and elderly 60 years and over. First-aid treatment is the same for all groups – put the collapsed person in the recovery position and get medical help fast.

Recovery position

Anyone who collapses should be laid on their side, leaning forwards. Make sure their airway – neck and throat – is not obstructed. If possible, keep their head lower than, or at the same level as, their heart. Always seek professional medical help immediately when anybody collapses.

Collapse in a young adult up to 40 years old

Probable

◆ Faint

Short-lived unconsciousness, caused by temporary reduction in blood supply to the brain. Caused typically by standing upright in warm or hot conditions. Lying flat will lead quickly to recovery.

◆ Epilepsy

- Often a known previous history of epilepsy.
- Aura or warning before a fit.
- Convulsive shaking of limbs.
- Tongue biting of frothing at the mouth.
- Recovery accompanied by an initial period of confusion or sleep.

◆ Drug or alcohol abuse

- Usually a known history of alcohol or drug misuse.
- Smells of alcohol.
- Neglected appearance.
- Pupils may be widely dilated or pinpoint sized.

- Inflamed veins or puncture marks on skin, made by a needle, usually at front of elbow, forearm or on back of hand.
- Empty pill packets or psychiatric history suggest drug overdose.

Possible

◆ Severe infection

The possibilities are considered in detail in *Fever*, pages 410.

◆ Pulmonary embolus

See page 210 .

A blood clot settles in the lung, cutting off blood flow. May be a rare but serious side effect of oral contraceptive use.

◆ Dehydration

See page 444.

Rare

◆ Pseudoseizure

Looks like a seizure, but is in fact enacted by the patient.

A form of dissociation, See page 372.

'General' Symptoms

◆ Addison's disease

Progressive, generalized weakness until some one-off stress causes collapse. See page 449.

◆ Other causes

The other causes of collapse will normally be accompanied by another symptom – see *Collapse with abdominal pain*, (opposite) *Collapse with shock or coma*, page 435.

Collapse in a middle aged adult

Probable

◆ Alcohol related

- Usually a history of alcoholism or problem drinking.
- Collapse occurs when intoxicated, alternatively:
- Abrupt withdrawal of alcohol results in a seizure.

Possible

◆ Heart rhythm disturbance

The heart beats abnormally fast or irregularly and circulation to the brain becomes insufficient and the person collapses.

An ECG will identify the abnormal rhythm and appropriate treatment is given. Warning symptoms include:

- Palpitations.
- Chest pain or shortness of breath.
- Family history of heart disease.
- History of high blood pressure or high cholesterol.

◆ Drop attack

This is usually a harmless condition typically occurring in middle-aged women in which the legs suddenly give way. There is no loss of consciousness. No treatment other than reassurance is needed.

◆ Partial seizures due to cerebrovascular disease

Usually occurs in a person with a history or risk factor such as smoking, high blood pressure, diabetes or high cholesterol. The collapse is a form of epileptic seizure, but may not involve unconsciousness. Part of the brain malfunctions and the person collapses. Treatment is aimed at the underlying cause, often with the addition of anti-epileptic medication.

◆ Other causes

The other causes of collapse will normally be accompanied by another symptom.

See *Collapse with abdominal pain*, (opposite), *Collapse with shock or coma* page 435.

Collapse in the elderly

Probable

◆ Sudden drop in blood pressure

On standing. Also known as orthostatic hypotension. The elderly person is normally taking medication for high blood pressure or their heart. When they stand up their blood pressure falls further, simply because of gravity, and they collapse. Treatment usually requires an adjustment or withdrawal of medication.

◆ Slow heart beat

Known medically as bradycardia. There are various patterns where the heart rate slows down or misses beats to the point where the brain is receiving an inadequate blood supply. An ECG or 24-hour ECG recording usually identifies the problem. Treatment may involve medication, or sometimes the insertion of a pacemaker.

Possible

◆ Other causes

The other causes of collapse will normally be accompanied by another symptom.

See *Collapse with abdominal pain,* below, and *Collapse with shock or coma* 435.

Collapse with abdominal pain

Often hard to diagnose, because the reasons for abdominal pain differ with age. The following is the obvious, but not an exhaustive, list of illnesses that can cause collapse in adults. Get medical help at once, otherwise shock and coma will follow.

Probable

The possibilities below all involve inflammation of internal organs, which can progress to rupture of the organ. It is frequently impossible to differentiate these causes without tests or surgery.

◆ Perforated peptic ulcer

There is erosion of the lining of the stomach or of the duodenum forming an ulcer. The condition is almost always associated with infection with bacteria called *Helicobacter pylori*. If the ulcer perforates, acid, food and blood gush into the abdomen.

• Commonest in middle age.

Gall bladder

Gall stones trapped in entrance to bile duct

Gall bladder   Duodenum

• A history of upper abdominal discomfort or indigestion.
• Dyspepsia: may be waking at night.
• Severe pain in the upper abdomen, apparently radiating into the back.

'General' Symptoms

- Vomit containing blood or particles looking like coffee grounds.
- Stools may be black, tarry-looking or bloody.
- A sudden severe worsening of pain with collapse suggests perforation.

◆ Pancreatitis

The pancreas lies at the back of the upper abdomen. There is usually existing gall bladder disease or a history of heavy drinking.

- Excruciating upper abdominal pain, worsening over a few hours.
- Pain in the back.
- Vomiting.
- Collapse.

◆ Gall bladder disease

Inflammation or obstruction of the gall bladder, usually connected with gall stones and commonest in middle-aged women.

- Pain felt in the upper right abdomen, under the ribs.
- Often a long history of discomfort on that side.
- Excruciating pain for hours at a time.
- Fever.

◆ Ectopic pregnancy

If a fertilized egg lodges in a fallopian tube, it can grow for a few weeks, eventually rupturing the tube, causing serious internal bleeding. This possibility should not be ignored in any fertile woman, even if there are no symptoms of pregnancy. Precise diagnosis is now relatively easy, thanks to sensitive pregnancy tests and ultrasound scanning.

- A missed period, tender breasts, nausea.
- Rapidly increasing lower abdominal pain, usually one-sided.
- Vaginal bleeding.

Possible

◆ Gastroenteritis

An infection of the bowels which, if severe, causes rapid dehydration as well as toxic effects from the actual infection.

- Cramping abdominal pains.
- Vomiting.
- Diarrhoea immediately, or after a few hours.

◆ Inflammatory bowel disease

Typically ulcerative colitis or Crohn's disease. Associated with:

- A long history of recurrent abdominal pains, diarrhoea.
- Bleeding or mucus in stools.

Rare

◆ Intestinal obstruction

Most often due to a trapped hernia or a growth in the intestine. A trapped hernia gives a tender swelling in the groin

- At first, cramping abdominal pains.
- Vomiting, swelling of the abdomen and constipation.
- Within hours, fever, generalized abdominal pains.

◆ Intestinal ischaemia

A clot blocks blood supply to the intestines. Most likely in the elderly, with pre-existing heart disease.

- Sudden abdominal pain.

- Diarrhoea, vomiting, blood in motions.
- Rapid progression to collapse.

Surgical removal of the clot can be successful, but it ought to be done early.

Collapse with shock or coma

An emergency. Making a precise diagnosis is less important than resuscitating the individual. As a medical term, 'shock' strictly means drastic reduction in blood flow around the tissues. Here the term is used in a less technical sense, so as to include a wider range of symptoms:

- Skin clammy, cold, pale.
- Thready, weak pulse.
- Cyanosis.
- Individual reaction can vary from confusion to coma.

Coma may here be taken as unconsciousness. In trying to work out the cause of collapse with shock or coma, also consider the possibilities in the two preceding sections.

Probable

◆ Stroke

Mainly affects the elderly. Caused by a blood clot or bleeding in the brain.

- Loss of consciousness.
- Paralysis of one side of the body.
- 'Sighing', rough breathing.

The diagnosis is usually confirmed by a CT scan. The outlook depends on the reason for the stroke and the individual's overall health. The longer the period of unconsciousness, the worse the outlook.

◆ Heart attack

A risk in the middle-aged and elderly.

- Sudden, crushing, central chest pain.
- Pain radiates up into jaws or down left arm.
- Breathlessness, sweating.

Collapse with coma in a heart attack victim usually means that the heart is severely compromised, and the outlook is generally poor.

◆ Heart rhythm abnormality

Very rapid, very slow or very irregular heart rhythms reduce the blood output from the heart. You may notice:

- Abrupt onset of thumping or fluttering in chest.
- Breathlessness.
- Shock.

◆ Blood loss

See also *Dehydration*, page 444.

Not always obvious, but easy to recognize if the blood loss is visible, for example in vomit, motions, from the vagina. A risk after injury, especially:

- Trauma to the abdomen, which can rupture the spleen.
- Fractured thigh bone with severe bleeding into muscle.

◆ Overwhelming infection

For complex reasons, a major infection, that gets into the blood stream, causes collapse via a drop in blood pressure. There will be the general symptoms of infection, such as:

- Fever, rigors, headache.
- Spontaneous bleeding and bruising.

◆ Severe pain

Severe pain from any source can cause collapse and coma as reflex actions.

Possible

◆ Diabetic coma

Diabetics can have two types of coma. Collapse due to low blood sugar gives:

- Sweating, light-headedness, irritability.
- Rapid progression to confusion, then collapse.

If blood sugar remains high for long, another, less sudden, form of collapse – ketoacidosis – can occur:

- Usually during another mild illness.
- Onset over a few hours or days.
- Dehydration, intense thirst, vomiting.
- Sweet smell on breath.

Both these conditions respond rapidly to the appropriate treatment.

◆ Alcohol/drug excess

See *Drug overdose*, page 398.

◆ Leaking aortic aneurysm

The aorta is the major artery leading from the heart, and carries its whole blood output. After years of service, its walls can swell out, weaken and then split, just like a car tyre may bulge and blow out. A not uncommon cause of sudden death, but there are sometimes warning symptoms:

- Unusual pulsation in the abdomen, in time with the heart beat.
- A lump you can feel in the abdomen.
- Onset of backache as the aorta starts to leak.

  Surgery is successful in early cases.

◆ Burns

Loss of body fluids invariably accompanies serious burns, with shock resulting both from this loss and from pain.

Rare

◆ Anaphylaxis

This term describes the worst form of severe allergic reaction. It is an unpredictable risk, to be borne in mind whenever someone is given an injection, but anaphylaxis can happen in response to foods and insect stings. Minor warning signs of allergic reaction are:

- Swelling of the lips.
- Itchy, raised skin wheals that come and go.

In anaphylaxis there is:

- Abrupt wheezing, progressing to cyanosis.

- Difficulty in swallowing, from swelling of the throat.
- Collapse.

Those fortunate enough to know that they are at risk should carry the appropriate medication, or a warning bracelet.

No appetite, or very poor appetite

Brief episodes of loss of appetite accompany our changing moods and minor infections. Indeed the regaining of appetite is among the earliest signs of recovery from these minor upsets, as is the disappearance of fever. If loss of appetite is accompanied by abdominal pain or weight loss (see these symptoms) then more unusual disease is a possibility.

Probable

◆ Minor feverish illness

- Fever, muscle aches, sore throat or cough.
- Appetite disappears suddenly.
- The return of appetite lags a day or two behind the disappearance of fever.

◆ Stress

Or worry. This all-too-standard ingredient of modern life can either stimulate or reduce appetite.

- Tense feelings in head, neck, shoulders.
- Irritability, mild depression.
- Mood and appetite recover rapidly when the source of stress is absent.

Possible

◆ Depression

See page 363. Suggested by prolonged loss of appetite as well as:

- Low mood.
- Loss of enjoyment.
- Expressions of despair, crying, poor self-image.
- Early morning wakening (or disturbed sleep pattern).

◆ Alcoholism

The high carbohydrate content of alcohol satisfies hunger and causes loss of appetite for normal solid food. Of course, drink is not at all nutritious, and eventually symptoms of vitamin deficiency appear, as well as those of alcoholism. Hence such symptoms as:

- Self-neglect, smell of drink.
- Memory disturbance, swings of mood.
- Sore mouth, cracks at corners of lips, recurrent infections.
- Dilated veins over the face.

◆ Hepatitis A

The combination of loss of appetite, fever for five to seven days, plus muscular aches and abdominal pains should arouse suspicion.

- Jaundice appears with yellowed eyes, dark urine.
- As the jaundice clears up, you begin to feel better.

'General'
Symptoms

Rare

◆ Cancer of the stomach

For reasons not understood, early cancer, especially of the stomach, can cause loss of appetite before other features appear. However, it is rare for loss of appetite alone to continue for long without the other symptoms described under *No appetite, losing weight*, below, and *No appetite, losing weight and chest pain*, opposite.

• Most common in the 45-plus age group.

• Persistent, otherwise unexplained, loss of appetite.

• Feeling of fullness very soon after eating a small amount.

• Otherwise unexplained symptoms, such as generally feeling unwell, tiredness, unusual bleeding, unusual pains.

◆ Heart failure

In certain forms of heart failure, loss of appetite is a noticeable symptom, probably related to congestion of blood in the liver. Among the many other symptoms which appear over days or weeks are:

• Breathlessness on exertion; tiredness.

• Breathlessness when attempting to lie flat.

• Pre-existing chest disease, such as chronic bronchitis, bronchiectasis or heart disease, typically angina.

• An early feature is swollen ankles, and eventually a swollen abdomen.

• Tenderness over the liver, reduction in the volume of urine.

No appetite, losing weight

This is a worrying combination. In the under-40s, the cause is usually a prolonged feverish illness or a psychological upset. In the middle-aged and elderly, more serious disease must be carefully considered. If you have noticed loss of appetite and weight loss, check whether you have any of the symptoms in the lists below. Then look them up elsewhere in the book, where they are featured under a heading of their own.

Probable

◆ Prolonged feverish illness

In children and young adults, loss of appetite and weight loss will accompany any moderately extended illness such as a bad chest infection or prolonged gastroenteritis. Both appetite and weight are rapidly regained after a couple of weeks.

In adults, a wider net has to be cast, in order to look for:

• Chills or night sweats.

• Recent abdominal surgery.

• Prolonged cough, diarrhoea, abdominal pains.

• Unusual bleeding.

• Changes in amount of urine.

Follow up these symptoms individually, looking at other pages in this book where they are discussed in detail.

'General' Symptoms

◆ **Duodenal ulcer**

Painless ulcers, though a little unusual, can cause:

• Hunger.

• Bleeding (from the ulcer), seen in vomit or revealed by your stools turning black.

◆ **Anorexia nervosa**

See page 396.

Possible

◆ **Emotional upset**

If severe enough, self-neglect may follow. Usually there is an obvious cause of stress.

• Other symptoms of emotional upset, such as swings of mood, irritability, crying, depression.

◆ **Cancer**

In the 40-plus age range these symptoms also require a careful check for other features suggestive of cancer such as:

• Unusual pains.

• Unusual bleeding from mouth, vagina, bowel, in phlegm, in urine.

• Swellings, lumps, enlarged lymph nodes.

• Malaise, tiredness.

No appetite, losing weight and chest pain

Though worrying, this combination is a little less so than simple *No appetite, losing weight*, opposite. Of course, any adult with these symptoms still needs careful assessment by a doctor, but there are relatively innocent causes:

Probable

◆ **Peptic ulcer**

The lining of the stomach and duodenum is washed by highly corrosive acid and salts. The digestive system has mechanisms to cope with this, but if the mechanisms break down, inflammation and eventually ulceration occurs. Smoking, drinking, worry and most anti-rheumatic drugs predispose to peptic ulcers. A high proportion are associated with bacterial infection in the stomach. Duodenal ulcers do not turn into cancers; gastric ulcers may become cancerous though there is debate about this. Twice as many men as women have ulcers.

◆ **Hiatus hernia**

A failure of the one-way valve mechanism that keeps stomach contents from regurgitating up into the oesophagus.

Often just a nuisance, but if long-standing, it can cause scarring of the oesophagus, interfering with normal swallowing of food. Weight loss then results.

• A condition of middle to later life, especially in the overweight.

• Burning pains.

'General' Symptoms

- Belching, especially on bending over or lying flat.
- Very commonly, the symptoms are worse during pregnancy.

◆ Oesophagitis

Inflammation of the oesophagus usually due to acid reflux from the stomach. The condition often co-exists with hiatus hernia.

- Burning pain behind the breast-bone (heartburn).
- Worse after hot or acid food.
- Pain may appear to spread across the chest, and up to the jaw.
- Improves with antacids or drugs which stop acid production.

Possible

◆ Gall bladder disease

This usually means gallstones, causing pain in the upper abdomen after eating, and resulting in disinclination to eat. See *Gall bladder*, page 433.

◆ Cancer of the stomach

See page 438. This has to be checked for in anyone over the age of 40 who develops these symptoms, especially for the first time. The stomach is examined by endoscopy – passing a flexible telescope or camera into the stomach. The earlier such symptoms are reported, the earlier the diagnosis and the better the chance of successful treatment.

Rare

◆ Lung cancer

90 per cent of lung cancers occur in smokers.

Peptic ulcer

Stomach

Duodenum

Ulcer

In addition to the three main symptoms there may also be:

- Breathlessness.
- Coughing of blood.

See details on page 209.

◆ Tuberculosis

Weight loss and loss of appetite, and sweating, are general features of this disease. Chest pain results from swelling of glands inside the chest. Cough is usually present sometimes with bloodstained phlegm.

See details on page 427.

'General' Symptoms

Abnormal hunger

Probable

◆ Indigestion

Food reduces the feelings of pain or emptiness caused by the excess acid present in indigestion. You feel like taking frequent snacks to relieve the discomfort.

- Burning sensation behind the breastbone.
- Burping, belching or other signs of wind.
- Persistent symptoms may signify a peptic ulcer.

◆ Low blood sugar

Very common in a mild form if you miss a meal. Diabetics, especially those on insulin, must be alert to the early symptoms.

- At first, you feel light-headed and have difficulty concentrating; also, irritability, headache.
- As it worsens, sweating, confusion, drowsiness.
- Symptoms rapidly eased by taking sugar.

Possible

◆ Overactive thyroid
- Weight loss,
- Sweating,
- Tremor of the hands.
- Often, bulging eyes.
- Hyperactivity, restlessness, nervousness.

Rare

◆ Intestinal worms

Very unlikely unless living or travelled in undeveloped countries. The worm infects humans via beef, pork or fish. Usually, no other symptoms until segments of worm appear in stools.

◆ Bulimia

Bulimia is binge eating, associated with Anorexia nervosa, page 396.

- Typically in young women worried about their weight.
- Excess dieting, interrupted by bouts of voracious feeding to the point of vomiting.

◆ Hypothalamic disease

Disease of the hypothalamus gland in the brain can gradually cause excess appetite and:

- Passage of enormous amounts of urine.
- Drowsiness, narrowing of visual field.

Putting on weight

The 'glands' so often blamed are rarely the culprits.

Probable

◆ Eating too much

This is not the same as overeating. Some individuals really do eat very little, yet gain weight. The reason is unknown. Being overweight is a major cause of ill health, if not outright disease, including osteoarthritis, heart disease, and diabetes.

- Worsens with age.

'General' Symptoms

- Fat is generally spread around the body.
- Honest, purposeful dieting achieves weight loss.

Possible

◆ Underactive thyroid

Slow, progressive weight gain See page 320.

◆ Drug related

The contraceptive pill is a commonly complained-about culprit. Typically, the pill results in less than 10 per cent increase in weight – often increasing mainly breast and hip size. Careful attention to healthy eating and using the lowest effective dosage of pill are the cornerstones of management. The other common culprit is steroid treatment, widely used in chest and rheumatic diseases, eventually causing the same symptoms as Cushing's syndrome – see page 320.

Rare

◆ Hormonal causes

Several unusual hormonal disorders, mainly in boys, cause obesity.

- Obese child is unusually small or unusually tall.
- Delayed puberty.
- Under-development of penis and testicles.

◆ Cushing's syndrome

Results from overproduction of natural steroids by the body.

- Gross obesity of body, with prominent purple stretch marks.
- Thin, stick-like limbs.
- 'Moon' face.
- Pronounced hump of fat on the back.
- Symptoms of diabetes.
- Thin skin, easy bruising.

    There are sophisticated treatments, depending on the cause.

Raging thirst

This is the counterpart to *Craving for water, feeling dehydrated*, page 444, and should be read in conjunction with that topic.

Probable

◆ Poor fluid intake

Circumstances which could make this a possibility are:

- Prolonged vomiting.

- Disabled individual: for example a stroke victim who must rely on others for drinks.
- Hot climate or excess exercise.
- Conditions that make swallowing difficult.

    The symptoms are:

- Dry mouth, low output of concentrated, dark urine.

- Skin becomes lax and loses its elasticity, eyes appear to sink.
- In babies, the soft spot on the skull becomes sunken.
- In extremes, apathy, confusion.

◆ Sweating

The fluid lost in sweat has to be replaced, otherwise thirst will follow. Fever, heavy exercise and hot weather might all cause profuse sweating. The symptoms are the same as for poor fluid intake.

◆ Diarrhoea

The body can cope with brief episodes of diarrhoea, but if it is prolonged, dehydration and thirst will follow.

Babies are particularly susceptible to the effects of diarrhoea, which is also often accompanied by vomiting at that age. A careful watch must be kept for signs of dehydration.

Possible

◆ Excess of diuretic drugs

These medications are widely used to treat heart disease. They rid the body of fluid: even so, thirst is not often a problem, unless doses are excessive, when you may see:

- Passage of large quantities of urine for hours after taking the diuretic.
- Increasing weakness over several days or weeks.
- Constipation.

◆ Bleeding

This has to be heavy and sustained to cause thirst. External bleeding is usually obvious, but internal bleeding may be another matter:

- Pallor, rapid pulse, collapse and thirst.
- Suspicious circumstances include:
- Recent abdominal injury (for example, a ruptured spleen).
- Recent severe abdominal pain (from, say, a perforated ulcer).
- Fractured thigh.
- Abdominal distension.

Rare

◆ Drug side effect

Many drugs cause a dry mouth; not, strictly speaking, true thirst – but the remedy is sips of fluid. Common drugs with this side effect are anti-depressants and drugs for urinary incontinence.

Raging thirst, high urine output

Probable

◆ Diabetes

See page 446. This combination of symptoms is the classical presentation of diabetes.

◆ Psychological

A vicious circle of drinking to excess followed by urinating to excess. Surprisingly common, especially in children, where consuming sweet drinks becomes their main source of comfort.

To diagnose, a doctor must exclude other causes.

Possible

◆ Chronic kidney failure

The passage of large quantities of dilute urine is an early sign of this problem. Often the sufferer is unaware of this; other symptoms are rather vague and may go completely unnoticed. Usually diagnosed on a blood test

- Excessive urine day and night.
- Malaise.
- As it worsens, thirst, mild anaemia, fatigue.

The outcome depends on the underlying cause, of which there are many.

Rare

◆ Hyperparathyroidism

The parathyroid glands lie in the thyroid gland in the throat; they control calcium balance. Too much calcium in the blood gives:

- Excessive thirst and urine output.
- Pains in bones, constipation.
- Kidney stones that may be painful.
- Depression, malaise.

Summed up by generations of medical students as 'Moans, bones and abdominal groans'.

◆ Diabetes insipidus

See page 446.

Craving for water, feeling dehydrated

Dehydration is the result of water loss exceeding water intake, remembering that water is lost not just in urine but in faeces (especially in diarrhoea), sweat (especially in heat exhaustion), blood (especially in haemorrhage) and via breathing. Thirst is frequently a symptom of dehydration; other signs, in order of severity, are:

- Dry tongue (but beware mouth breathers, whose tongues are dry anyway).
- Reduced output of urine, the urine being dark and strong-smelling.
- Dry, lax skin.
- Sunken eyes.
- In babies, a sunken soft spot in the skull.

- Eventually apathy, confusion, collapse.

Depending on the cause, dehydration can develop over any length of time, from days to weeks, unless there has been a large and sudden loss of fluid. It is important to realize that babies and elderly people can dehydrate in a matter of hours, typically from diarrhoea and vomiting, and may not show any symptoms, apart from restlessness, until fluid loss is extreme.

Probable

◆ Vomiting

Whatever the reason for the vomiting, eventually dehydration results simply because insufficient water is being kept down. In both children and adults, the usual cause is gastroenteritis, otherwise known as gastric 'flu or tummy upset, with:

- Abrupt onset of vomiting.
- Chills, muscular aches.
- Diarrhoea may accompany these, or begin a few hours later.

Provided adequate fluids are taken frequently in small amounts, there will usually be enough fluid retained within the body to prevent dehydration.

Proprietary glucose and electrolyte re-hydration solutions are very useful in helping to avoid dehydration, especially in babies and small children. In practice, dehydration is an uncommon risk except in babies, who should be carefully watched.

◆ Diarrhoea

A few episodes of diarrhoea cause no harm. Profuse, watery diarrhoea is a different matter because if that continues for more than a few days dehydration becomes a real risk, especially in the very old and the very young.

◆ Sweating

In a hot, dry atmosphere it is possible to lose large amounts of fluid by sweating without noticing it. Those who run for pleasure should also remember this and take fluids regularly, even when on the move.

Early features would be:

- Muscle cramps.

- Thirst, but not as a prominent symptom.
- Weakness, vomiting.

◆ Decreased fluid intake

If disease interferes with swallowing dehydration, and indeed starvation, are risks, unless arrangements are made to enable feed to be taken some other way. The same applies to anyone unable to take sufficient fluid because of confusion, stroke or unconsciousness. The symptoms of dehydration can become confused with the symptoms of their disease, leading to a vicious circle. Look for:

- Low urine output.
- Increasingly lax skin.
- A tongue so dry it begins to crack.
- Increasing confusion.

Possible

◆ Overuse of diuretics

These invaluable and widely-used drugs cause an increased urine output. They are used to treat heart failure or high blood pressure. When used over long periods, they can cause slow dehydration. You may come to accept as normal a dry mouth or increased thirst.

It is rare for diuretics to cause rapid dehydration, except through deliberate overdose, for example when used as a slimming aid, or in high dosage to relieve serious heart failure, when it is normal to monitor their effect with blood tests.

The symptoms would be those of dehydration, as listed above, with:

- General weakness, also muscle weakness.

- If very severe, apathy and vomiting.

◆ Diabetes

In this condition, excess sugar in the blood stream starts to 'leak' through the kidneys, dragging large quantities of water with it. Water laden with sugar leaves the body in the form of large quantities of urine, day and night, giving the combination of thirst and dehydration.

Other features might include:

- Tiredness or weakness.

- Vague feeling of ill-health.

- Weight loss.

- A sweet smell on the breath.

- Eventually, confusion and coma.

This would be the typical presentation of type 1 diabetes in a child or young adult (the type which requires insulin treatment).

In middle-aged or elderly people, type 2 diabetes (usually managed with diet and initially tablets) is very much commoner: the onset is usually less dramatic and slower, sometimes with rather vague symptoms or no symptoms at all. In both cases a blood test rapidly confirms the diagnosis.

Rare

◆ High blood calcium

Occurs mainly in association with diseases that affect the bones and tends to be part of a rather vague, gradually developing picture which might include:

- Weakness, drowsiness, nausea, vomiting.

- Pains in the abdomen, constipation.

- Diagnosis of this condition constitutes a medical detective story.

◆ Diabetes insipidus

This results from damage – typically as a result of head injury, tumours or meningitis – to the part of the brain that controls water balance (the pituitary gland).

- Passage of gallons of urine a day.

- A huge compensating thirst.

If you have this condition, now readily treatable, every medical school for miles around will be asking you to appear as a case in their students' examinations.

Hiccups

Hiccups result from a sudden contraction of the diaphragm, the sheet of muscle which separates the chest from the abdomen. It is an uncontrollable reflex action, like blinking. The chance of hiccups being the only symptom of illness is remote, even if hiccups are unusually persistent.

Pains in various parts of the body

A precise definition is essential. Considered here is recurrent, generalized pain as opposed to pain in a specific part of the body. Such generalized pains can include the vague aches and pains which plague most people from time to time, and which may well have a psychological origin.

Generally speaking, pain as a symptom of serious underlying disease is obvious when it strikes.

Probable

◆ Depression

The pains tend to be the same minor ones everyone experiences, but they take on an exaggerated significance for the depressed person who has a lower tolerance of irritation.

- Low mood.
- Los of enjoyment.
- Disturbed sleep, poor appetite and weight loss.
- Crying, negative feelings.

◆ Hypochondria

If you have bought a copy of this book, you probably need no one to define for you the agonies of occasional hypochondria. It is a universal human condition, and if you do automatically think the worst of every symptom, this book ought to give you some relief. Persistent hypochondriacs – the ones who see their doctors as often as once a week – are another matter, characterized by:

- Lack of insight.

- Resistance to reasoned explanation or proof, after investigation, that they are healthy.
- Often, a long history of neurotic behaviour.

Hypochondria is sometimes not as benign as it seems. Those who constantly complain of sundry symptoms can be so preoccupied that they neglect the early symptoms of true disease. Everybody eventually dies of something – the hypochondriac included.

Possible

◆ Diabetes

Diabetes affects the working of nerves all over the body and can cause widespread nerve disturbance. Sometimes neuropathic pain (pain derived from damage to nerves) can be the presenting symptom of diabetes.

- Pain, tingling of lower limbs especially feet.
- Pain worse at night.
- Other symptoms of diabetes.

Neuropathic pain is commoner with poor blood glucose control. Once established, the symptoms are difficult to control, though they often give way to loss of sensation (anaesthesia). Early attention to improving blood glucose control is therefore crucial.

◆ Polymyalgia rheumatica

A disease affecting the elderly. It comes on over a period of a few weeks giving pains in any muscles, but particularly:

- Across the shoulders.
- Tenderness at the temples.
- Vague malaise, occasional fever.
- Weight loss.

Diagnosis confirmed with a simple blood test. The symptoms very rapidly improve with steroid medication which usually needs to be continued for two years or more.

◆ Pernicious anaemia

General features of anaemia, see page 390, plus:

- Tingling, numbness of limbs, hands or feet.
- Unsteady walking.

- Sore tongue.
- A hint of jaundice or yellowed skin.

Vitamin B12 injections treat both the anaemia and the pains.

Rare

◆ Sickle cell disease

In which haemoglobin, the blood's oxygen carrier, is abnormal. Found in people of African origin.

- Normal, pain-free existence interrupted by bouts of pain in limbs, abdomen.
- Pains set off by infection, surgery under anaesthetic, pregnancy.
- Screening is simple.

Feeling the cold

Probable

◆ Natural tendency

In the great majority of cases, sensitivity to cold is a natural feature of the constitution: you may well have always suffered from numb and/or bluish fingers and toes (see also *Bluish skin*, page 74). The elderly often find that they 'feel the cold'. Similarly, babies have a reduced ability to compensate for low temperature, making adequate room temperature and warm clothing essential.

Possible

◆ Raynaud's phenomenon and disease

Common conditions in which the circulation of the fingers and toes over-

reacts to changes in temperature.

- Fingers and toes always feel cold; go white or blue easily.
- Pain and redness are evident as they warm.

Severe forms of Raynaud's can cause ulceration of fingers and toes. The problem may occasionally arise as a side-effect of taking beta-blockers for high blood pressure, or of working with vibrating equipment; it might also be a complication of a connective tissue disorder, such as sytemic lupus erythematosis, see page 417.

◆ Underactive thyroid

Slowly increasing sensitivity to the cold is one of the classic features of this easily treated disorder. See page 320.

Rare

◆ **Addison's disease**

A gradually-developing hormone deficiency causing generalized weakness and lack of resistance to physical stress, including low temperature. People with Addison's look strikingly pale.

Swollen lymph nodes

The lymphatic system, which includes the lymph nodes, liver and spleen, is in the front line of defence against infection and, indeed, other threats to the system. Temporary swelling for a week or two is, therefore, of little significance, being a feature of many minor viral illnesses and injuries. However, there is no escaping the fact that prolonged swelling of lymph nodes can be a sign of several serious conditions.

Frequently, these conditions are treatable, especially at an early stage, making it essential to report persistently swollen lymph nodes.

Blood tests and lymph node biopsy are usually needed to confirm the diagnosis.

Probable

◆ **Glandular fever**

An extremely common infection in teenagers or young adults, with a combination of severe sore throat, swollen glands and tiredness. A blood test confirms the diagnosis. No specific treatment, but be reassured that you will eventually make a full recovery.

◆ **Tonsillitis**

Just a sore throat can cause massive swelling of lymph glands below the chin. This can be particularly dramatic in children; see page 116.

Possible

In most of the following, the lymph nodes gradually enlarge and remain enlarged:

◆ **Hodgkin's disease**

A particular type of cancerous condition of the lymphatic system and lymph glands (lymphoma). Typically occurs in young adults.

• Painless.

• Rubbery feel to lymph nodes.

• Lymph nodes grow steadily over a few weeks or months.

• Tiredness, sweats at night.

Swelling of the neck glands is the most likely symptom to be noticed.

Diagnosis requires biopsy of a gland.

◆ **Other lymphomas**

There are several other types of lymphoma distinct from Hodgkin's disease. Theses lymphomas typically affect an older age group – 35 plus. Symptoms are similar to those in Hodgkin's disease, with:

• Widespread, painless swollen lymph nodes.

• Weight loss, sweats at night.

Treatment depends on the cell type of lymphoma – determined by blood test,

'General' Symptoms

plus bone marrow and lymph node biopsy. The outlook is very variable dependant on the cell type involved. Treatments range from simple observation to radiotherapy and chemotherapy.

◆ Cancer

By the time it causes generalized swelling of nodes, the cancer will be so advanced that it is bound to be obvious from other features. More important from the point of view of early diagnosis is enlargement of a single group of lymph nodes, which may signal the presence of an early cancer in such sites as the breast or the thyroid gland before there are other obvious features. The sites most noticeable are:

- Neck (cancers of lung, thyroid, nose and stomach).
- Groin (cancer of bowel, womb, prostate).
- Armpit (breast cancer).

◆ Toxoplasmosis

An infection acquired through eating infected meat, or sometimes via cat droppings. If caught during pregnancy, it sometimes causes brain and eye damage in the baby.

- In mild cases, generalized, painless, swollen lymph nodes.
- Possibly fever, weakness as well.

◆ Tuberculosis

The usual glands involved are those around the neck. The swelling is painless and accompanied by general features of

TB such as:

- Prolonged malaise.
- Weight loss.
- Cough, possibly with blood in sputum.

◆ Leukaemia

Leukaemia can present with widespread swollen nodes, both in childhood and adulthood. In children, presentation tends to be more dramatic with:

- Abnormal bleeding, sore throat, malaise.
- Fever, anaemia.
- Enlarged liver, spleen.

In adults the disease tends to have a much slower onset, with:

- Enlarged lymph nodes as a main feature.
- Possibly effects of anaemia, and recurrent infection.

Leukaemia in childhood often carries a good outlook with treatment providing excellent prospects of remission or cure. Prognosis in adults depends on the type of leukaemia – chronic lymphatic leukaemia, which is the commonest type, carries a good outlook and often requires no treatment; other types are more insidious, with a much worse outlook.

Rare

◆ Sarcoidosis

A condition of unknown origin, often picked up by chance from seeing enlarged lymph glands on a chest X-ray. Usually benign, but may cause:

* Rashes, joint pains.
* Malaise.
* Large, painful red lumps on shin.
* Painful, red eye.
* Breathlessness.

◆ Secondary syphilis

A sexually transmitted infection, numerically very uncommon; risk increased with multiple casual partners or sex with a sex industry worker, especially abroad.

* The initial sign is a painless sore on the genitalia.
* General lymph node swelling after several months.
* Wart-like growths around genitalia.
* Vague malaise.

Diagnosis is by blood test; antibiotic treatment is effective and essential in order to prevent progression to serious nerve disorders, possibly years later.

◆ Yaws

A syphilis look-alike found in the tropics. Unlike syphilis, it is spread by poor hygiene, rather than sexually transmitted.

* Ulcerating skin rash, mainly on palms and soles of feet.
* Widespread enlargement of the lymph nodes.
* Treatment prevents disfiguring destruction of bone.

◆ Cat scratch fever

An interesting, and probably under-recognized, reason for enlarged glands. Said to be one of the commonest causes of persistently swollen glands in the USA. Contact with kittens may pose an increased risk.

* At first, just broken skin from the scratch.
* After a week or two, a small red lump appears.
* Swollen local glands, for example, in armpit.
* Glands enlarge, and may discharge pus.
* Illness settles over a few weeks.
* Can be cleared up with antibiotics.

A

H

M

P

W

X

Y

Z

Also from Kyle Cathie...

ISBN 978-1-85626-655-0

ISBN 978-1-85626-567-6

ISBN 978-1-85626-500-3

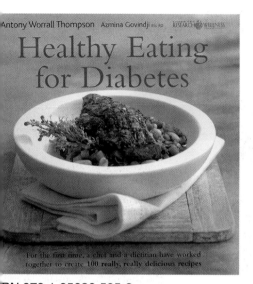

Antony Worrall Thompson Azmina Govindji BSc RD RESEARCH WELLNESS

Healthy Eating
for Diabetes

For the first time, a chef and a dietitian have worked
together to create 100 really, really delicious recipes

ISBN 978-1-85626-505-8

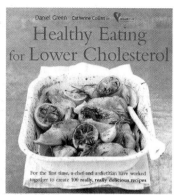

Daniel Green Catherine Collins RD

Healthy Eating
for Lower Cholesterol

For the first time, a chef and a dietitian have worked
together to create 100 really, really delicious recipes

ISBN 978-1-85626-679-6

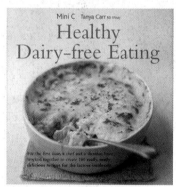

Mini C Tanya Carr RD RNutr

Healthy
Dairy-free Eating

For the first time, a chef and a dietitian have
worked together to create 100 really, really
delicious recipes for the lactose intolerant

ISBN 978-1-85626-622-2

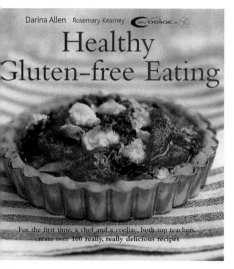

Darina Allen Rosemary Kearney Coeliac UK

Healthy
Gluten–free Eating

For the first time, a chef and a coeliac, both top teachers,
create over 100 really, really delicious recipes

ISBN 978-1-85626-542-3

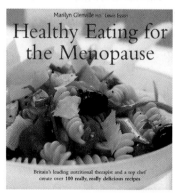

Marilyn Glenville PhD Lewis Esson

Healthy Eating for
the Menopause

Britain's leading nutritional therapist and a top chef
create over 100 really, really delicious recipes

ISBN 978-1-85626-547-8

FREE

YOURSELF FROM

SMOKING

A 3-POINT PLAN
TO KILL NICOTINE
ADDICTION

KRISTINA IVINGS

ISBN 978-1-85626-657-4